Stigma and Social Exclusion in Healthcare

Edited by
Tom Mason,
Caroline Carlisle,
Caroline Watkins
and Elizabeth Whitehead

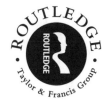

London and New York

First published 2001
by Routledge
11 New Fetter Lane, London EC4P 4EE

Simultaneously published in the USA and Canada
by Routledge
29 West 35th Street, New York, NY 10001

Routledge is an imprint of the Taylor & Francis Group

Typeset in Sabon by Taylor & Francis Books Ltd
Printed and bound in Great Britain by Biddles Ltd, Guildford and
King's Lynn

British Library Cataloguing in Publication Data
A catalogue record for this book is available from the British Library

Library of Congress Cataloging-in-Publication Data
Stigma and social exclusion in healthcare / edited by Tom
Mason ... [et al.].
p. cm.
Includes bibliographical references and index.
1. Medical care–Social aspects–Great Britain. 2. Stigma (Social
psychology)–Great Britain. 3. Health services accessibility–Great
Britain. 4. Social isolation–Health aspects–Great Britain. 5. Social
medicine–Great Britain. I. Mason, Tom.

RA427 .S725 2001
362.1'0′′′′941–dc21
                                                    2001019139

ISBN 0–415–22199–4 (hbk)
ISBN 0–415–22200–1 (pbk)

Contents

vi   *Contents*

Illustrations

Tables

Figures

About the editors

Tom Mason PhD, BSc (Hons), RMN, RNMH, RGN has worked in the field of mental health for over twenty-seven years, seventeen of which were spent in clinical practice with the latter years in the academic positions of research fellow and senior lecturer. He has published more than fifty articles on a variety of subjects relating to forensic mental health, and has co-authored and co-edited six previous books (*Seclusion and Mental Health*, Chapman and Hall, with Ann Alty; *A Sociology of the Mentally Disordered Offender*, Longman, with Dave Mercer; *Critical Perspectives in Forensic Care*, Macmillan, with Dave Mercer; *The Management of Violence and Aggression*, Churchill Livingstone, with Mark Chandley; *Forensic Mental Health Care*, Churchill Livingstone, with Dave Mercer, Mick McKeown and Ged McCann; and *Behaviour, Crime and Legal Processes*, John Wiley, with James McGuire and Aisling O'Kane). He has a longstanding interest in the emotional impact of isolation, both voluntary and involuntary, and the processes by which stigmatised individuals become socially excluded. He is currently professor of forensic nursing at the Caswell Clinic and the University of Glamorgan in South Wales.

Caroline Carlisle PhD, MSc, BA, RGN, RM, DNCert, DipCouns, RNT currently holds the Rathbone Chair in Community Nursing at the University of Liverpool. After initial registration as a nurse, her clinical practice has been mainly in the field of community nursing and midwifery. Since the mid-1980s she has worked closely with people affected by HIV and AIDS, and is currently engaged as a counselling therapist with an HIV and AIDS voluntary organisation on Merseyside. Her main research activity relates to sexual health and her doctoral work focused on psychosocial issues related to family caregiving in HIV. This PhD thesis presented a model of caregiver experience in which stigmatising attitudes played a major part in the social exclusion of those affected by HIV. She publishes widely on a variety of subjects relating to her professional field.

Caroline Watkins PhD, BA (Hons), RGN qualified as a nurse in Liverpool over twenty years ago and has been an active researcher for fourteen years. She is currently Senior Lecturer in the School of Nursing, Midwifery and Health Visiting, Manchester University; the North West Regional Stroke Task Force Coordinator (charged to raise the profile of quality stroke care); and a Director of Liverpool Crossroads (a voluntary organisation supporting carers). Guided by her expertise in nursing, psychology and social services, she aims to improve the integration and quality of care provided in acute and primary care settings. The Stroke Research Unit at University Hospital Aintree, which she set up with Dr Anil Sharma, is regarded locally, nationally and internationally as a centre of excellence for stroke care and stroke research. She has many other areas of clinical and research interest, including older people (e.g. falls and mobility issues), occupational problems (e.g. team working), and alternative approaches to education (e.g. problem-based and inter-professional learning, and the development of behavioural observational skills in ward nurses). She has an established publication record and is Junior Secretary to the internationally renowned Society for Research in Rehabilitation. She has always maintained close links with clinical environments and with practising clinicians. The psychological impact of stroke, adjustment to and treatment of such problems form the main focus of her current research activity.

Elizabeth Whitehead PhD, BA (Hons), RGN, RM, RHV, ONC has been nursing for more than twenty years in clinical practice before moving into academic posts in 1997. She worked as a midwifery sister in Liverpool Maternity Hospital in the early 1980s, and then as a health visitor in the inner city in the late 1980s and early 1990s. Her first academic appointment was as Lecturer in Health Visiting and Sociology, and she now works as Senior Lecturer at Chester College of Higher Education. She was awarded her PhD in the field of teenage pregnancy and stigma from the Department of Sociology at Liverpool University and is currently working on the issue of terminations and adolescent pregnancy. Her main publications are on teenage pregnancy and social exclusion, and her main professional interests revolve around issues of marginalisation and the sociology of health.

Contributors

Dr Gus A. Baker: FBPsS, BA (Hons), MSc, PhD, Consultant Clinical Neuro-psychologist and Senior Lecturer in Neuropsychology, The Walton Centre for Neurosurgery.

Caroline Benjamin: RGN, BSc, MSc, Macmillan Genetic Associate, Merseyside and Cheshire Clinical Genetics Service, Alder Hey Children's Hospital.

Eric Blyth: BA (Hons), MA, CQSW, Professor of Social Work, University of Huddersfield.

Kathy Corrin: RSCN, BA (Hons), Dip. N., Service Manager Outpatients, Royal Liverpool Children's NHS Trust, Liverpool.

Clare Croft-White: BA, MBA, Independent Consultant, London.

Jon Derricott: RGN, RMN, Freelance Trainer and Writer, Liverpool.

Tom Donovan: BA (Hons), RMN, RGN, DN Cert., PWT, Cert. Ed., Macmillan Lecturer/Practitioner in Cancer Nursing, Department of Nursing, University of Liverpool.

David Evans: RN, BA (Hons), PGDip. Psychol. Couns., PGCE, MPhil, Educational Consultant in Sexual Health (freelance).

Mike Farrell: BSc (Hons), RGN, RSCN, Dip. Health Studies, ENB Higher Award, Lecturer/Practitioner in Child Health, Department of Nursing, University of Liverpool.

Dr Bernard Gibbon: MSc, PhD, RMN, RGN, RNT, Head of Department, Primary and Community Nursing, University of Central Lancashire, Preston.

Dr Janet Heyes: FRCGP, General Practitioner (ret'd), Liverpool.

Neil Hunt: MSc, RMN, Lecturer in Addictive Behaviour, Kent Institute of Medicine and Health Sciences; Director of Research, KCA, University of Kent and Canterbury.

Professor Ann Jacoby: BA (Hons), PhD, Professorial Research Fellow in Medical Sociology, Department of Primary Care, University of Liverpool.

Brenda Jacono: RN, BN, MSc, Professor at the School of Nursing, St. Francis Xavier University, Canada.

John Jacono: RNMS, SRN, Reg. N. (ONT), BA (Hons), PhD, Professor at the School of Nursing, St. Francis Xavier University, Canada.

Sue Kaney: BA (Hons), M.Clin. Psychol., C. Psychol., Lecturer in Health Psychology, Department of Clinical Psychology, University of Liverpool.

Emily McArdle: BSc (Hons), MRCSLT, Principal Speech and Language Therapist, St Catherine's Hospital, Wirral.

Mick McKeown: BA (Hons), DPSN, RGN, RMN, Lecturer, Primary and Community Nursing, University of Central Lancashire, Preston.

Dave Mercer: BA (Hons), MA, RMN, PGCE, Lecturer in Nursing, Department of Nursing, University of Liverpool.

Ruth Moore: BSc (Hons), PhD Research Student, School of Human and Social Sciences, University of Huddersfield.

Georgie Parry-Crooke: AcSS, Senior Lecturer, School of Social Sciences, University of North London.

Dr Rachel Perkins: BA, MPhil (Clinical Psychology), PhD (Psychology), Clinical Director and Consultant Clinical Psychologist, Rehabilitation and Continuing Care Service, South West London and St George's Mental Health NHS Trust, Tooting, London.

Julie Repper: MPhil, BA (Hons), RMN, RGN, Research Student, University of Manchester.

Bob Sapey: MA, CQSW, Lecturer in Social Work, Department of Applied Social Science, Lancaster University.

Pete Shaughnessy: Member of Mad Pride.

Tuxephoni Simmonds: RN, BN, Forensic Correctional Nurse, Alberta Justice Department, Calgary.

Dr Mary Smale: BA, Cert. Ed., PhD, Breastfeeding Counsellor and Tutor, National Childbirth Trust; Honorary Research Fellow, Mother and Infant Research Unit, University of Leeds.

Dr Mark Stowell-Smith: BA (Hons), MSc, PhD, Psychotherapist, Psychological Therapy Service, Whiston Hospital, Merseyside.

Tony Wright: Dip. Couns., MA, Counsellor, Christopher Grange Counselling Service, Liverpool.

Foreword

Stigma and social exclusion: narratives and agendas

Graham Scambler

Periods and times can sometimes be characterised in terms of the concepts that hit and hold their place in the media headlines, and 'social exclusion' is such a concept. Emerging on the eve of the millennium, it is still around, representative of New Labour's commitment both to the disadvantaged and to the promise of (Clinton-like) 'Third Way' solutions to their problems. Too many people, it is said, have been left behind or excluded from society; social exclusion, moreover, brings with it unacceptable burdens of stigma, hopelessness and misery. Ways must therefore be found to make society more inclusive, to ensure that all citizens – the poor, the sick and the undervalued and unwanted – are brought back into the mainstream. It is impossible to deny either the desirability of inclusion over exclusion, or the virtue of policies designed to enhance the former at the expense of the latter. But there is political rhetoric as well as conviction here, structure as well as agency; there are agendas to disentangle.

One issue is the extent to which Prime Minister Blair's narrative or ideology of the 'Third Way' is functionally equivalent to Thatcherite neo-liberalism. One obvious point of concern is New Labour's degree of willingness to encourage the growth of deregulated (global) private enterprise, consumerism, clientism (displacing the citizenship associated with the postwar welfare state) and processes of individualisation, all of them associated with a widening and deepening of inequality, and therefore with an increase in the numbers of those excluded. A second, related issue is New Labour's apparent propensity to go on to hold individuals responsible for their own exclusion; one wonders, for example, whether its acknowledgement of the salience of household income differentials for health inequality will not, even in a projected second term in office, lead to effective government fiscal and other interventions to reduce differentials, but rather to a system of moral and political sanctions for those unwilling/unable to act to improve their own lot (e.g. the spread of US-style 'workfare').

One of the virtues of this volume is that it both raises macro issues like these, and also considers – and in detail – the ramifications of social exclusion, not only for social scientists and others wishing to describe and account for it, but for front-line workers charged with combating it on behalf of their clients. This makes for a rich, thought-provoking text. There is a brief discussion of some of the theoretical issues raised by the concept of social exclusion, issues not always addressed in what is a new, already abundant and often faddish and naïve literature. The comprehensive middle section is devoted to a series of concise, substantive, 'practice-oriented' attempts to draw out the significance of stigma/social exclusion across a range of specific topic areas – from teenage pregnancy to epilepsy to class-related health inequalities – under the rubrics of 'difference', 'deviance' and 'dilemmas'; the knowledgeable authority of the contributors is impressive. And finally, the editors do not shirk the unenviable task of outlining a manifesto for change: it is a manifesto, moreover, which seems to grow naturally out of the bulk of the preceding analyses in (1) its recognition of the macro- as well as micro-politics of exclusion, and (2) its determination to shape practical responses.

Stigma and Social Exclusion in Healthcare will be widely referred to, both because of its topicality and coherence and because it has 'something for everyone'. But this short Foreword gives me an opportunity to raise one further matter, largely and understandably beyond the brief of this volume, although it is touched upon. This is that the social structures we all of us – most of us more unwittingly than wittingly – reproduce day-to-day to sustain and favour the (increasingly global) rich and powerful while permitting the lot of the 'new poor' to deteriorate, and not only in relative terms. These are not my concepts of choice, but it is surely right to recognise that the emergence of late of a national, even a regional, 'underclass' is not unrelated to the new-found prosperity of a global 'overclass'. To understand why the poor and powerless *are* poor and powerless (and a whole family of 'life events' with their associated stigmas derive from enduring relative material deprivation), it is essential to study the rich and powerful. It is an argument, of course, which leads naturally to an analysis of the world system rather than of a single nation-state like Britain. There is an urgent need, in other words, to delve beneath the surface and investigate the role of social structures in occasioning and perpetuating disadvantage. This, it seems to me, is a sociological task and one at which we are not currently excelling. The theoretical observations and pragmatic thrust of *Stigma and Social Exclusion in Healthcare* carry messages for all of us; academics, policy-makers, front-line workers and those presently facing the cruel miseries of exclusion.

Preface

In undertaking this current editorial work we have been motivated by two dominant themes. The first concerns a micro-level aspect which involves the many individuals that have been, are now, and will be in the future both excluded and marginalised. The second concerns the macro political forces that have been exercised to create the conditions that have led to the exclusion, or inclusion, of individual members of society.

Most healthcare workers enter their respective professions with the intention of assisting those who are unfortunate enough to require their services. This motivation is usually grounded in compassion, and driven by a desire to care for those afflicted. Although we cannot guarantee that this is the basis of all healthcare delivery, as the infamous cases of Beverly Allit and Harold Shipman testify, we can feel reasonably confident that the majority of professionals operate with the best interests of the patient in mind. It may, therefore, seem odd that a major part of this book is concerned with how healthcare workers may contribute to the stigmatisation and social exclusion of those they intend to help. The processes by which this occurs are often subconsciously derived and we are not overtly aware that we are contributing to this unwanted condition. Furthermore, the hierarchical nature of healthcare professions and services provides fertile ground in which we may well stigmatise and exclude fellow workers, intentionally or unintentionally. If we wish to change this state of affairs, then we need to be aware of how these processes operate and how we can begin to change professional practice.

There is a call from many groups within society to re-examine the conditions that have led certain members to become socially excluded. These groups include those involved in education, those concerned with charitable organisations, those from ethnic minorities, those from various churches, and those from politics. We would like this book to be read as a text which joins this chorus, but which focuses on those stigmatised and excluded in the healthcare setting. Furthermore, we would feel that a major aim of the book would be achieved if healthcare professionals were enthused to voice, even louder than they already do, their concerns regarding the marginalised patient. The reasons for the concerns of all the foregoing groups regarding the impact of social exclusion are the same. That is, the corollaries of being socially excluded actually exacerbate the original problems that led to the exclusion. Thus it is a spiralling problem.

On a broader level the modern notion of social exclusion can be rooted in the Black Report (DoH, 1983). This report portrayed a Britain that, in terms of social concerns, economics and health, was divided into two halves; those who were excluded from and those who were included into mainstream society. A later report by Margaret Whitehead, *The Health Divide* (1985), reinforced and expanded the Black Report and gave an evidence-based analysis of the stakeholders from politics, economics and health, and concluded that Northern Britain suffered greater inequalities than their Southern counterparts. Although the Black Report had been commissioned by the government of the day, led by Margaret Thatcher, its results were so disturbing that the recommendations were not acted upon. In the years following the publication of the Black Report we have seen that the United Kingdom has many groups and individuals who are disadvantaged, stigmatised and excluded from our society. Two further reports have added weight to this argument, in terms of health, and indicate that we face enormous challenges in our endeavours to overcome these differences. These reports are *The Health of the Nation* (DoH, 1994) and *Our Healthier Nation* (DoH, 1998). Furthermore, as we move further within the confines of Europe, we see that in comparison with many of our European neighbours we have fallen behind in many areas of health. Finally, the Social Exclusion Unit, which is a product of the current Labour government, casts a wide net in its attempts to understand and advise on the dynamics of social exclusion. The work of the SEU is summarised in the report by Sir Donald Acheson (*Independent Inquiry into Inequalities in Health Report*: Acheson, 1998) and makes a strong statement regarding the need to address those areas of British society that contribute to the exclusion process.

This brings us to the prime need for this book. It would appear that one of the main mechanisms for providing the circumstances and context in which prejudices, bigotry and dogma may be brought under the lens of scrutiny is to create the conditions of critical evaluation. We hope that this book contributes to that process.

References

Acheson, D. (1998) *Independent inquiry into inequalities in health report*, London: The Stationery Office.

Department of Health (1983) *Inequalities in health (Black Report)*, London: HMSO.

—— (1994) *The health of the nation*, London: DoH.

—— (1998) *Our healthier nation*, cm3852, London: The Stationery Office.

Whitehead, M. (1992) *Inequalities in health: the health divide*, London: Penguin.

Acknowledgements

As always, there are many people who have assisted us in this book but too many to mention individually. They know who they are and we thank them.

Special thanks go to all those at Routledge who have supported us along the way and guided us so carefully. Also a special thanks go to all the contributors who produced their chapters promptly (well, nearly) and professionally. Finally, we would like to extend a very special thank you to Jackie Lucock, who masterfully coordinated, cleverly coerced, and magnificently harmonised the entire project.

1 Introduction

*Tom Mason, Caroline Carlisle, Caroline
Watkins and Elizabeth Whitehead*

Introduction

By and large people are social animals, with only a few life-long excep-
tions of hermit existences. Although most people do enjoy their own social
space, time alone and moments of peace, quiet and solitude, there is a
strong inherent drive for the company of others. This instinctual urge may
be a primitive artefact when pre-historic human groups herded together
for safety and protection, or it may be a socio-psychological coupling that
is rooted in the drive for procreation. Whatever its heritage, the idea of
belonging to a particular social group of our choice is deep-seated indeed.
When denied that company, either through forced solitary confinement,
exile or banishment, it is often considered a cruel and unkind act of
punishment. Consider the testimony of those who were politically exiled,
such as Alexander Solzhenitsyn, or those forced into solitary confinement,
such as the Beirut hostages, or those transported to foreign lands as
punishments for criminal acts, and bear witness to the pain and torment of
their troubled emotions on being excluded. It is almost as if the overwhelming need to feel socially included has, as its binary opposition, its
most potent punitive counterpart, that of social exclusion.

From a global perspective we all share the same planet, and should we
come under interplanetary attack from some distant cosmological force
we would, no doubt, bind together to fight this common enemy.
However, we are all aware of the global fragmentation into continents,
countries, clans and creeds as barriers, borders and boundaries are
erected to separate and divide. Then, within these states, fractions may
develop to cause North and South differences or East and West discrepancies, leading to further conflict and tensions. Even within cities, we
know of areas of affluence and areas of poverty, areas which are predominantly one culture or another. Furthermore, we are all probably aware of
the disunity that can exist in small environmental areas such as streets,
playgrounds, wards or units, as gangs, cliques and clubs form to isolate
the in-group from the out-group (see page 35). It would seem to be a
human social characteristic to splinter into smaller groups and to sever

ourselves from the main social body. Although, as already mentioned, this may have some properties remnant of the primitive past, in contemporary times it can, and does, lead to pain and suffering. From the Holocaust to ethnic cleansing, and from the bullied child in school to the discredited patient in the clinic, the human capacity to hurt, and be hurt, knows no bounds.

From a national perspective, in Britain, we can note the many tensions that exist between the nationalistic fervours of Scotland, Ireland, England and Wales; between the islanders and mainlanders; between those north of Watford Gap (a service station on the M1 motorway) and those south of it; and both between our cities and within them. It is not surprising that British society is deeply concerned with the levels of ethnic, racial and religious intolerance that underpins many of our social problems. In many ways the strategies by which we exclude each other are both sophisticated and simple, and yet so deeply entrenched in our social psyche as to be obscured and veiled. Through the exploration of our own roles and functions, and reflexively considering our own values and prejudices, we believe we can alter our human action. In order to progress we need to have the ability and maturity to question ourselves so as to change our behaviours towards each other. In this book we narrow our focus to concentrate our attention on the nature of stigma and social exclusion in healthcare settings.

Stigma and social exclusion: its impact

Stigma has its roots in 'differences'. The pain and emotional hurt experienced by the stigmatised person is linked to others' pity, fear, disgust and disapproval of this difference, whether that difference is one of personality, physical appearance, illness and disability, age, gender or sexuality.

Stigma can be defined as an attribute that serves to discredit a person or persons in the eyes of others (Franzoi, 1996). Attitudes towards these discreditable attributes vary through time, so for example the stigmatising impact of being an 'unmarried mother' has gradually lessened over the past few decades. Stigma is also culturally defined, and variation is evident in the ways in which particular attributes are either accepted or otherwise between culturally diverse groups. The practice of tribal scarring in particular cultural groups highlights this point. Similarly, healthcare provides examples of how politically correct terminology has entered the vocabulary, partly as an attempt to demonstrate acceptance of differences; hence we now refer to 'gender realignment' instead of 'sex change', and 'Down's Syndrome' instead of 'mongol'. Changes in vocabulary and the passage of time, however, cannot fully eradicate stigma and alter complex cognitive behavioural aspects of stigmatising attitudes. Indeed, when defining issues of 'deviancy', healthcare provision and medical diagnosis can shape and promote images of stigma bearers. So, for example, blindness may be defined in terms of the impact on people's personality and psychological adjustment rather than as a technical handi-cap which can be compensated for by acquiring new techniques.

The impact of stigmatising attitudes on the stigmatised individual can vary in form and intensity. Much of the behaviour, however, towards the stigmatised serves to emphasise 'difference', and thus there are forms of discrimination and prejudice which can be identified in the interactions between the 'normal' and the 'discredited' (Goffman, 1990). Discrimination and prejudice in any form serve to separate and exclude individuals from society and from many of the benefits of society, such as equitable access to services like housing, education, health and social support. Discrimination in this way is a form of social exclusion.

At an individual level the impact of stigma and social exclusion can be devastating, leading to low self-esteem, poor social relationships, isolation, depression and self-harm. Groups as well as individuals can be stigmatised and prejudicial behaviour towards them based on race, sexual orientation, culture and religious belief is experienced at an individual as well as a group level. One of the largest potentially stigmatised groups is that of the 'kingdom of the sick' (Sontag, 1978) and it is no coincidence that many of the chapters in this book address those individuals affected by illness and disability. The impact of stigma on those individuals who are already coping with acute or chronic health problems can be profound, and we hope that this book will serve to raise the awareness of all healthcare professionals, and provide some insight into the experience of stigma and social exclusion for people affected by physical and mental health problems.

Contextual framework

As we noted earlier, there appears to be a very distinct human capacity to form groups, and in forming such groups certain social structures become apparent (Simmel, 1950). For example, a group identity is formed by which individual members can distinguish themselves from others (Hughes, 1945). This identity is underpinned by a set of values and normative prescriptions that govern the rules of behaviour for that particular group. For example, if a group values the belief in the superiority of their skin colour and the purity of their blood lineage, those values may form the normative prescription of excluding other groups from inter-marrying. Such prescriptive rules may manifest themselves as banning their children from mixing with, or dating, others from different ethnic/cultural backgrounds, or may incorporate stigmatising strategies of ridiculing, de-valuing and dismissive commentary. These latter strategies are employed by many members of a particular in-group who denigrate and disregard those in the out-group (Redfield, 1960). This can be seen when children form groups in the school setting as much as it can be seen in national racist humour that disparages other national groups (Coleman, 1961).

The major function of these stigmatising strategies is to establish the 'them and us' principle (Foucault, 1973). The complex interpretation of this principle is beyond the scope of this book but suffice to say that it is concerned with establishing those deemed within a value structure which is considered good and in favour, and those considered bad and out of favour (Foucault, 1973). This principle, once established, allows for any amount of stigmatisation and social exclusion, which is then justified and sanctioned by the prejudiced view that distinguishes the difference: i.e. 'them and us'. Few better examples of this principle, although extreme ones, are found than in the extermination of many millions of people throughout history under the name of ethnic cleansing. Although we would reiterate that these are extreme examples, they typically begin with the same stigmatising processes as do the street gangs, the playground bullies and the workplace cliques. The difference is merely one of degree.

The final context that we wish to mention here concerns the social pressures that are wielded not only to exclude certain individuals from the in-group but also to include chosen members. Peer group pressure is a well-known social phenomenon that is employed to compel people to conform to a set of values. To create the feeling that a person belongs to, or is identified or associated with, a particular group is a powerful mechanism of communication, and can be as effective in rewarding conformist behaviours as well as punishing 'aberrant' ones. Once established as a member of any particular in-group it is often difficult for individuals either to extricate themselves from that group or to change group thinking. In short, the group socialisation process becomes a self-reinforcing circuit of control. In the healthcare setting this can lead to all manner of disturbing actions towards vulnerable groups, as witnessed in the numerous inquiries into allegations of abuse. For example, there are numerous reports concerning abuse by staff in learning disability hospitals (for example HMSO, 1972), reports on allegations of abuse by nurses of mentally disordered offenders (HMSO, 1992), and reports on the killing of patients by registered practitioners (for example the Beverly Allitt Report: HMSO, 1994). Furthermore we will no doubt have reports on the Bristol child cardiac inquiry, the case of general practitioner Harold Shipman, and the Alder Hey children's organ removal scandal. What all these examples share is a belief in being a member of an 'in-group' with the power to stigmatise or socially exclude others. Healthcare settings can be very dangerous places!

Healthcare contexts and stigma/prejudice/social exclusion

These examples of stigma and its impact on or within healthcare systems have mainly identified specific situations or problems which are potentially observable. However, there are more subtle processes which are not so directly observable, but which nevertheless impact on and relate to the partial or impartial provision of healthcare. These issues originate from healthcare's tendency to focus on illness and the prevention of illness which are suggested here as being the origins of stigmatising processes. Supporters of the biomedical model may push forward the medical profession's knowledge as the only right explanation, using language to bolster these ideas – 'doctor knows best', 'a little knowledge is a dangerous thing' – so that these ideas are seen as the only 'reality' and others find it difficult to disagree (Berger and Luckmann, 1966). Furthermore, health professionals frequently, but mistakenly, think that lay health beliefs 'are at best watered down versions of proper professional medical knowledge (i.e. no more than old wives tales)' (Stainton Rogers, 1991: 3).

However, it is important to recognise that biomedicine is only one of many differing explanations. Illness itself is merely a matter of definition, which could be illustrated by the following:

> The fracture of a septuagenarian's femur has, within the world of nature, no more significance than the snapping of an autumn leaf from its twig; the invasion of the human organism by cholera germs carries with it no more the stamp of 'illness' than does the souring of milk by other forms of bacteria ...
>
> (Sedgewick, 1982: 30)

That is, illness is only what it means to the individual, and its implication for the person themselves is socially defined. There may be a number of explanations ('sub-universes of meaning') which compete with each other, both within society and within the individual (Berger and Luckmann, 1966). Therefore it is imperative that lay beliefs are recognised, and that both illness and health should be seen as normality and consequently as being within a normal person's control (Dingwall, 1976), such that healthcare professionals are not viewed as the only source of knowledge.

Healthcare professionals must be challenged to take account of these lay beliefs, which may differ – even within an individual – according to the particular event and time point within their life. People choose from a range of conflicting attitudes, and this choice depends upon situational demands, mood, and perceived importance at that moment. People are endeavouring to 'create order out of chaos, and moment to moment make sense of their world amid the cacophony' (Stainton Rogers, 1991: 10).

Consequently, when healthcare professionals are trying to explain (as they are charged to do) what factors have contributed to a person's illness and to discover what will enable them to recover, they must examine personal accounts. This is starkly apparent in those who have recently suffered a stroke, where it is the person's own ideas of what will help them to get better and what will happen to them in the future that determine their short- and long-term feelings of wellbeing.

It is increasingly apparent that we need a system which allows people to be recognised as having their own ideas and opinions, which may or may not be directly in line with medical philosophies; as having their own ways of motivating themselves; and as needing to be allowed some choice and also some control over their own bodies, treatments and futures.

Taking account of people's own ideas and aspirations poses a challenge to healthcare professionals who have developed in a society which encourages conformity. There are strong expectations of participation in healthcare treatments (e.g. rehabilitation, medication, alterations in lifestyle, etc.) and strong penalties for non-participation (e.g. smokers being refused coronary artery bypass operations). Yet what we are suggesting is that healthcare professionals should be able to operate in a non-judgemental way, responding to people's individual needs. However, at present, few mechanisms are in place to equip staff with these skills, either during their training or even after they qualify. Until suitable mechanisms are identified and instigated, the stigmatising nature of healthcare will be potentiated by the very people who should be educating others to take non-judgemental account of difference and diversity.

Healthcare professionals are in a unique position with regard to those who have recently acquired a disability. The attitudes of staff can not only determine how the person with the new problem feels about themselves, but also how others react to their problem. It is foolish to expect that these staff know instinctively how to react to particular situations or people. It is therefore imperative to develop the ability of staff to reflect on their own attitudes and prejudices in order to minimise them and to develop strategies to overcome them.

Furthermore, the inability to provide individualised care and the potentiation of stigmatising attitudes are compounded and exacerbated by the healthcare system itself. Resources are allocated based not on the requirements of individuals themselves, but on the needs of whole groups. People are thus, by necessity, labelled as having a specific problem in order to be judged in need of a particular type of care or treatment. Any move to avoid labelling people may result in non-allocation of services.

The government has recently recognised that mechanisms need to be put in place to ensure that everyone has equitable and rapid access to the required services. However, caution should be taken in the development of such mechanisms to ensure that the very nature of the system does not exacerbate the problems of stigma, prejudice and social exclusion which currently abound.

Government concerns and social exclusion

The Independent Inquiry into Inequalities in Health Report (the Acheson Report; Acheson, 1998) is one of the most significant expressions and statements of concern regarding social exclusion that is experienced in

Britain today. This report has become the benchmark for understanding, first, the nature of social inequalities in Britain, and second, the manner in which future analysis, research and policy formulation should be undertaken. It argues that the scientific evidence indicates that the adopted socio-economic model is the most appropriate, and highlights three layers of health determinants that are dependent upon each other: first, the individual lifestyle which is concerned with cultural constrictions and socialised behaviours; second, social and community networks as a form of peer group pressure; and third, general socio-economic and environmental conditions. Acheson goes on to argue that the main areas for increased scrutiny and developmental considerations are:

- policies that are likely to have an impact on health inequalities;
- a high priority being given to health of families with children;
- further steps to improve the living standards of poor households.

What we see here is a focus on the accepted relationship between individual action, social networks and economic conditions. These, argues Acheson, can combine to form either a positive way forward or, if negatively coalesced, a downward spiral of conditions of poor health.

The Social Exclusion Unit (SEU), subsequent to the Acheson Report, continues to promote and evaluate research and put forward recommendations to impact on policy. Examples of this are the *Truancy and Social Exclusion Report* (SEU, 1998a) and the *Teenage Pregnancy Report* (SEU, 1999a). Both of these reports deal extensively with their issues and form platforms for further policy expansion, and they are an excellent source of evidence to support practice development.

Ultimately, social exclusion is about an individual or a group of people suffering within mainstream society due to the fact that they are disadvantaged in some way. The stigma that is anticipated and experienced from being socially excluded due to healthcare issues is the main focus of this book, and we are concerned with the impact that healthcare workers can have, both positively and negatively, on this stigma.

As we point out in Chapter 3, we live in a dynamic society that is constantly changing, often relatively quickly (as with the advancement of technology) but sometimes quite slowly (as with nationalistic prejudice). In terms of stigmatised groups we may well experience the demise of one form of social exclusion but readily witness the rise of another. If we can learn to anticipate the targets and processes of social exclusion, then we may be in a better position to prepare and curtail their impact. An example of this is the government's urgency to address the exclusion felt by those people who do not have access to computers by ensuring that new technology is available in schools and libraries, and that the teaching resources are available for children. At one time computers were a luxury, a commodity of the rich; now they are fast becoming the mechanism of social communication. In a few years from now those who do not have access to a computer will become, at one and the same time, deaf, dumb, blind and ignorant. They will become the next generation of socially excluded.

The need for this book

The launch in 1997 of the government's Social Exclusion Unit raised public awareness of the need to acknowledge and address the challenges which face many socially excluded groups within society. A recent review of the SEU has highlighted its success (SEU, 1999b) and outlined the remit of 18 Policy Action Teams (PATs) which have been set up to coordinate and report on issues within the SEU. Healthcare professionals now have access to some of the work completed by the SEU, including reports on sleeping rough (SEU, 1998b) and teenage pregnancy (SEU, 1999a), and the first PATs' reports such as *Young People* (SEU, 2000). Given this increased political emphasis on social exclusion, an exploration of the experiences and needs of individuals who experience social exclusion through stigmatising attitudes is timely. This book focuses explicitly on the needs of healthcare professionals for knowledge and awareness of this topic in relation to specific patient and client groups.

Structure and rationale for the book

The book is divided into three parts. Part 1 is comprised of three chapters which focus on the theoretical underpinnings of stigma and social exclusion. Part 2, the largest section of the book, involves twenty-two chapters from practice areas which can have strong associations with stigmata. In dealing with the process of social exclusion we have grounded the structure of Part 2 in the works of Goffman's (1990) three types of stigma: (a) physical, (b) character and (c) racial; and Jones *et al.*'s (1984) six dimensions of stigma: (a) concealability, (b) course, (c) disruptiveness, (d) aesthetics, (e) origin and (f) peril. Drawing these strands together and bringing them into a contemporary focus, we have compartmentalised the concepts into Difference, Deviance and Dilemmas, and these form the sections of Part 2. However, we are fully aware that there are many areas of overlap between these broad perspectives and, indeed, that a stigmatised person may well be located in any permutation of these groups. This is part of the complexity of human affairs, and no attempt has been made to suggest that a clear delineation exists between them. Finally, Part 3 consists of one small but important chapter that points to the future and offers us a way forward.

The practice areas of Part 2 were chosen because of their commonality in healthcare settings and their dynamic status as changing modes of exclusion. They have been placed within the broader areas of Difference,

Deviance and Dilemmas in relation to their general 'fit' within Jones *et al.*'s (1984) six dimensions. Thus the chapters in Section 1 of Part 2 (Difference) are mainly concerned with issues of 'concealability' and 'course'. 'Concealability' refers to the extent to which a person engages in strategies whereby they hide their stigma so as not to reveal it to the world. For example, unwanted pregnancies may be hidden by clothing until the woman's growing abdomen reveals to the world her underlying condition. 'Course' relates to the progress of the stigmatising condition and the extent to which the person has some control over its advancement. There are often tensions between visible versus hidden conditions and the extent to which their course affects the person's life and those of related others. The chapters in the second section (Deviance) are focused on 'disruptiveness' and 'aesthetics'. By 'disruptiveness' we mean that property of a stigma which hampers, obstructs and curbs the interpersonal relationships of the stigmatised person and 'aesthetics' refers to the response of community members to the presented stigma: clearly, but sadly, a disfigured face causes greater social stress than does a blemish that is hidden by clothing. Finally, Section 3 (Dilemmas) deals with 'origin' and 'peril'. The former concerns the extent to which the stigmatised person is deemed responsible, which can be real or symbolic, for their condition, while the latter relates to the threat, or danger, that the stigma poses to the life of the person.

Within the above structure lies the rationale for the book. We are, first and foremost, socialised members of society, and we know, understand and operate according to the rules of our culture. We learn these rules as we grow through childhood into adulthood, by which time we may well have chosen to become healthcare professionals with our own code of rules, norms and values. However, the extent to which these social and professional codes of conduct clash, overlap and influence each other is highly complex and confusing. Although we may like to believe that we can separate and bracket out our personal views from our professional ones we have many examples where, maybe subconsciously derived, they in fact fuse together and are manifested in our actual behaviour. Thus, even healthcare professionals can contribute, knowingly or unknowingly, to the creation and maintenance of stigma and social exclusion. This book is concerned with examining some areas in which this occurs.

We believe that, through examining these areas, highlighting our own roles in stigmatising certain conditions, and reflecting on our practice, we can change that action. Thus we hope to assist others, as well as ourselves, in contributing to reduction of the pain and suffering associated with stigma and social exclusion.

A brief summary of the chapters

Chapter 2 reviews the major works on stigma, marginalisation and social exclusion from varying perspectives including sociology, social psychology, media studies, politics and anthropology. In Chapter 3 the focus is on the changing dynamic of stigma as it is modified across cultures, contexts and time, and contemporary issues that contribute to creating stigma in health-care settings are highlighted. We make the case in Chapter 4 for viewing health services as an important location for the experience of, and applica-tion of, stigma. We see nurses as having a pivotal role in both being a party to the stigmatising process: as instigators of stigma; occasionally as a stigmatised group themselves both within professional hierarchies and by association with highly stigmatised groups; and as being in a prime posi-tion to challenge stigma in practice or in politics.

In Section 1 of the practice areas, the authors deal in Chapter 5 with congenital disfigurement as a particularly traumatising event for both the parents and other family members and the affected child itself. In Chapter 6 there is a focus on aspects of stigma associated with genetic conditions which are often feared far beyond their capacity to affect future genera-tions. Deafness is the focus of Chapter 7, as it forecloses on a large area of human perception and can seriously damage the communicative process. As we learn to speak through hearing the spoken word, it is not surprising that those with this disability often have a speech impediment, and as a result may by association be incorrectly labelled as mentally impaired. With blindness, in Chapter 8, the stigmatisation process is overt, and this area of professional practice revolves around notions of dependence and independence. Obviously, people who are blind cannot 'see' the socially stigmatising behaviours that accompany their condition, but they most certainly 'feel' their effect. Differing levels of sight restriction may evoke different levels of marginalisation with the concomitant identification of 'problems' by health professionals who may well misjudge their impact. In Chapter 9, speech impediment as a stigma is considered. This area of healthcare falls roughly into expressive problems and receptive ones, with a frequent confusion between the two for those attempting to communi-cate with people with such conditions. In Chapter 10, the lack of knowledge of sexuality in healthcare is considered to be of growing concern and the salient issues are outlined accordingly. Assumptions of heterosexuality in all patients often govern the professional response to them. In Chapter 11, the specific stigma of HIV is discussed in relation to the political aspects of marginalisation of positive people. The penultimate chapter in this section, Chapter 12, deals with our understanding of epilepsy and the social response to it. Despite modern treatment and understanding of epilepsy, society generally remains wary and fearful of this condition in its more manifest states. Finally, in Chapter 13, burn injuries and their associated stigma are discussed. Burn injuries can be a significant cause of physical disfigurement and incapacity and, as a result of physical disfigurement, affected individuals might experience a range of negative social responses resulting in loss of personal self-esteem.

In Section 2 of Part 2, relating to deviance, Chapter 14 is concerned with the use of language and mental illness. In many ways, particularly for sociological theorists, mental illness is the archetypal case for the study of deviance and associated social relations. The institutions of psychiatry (especially forensic psychiatry) have had a particularly chequered history in dealing with minority groups, no more so than in contemplation of the notion of race, the central theme of Chapter 15. In the following chapter, Chapter 16, mental disorder and offending become the focus of attention, and the case of paedophilia is employed to bring into stark relief the tensions between society and mental health professionals. The notion of *Not in My Back Yard* (NIMBY) as a formal and informal societal response to locating the mentally ill in community settings remains problematic. Chapter 17 is written by a user of mental health services and is a powerful example of the role that professionals can play in creating stigma. In Chapter 18, drug abuse is the focus of attention as it is inextricably entwined with wider social, economic and political factors. Whereas the ingestion of some drugs is socially legitimated within limits (e.g. alcohol and tobacco), others such as cannabis are considered illicit. Although changing mores provide a platform for changing laws, it is the social domain that usually requires an alteration in its perception of the drug that precedes such legislative manoeuvres.

In Section 3 of Part 2 the central concern is with dilemmas, and Chapter 19 focuses upon homelessness and the marginalisation of homeless people in society. Chapter 20 deals with infertility. The procreation of our species lies at the very heart of human survival and thus forms the basis of the continuation of mankind, albeit in an evolutionary framework. The need to fulfil reproductive roles, within the normative values of each given society, is a central component of social status and is highly rewarded when appropriately fulfilled. However, when this ability to procreate is curtailed, for whatever reason, despite platitudes to the contrary, it can be a seriously stigmatising event. Chapter 21, on teenage pregnancy, deals with the social convention which suggests that having children ought to be undertaken in the confines of marriage and with the pregnancy being, if not planned, at least approved of. However, when young women in their teenage years become pregnant, the social response is often felt as negative and humiliating. Breastfeeding, not readily acknowledged as fertile ground for stigma and social exclusion, is focused upon in Chapter 22 to reveal a powerful force which can, indeed, create the conditions of marginalisation. Chapter 23 is concerned with terminal illness in children. It is hard to imagine that children with a terminal illness (and their families) can be 'victims' of stigma. Yet the threat of a child's death is one of the most feared life experiences. Young children are a particularly vulnerable group in society, as they tend to hold adults in parental awe, are socialised into doing what they are told to do, and form bonds of trust with 'grown-ups' who 'know best'. When the taboo of child abuse is broken it is viewed as a particularly stigmatising event which can destroy whole families, communities of friends, and the victims of such abuse. In Chapter 24 victims of stroke are the central theme. For those patients suffering from stroke there is a complex interplay of physical and cognitive deficits which, when they become apparent, can produce a wide-ranging set of problems such as loss of confidence and withdrawal. Older people are the main topic of investigation in Chapter 25. Older people are often stigmatised as being old-fashioned, out of touch, and not up-to-date irrespective of their wealth of experience and knowledge. Coupled to this marginalisation process is the misconception that old people are by association cognitively impaired. Finally in this section, Chapter 26 focuses on physical disability as stigma. For those persons with a physical disability there is often the accompanying suggestion that they are not in control of their mental faculties, which causes a great deal of anger and frustration on their part. Persons with a physical disability are often dismissed as having little to contribute to society and are patronised with superficial attempts at empathy.

Part 3 of the book is comprised of a single chapter which deals, first, with formulating a manifesto for change and a strategy for influencing policy development. This is a vitally important area which requires careful consideration if progress is to be made. Second, we draw all the major themes of the book together and offer a final conclusion on the issues of stigma and social exclusion.

Socially excluded groups tend to exist because of socialised attitudes governing prejudicial behaviour against them. Changing this state of affairs is notoriously difficult and an extremely protracted undertaking. Furthermore, legislation regarding such prejudices usually follows long campaigns against this kind of behaviour and its place in the latter part of our text reflects that it emanates from, rather than precedes, stigmatisation.

References

Acheson, D. (1998) *Independent inquiry into inequalities in health report*, London: The Stationery Office.

Berger, P. and Luckmann, T. (1966) *The social construction of reality*, London: Allan Lane.

Coleman, J.S. (1961) *The adolescent society*, New York: Free Press.

Dingwall, R. (1976) *Aspects of illness*, London: Martin Robertson.

Foucault, M. (1973) *The birth of the clinic: an archaeology of medical perception*, New York: Vintage Books.

Franzoi, S.L. (1996) *Social psychology*, London: Brown & Benchmark.

Goffman, E. (1990) *Stigma – notes on the management of spoiled identity*, third edn, London: Penguin.

HMSO (1972) *Report into conditions at Farley Hospital*, London: HMSO.

—— (1992) *Report of the Committee of Inquiry into complaints about Ashworth Hospital*, London: HMSO.

—— (1994) *The Allitt Inquiry: independent inquiry relating to deaths and injuries on the children's ward at Grantham and Kesteven General Hospital during the period February to April 1991*, London: HMSO.

Hughes, E.C. (1945) 'Dilemmas and contradictions of status', *American Journal of Sociology*, March: 353–9.

Jones, E.E., Farina, A., Hastorf, A.H. *et al.* (1984) *Social stigma, the psychology of marked relationships*, New York: W.H. Freeman.

Redfield, R. (1960) *The little community*, Chicago: University of Chicago Press.

Simmel, G. (1950) *Sociology*, New York: Free Press.

Social Exclusion Unit (1998a) *Truancy and social exclusion,* London: The Stationery Office.

—— (1998b) *Rough sleeping*, London: SEU.

—— (1999a) *Teenage pregnancy*, London: SEU.

—— (1999b) *Review of the Social Exclusion Unit*, London: SEU.

—— (2000) *Young people: a report by Policy Action Team 12*, London: SEU.

Sontag, S. (1978) *Illness as metaphor*, London: Penguin.

Stainton Rogers, W. (1991) *Explaining health and illness: an exploration of diversity*, London: Harvester Wheatsheaf.

Part I
Theoretical underpinnings

2 Historical developments

*Elizabeth Whitehead, Caroline Carlisle,
Caroline Watkins and Tom Mason*

Introduction

Today, the term 'stigma' may well carry a negative connotation but, etymologically, the origins of the semantic derive from the Greek word referring to a tattoo mark. More specifically, this was the branding of a name with the use of a hot iron impressed on people to show that they were devoted to the services of the temple. Later this religious message was somewhat secularised to designate the marking of an individual as a slave or criminal, which is an early indication that the concept of stigma is not static and fixed but one that is influenced by the social changes over any given epoch. This changing dynamic of stigma and its corollary, social exclusion, will be emphasised throughout this book. Even in contemporary times society's beliefs and attitudes continue to influence the meaning of stigma as we understand it in terms of our own culture and societal context. The profound and dramatic world events that shake the foundations of a society cause its individuals to reconsider, reflect, and re-prioritise what is considered as really important to their individual communities. It is at such times that notions of stigma and social exclusion are shaken and re-formed, and the boundaries defining what was considered to be obviously deviant at another period of our time become blurred and indistinct. Such social movement emanates from the normative prescriptions according to a society's structure, function and influences, logically leading to questions relating to the causes of such changes. It is suggested that, while some situational conditions move to a state in which they appear to carry less potential to create stigma, others arise to increase the likelihood of creating difference. There are also strong cultural differences in what is considered a stigma, as well as regional variations within wider social contexts. From national values to gang-cultural codes, the variety of rules and taboos which may be transgressed can all elicit the process of marginalisation and contribute to the formation of stigmatised conditions.

However, it is not only the derivation of the word that is of interest but also the accompanying semantics by which we come to know what it means to be stigmatised. Most of the readers of this chapter will already have had experience of attempts to change the words that attend to a particular stigmatising condition. For example, the term 'lunatic' was considered a pejorative label and was changed to the more acceptable term of 'mentally ill', the term 'mentally handicap' became 'learning disability', and the Spastics' Society changed its title to Scope. These examples, and many more, attest to the fact that alongside the terminology that is used to give meaning to the subject there may develop a whole range of prejudice, intolerance and preconception contributing to the marginalisation of those with the 'appropriate' label.

Stigma and social exclusion within a historical context

The move towards the acceptance of a certain form of behaviour, a particular ethnic group or a specific physical abnormality is dependent upon the development of a society's cultural heritage, which may be determined by key historical and social landmarks creating the values of that society. The origins of such stigmatisation lie in the group feeling threatened by an individual, or a number of individuals, who are perceived to disunite, undermine and contaminate the larger society. Such reactions not uncommonly arise from a fear of the unknown and the unfamiliar. This is clearly a sociological area of study, but it also has strong links with both social psychology and anthropology. The historical developments will be dealt with in an overlapping style, reflecting their emergence from a number of perspectives.

Deviance

Stigma is not an isolated sociological concept but one that is more closely wrapped up with many other aspects of the human condition, leading to prejudices and marginalisation. These often produce derogatory identification terms such as deviance, which, like stigma, is a fluid concept and, again, one that changes over time. Therefore, deciding what is deviant and what is not is a process that can only be defined by a particular society at a given point in its social development. Deviance may be considered as a form of social behaviour, as defined by that group for their purposes and function. It is the social group itself that defines its norms and decides what forms of behaviour lie outside of those regulatory frameworks. In its relationship with stigma, deviance is most closely associated with Goffman's concept of 'moral behaviour' (Goffman, 1990). For example, when society chooses to stigmatise on moral grounds it is actually making a statement regarding what it believes to be considered as deviant. As deviant behaviour is culturally relative, that which is considered to be deviant in one culture may not have the same structural components as in another. For example, marriage for thirteen-year-old girls among the Muslims of Pakistan is an accepted, and welcomed, cultural practice. In Britain this is not accepted, and marriage is illegal until the age of sixteen years.

Durkheim and deviance

The significance of the French sociologist Emile Durkheim's (1858–1917) work on deviance lies in the influence he was to have on later sociologists. Taken as a whole Durkheim's sociological work may be considered as nothing less than the construction of what later philosophers would call 'a scientific research programme'. This can be said to have three central components: (a) a 'hard core' comprised of metaphysical beliefs; (b) an intermediary 'protective belt' of positive and negative heuristics; and (c) outlying theories for numerous sub-disciplines which make empirical statements, predictions and interpretations of differentiated sectors of the real world. In short, Durkheim produced a sociological research programme that had the central components of the natural scientific method and ensconced sociology alongside such other procedural sciences. His notion of deviance is closely linked to social and religious community and, although he earlier believed that social malaise was responsible for the condition of deviance, he came to feel that society itself had lost its moral code, thus isolating individuals and marginalising them as deviants. What is important is that this 'positioning' of deviance as being at one level the responsibility of the individual and at another the fault of society is reflective of our contemporary British community and its reaction to what it considers as deviance.

Symbolic Interactionism

Durkheim's positivist methodology was a constant striving to demonstrate that sociology should be acknowledged as an empirical science as governed by natural laws, although later thinkers in sociology felt that this was a fruitless endeavour. Symbolic Interactionism originates from a particularly fertile and exciting time in American sociology, which can be located in the early 'Chicago School'. The Chicago School, particularly in the inter-war years, can boast a number of prominent Symbolic Interactionists such as George Herbert Mead, Charles Cooley, Howard Becker and Erving Goffman (Burns, 1992). The concept of Symbolic Interactionism rests on one individual being able to imagine the social role of another, and on our ability to imagine ourselves as acting in other social roles. Furthermore, the reflexive adoption of the role of the other will depend upon our capacity for an internal dialogue with ourselves regarding what the constituent parts of that role may be. Herbert Blumer and others have analysed the complexities of this reflexive process, and the three main principles of Symbolic Interactionism as put forward by Blumer are:

- human beings act towards things on the basis of the meanings that things have for them;

- these meanings arise out of social interaction;
- social action results from a 'fitting together of individual lines of action'.

Thus there is a close relationship between the individual, the group, and the wider social context in which they operate. Outside of this, a deviation leads to the production of stigma (Blumer, 1956).

Labelling theory

The importance and relevance of Howard Becker rests on his contribution to the study of deviance and his formulation of labelling theory. Unlike many of his predecessors, Becker's approach to deviance was not put forward as a pure theoretical concept but rather as a dynamic force which occurs within a framework of sociological interaction. In this context, deviance is a product of the social world and the effect of the operationalisation of the values, and their meaning, in which Symbolic Interactionism is concerned. In terms of social exclusion the following extract from Becker's *Perspectives On Deviance: The Other Side* (Becker, 1963) outlines the relationship between the labelling of deviance and the social group which is applying it.

> Social groups create deviance by making the rules whose infraction constitutes deviance, and by applying those rules to particular people and labelling them as outsiders. From this point of view, deviance is not a quality of the act the person commits, but rather a consequence of the application by others of rules and sanctions to an 'offender'. The deviant is one to whom that label has successfully been applied; deviant behaviour is behaviour that people so label.
>
> (Becker, 1963: 3)

Thus we can see the concepts of labelling theory and stigma as being highly relevant to the healthcare settings of today in which many conditions are seen as deviant forms of behaviour. As labelling theory is constructed around how relationships are formed by the influences of society and specific groups within that community, this is a particularly relevant perspective for understanding the role of healthcare workers in contemporary practice.

Erving Goffman

Contemporary sociological analysis of stigma and social exclusion has its origins in the work of Erving Goffman (1922–82), who in turn was influenced by others such as Durkheim. When the first edition of his work on *Stigma: Notes on the Management of Spoiled Identity* was published in

1963 (Goffman, 1990), both the academic and the lay reader were for the first time provided with a comprehensive sociological map of the concept of exclusionary techniques. Although an absolute definition of stigma is difficult to encapsulate, the following attempt by Goffman is an excellent starting point on which to base further sociological exploration.

> While the stranger is present before us, evidence can arise of his possessing an attribute that makes him different from others in the category of persons available for him to be, and of a less desirable kind – in the extreme a person who is quite thoroughly bad, or dangerous, or weak. He is thus reduced in our minds from a whole and usual person to a tainted discounted one. Such an attribute is a stigma.
>
> (Goffman, 1990: 12)

This extract focuses Goffman's understanding of stigma from the viewpoint of society and shows how the individual can socially emerge as different. His concern with understanding how and why some members of society choose to stigmatise a particular social group is important in understanding the reasons for the stigmatising process. A notable achievement of this work is that it provokes the reader, irrespective of their sociological background, to critically consider the dynamics of stigma from either an experiential or a theoretical perspective. The value of this is that it is a proven framework for generating research and analysis on the attitudes of society towards marginalised individuals and groups. The significance of Goffman's analysis is that it has remained a text of shared identification and meaning for people across many societies, and pivots on personal accounts and lived experiences of being, and feeling, excluded. There are a significant number of vignettes in Goffman's text that are personal experiences from stigmatised individuals, and these personal accounts ground the book in the lifeworld of the marginalised 'other'. Deeply rooted in Goffman's work is his identification of moral career as an emergent concept within the creation of difference and the shared learning experiences of particular stigmatised individuals within a wider marginalised group. Goffman highlights the following example.

> This illustration is provided by a homosexual in regard to his becoming one: I met a man with whom I had been at school. He was, of course, gay himself, and took it for granted that I was too. I was surprised and rather impressed. He did not look in the least like the popular idea of a homosexual, being well built, masculine and neatly dressed. This was something new to me. Although I was perfectly prepared to admit that love could exist between men, I had always been slightly repelled by the obvious homosexuals whom I had met

because of their vanity, their affected manner and careless chatter.
These, it now appeared, formed only a small part of the homosexual
world, although the most noticeable one...

(Goffman, 1990: 53)

The gay person in Goffman's text highlights the complex world of
'difference' and 'sameness' as dilemmatic relations within the concept of
stigmatisation. The gay speaker understands all too well that he will be
stigmatised as different, as odd; and yet within the notion of being
different he also wishes to be seen publicly as the same, as 'normal',
within his own group. In historical terms this early understanding was
central in identifying the tensions and contradictions between a desire to
be the same as others within a marginalised group and an acknowledgement of difference between them and the wider, more powerful,
normative society.

Understanding social exclusion and its analysis as a major thread of
social interaction of contemporary society is of fundamental importance.
Goffman, and later others, provide the framework and signposts to
address the issues of why some individuals experience perceptions of
stigma. When a person becomes the perpetrator of stigmatisation towards
others, that individual, according to Goffman's analysis, will experience a
number of emotional reactions. According to Goffman, those individuals
who stigmatise others believe them to be of less value, bad or dangerous. It
is very difficult to conceal such feelings of extreme condemnation, and
while there are those whose prejudice is subconscious there are other
perpetrators of stigma who indeed consciously wish for their feelings to be
overtly known. Although Goffman did not develop a sophisticated analysis
of the power relations within institutional and social structures, his work
most certainly set the scene for others to do so.

Edward Jones and his co-authors

Another influential historical contribution comes from Edward Jones and
his colleagues whose work post-dates Goffman by twenty years. Our own
book is enhanced by the diverse disciplines of those authors who also
have the benefit of the work of Goffman, and also of other writers since
his classical work was published. Jones *et al.*'s *Social Stigma: The
Psychology of Marked Relationships* (1984) has made a significant contribution to the research and subsequent understanding of the nature and
social impact of stigmatised individuals. Edward Jones, as the editor of
the book, wrote:

[We] intend to focus in this book on a particular category of social
relationships – those in which one participant has a condition that is
at least potentially discrediting. We shall be concerned with the cogni-

tive and affective underpinnings of such relationships and with the behavioural problems they entail. We shall also be concerned with the course and development of such relationships over time...

(Jones *et al.*, 1984: 6)

We can see from this focus that Jones *et al.*'s main concern was to be the impact of the stigmatising condition on the mental state of the person concerned, and the overall impact that this was to have on their functioning in the wider society. This is of central concern for healthcare workers who often interface with such persons and have a role to play in understanding its wider influence on social and behavioural problems. This fundamental contribution which emanates from the work of Jones and his colleagues can be located under the rubric of affective psychology. In this, the personal experiences of marginalised individuals are very much associated with emotional feelings of depression, anger and humiliation.

In this historical development the contributors, representing many disciplines, examine stigma and social exclusion from broad perspectives, with Jones's overall analysis being concerned about social relationships that involve at least one person who is vulnerable to being labelled as deviant and thus being stigmatised. Thus the significant value of Jones's contribution is the relationship between societal values and the perceptions of the marginalised individual as a devalued person. Therefore it is the feeling of stigma as perceived by vulnerable individuals which in this context deals with the personal responses of fear, anger, worthlessness and depression etc. The emotional impact of these engendered feelings, whether or not explicitly evoked by the societal response to the stigma, is implicitly felt as a corollary of those social expectations. The result of this, according to Jones *et al.*, is the development of a mental strategy to deal with the social implications of the stigma. These he terms the 'six dimensions' of (a) concealability, (b) course, (c) disruptiveness, (d) aesthetic qualities, (e) origin and (f) peril. We can now look at these dimensions in a little more depth.

Concealability

In social terms this refers to whether the stigmatising condition is hidden or visible and deals with the question of to what extent its visibility is controllable by the recipient, or the wish to control it is desirable. For example, an unwanted teenage pregnancy may be hidden up to the point when the girl's growing abdomen indicates otherwise, although she may have the desire to conceal her condition for longer. Similarly, someone with an early diagnosis of cancer may well be able to conceal this until external physical signs become apparent, although they may, again, desire that they could withhold the information from the outside world. In both states there is a cut-off point at which the person inevitably reveals their condition irrespective of their desire to hide it.

Course

This is concerned with the pattern of change in relation to social expectations of the condition, and examines what the anticipated social consequences of the outcomes are. Once the person reveals that they have a particular condition which may well lead to stigmatisation, this may well have an impact on their social relations. It is not uncommon, for example, for someone with an unwanted teenage pregnancy to remain socially excluded until after the baby's arrival. Similarly, someone who has a disfiguring disease may well withdraw from social interaction as the course of the condition progresses.

Disruptiveness

This refers to the extent to which the condition blocks or hampers social interaction or communication with the social network. This moves beyond the fatalistic course of events described in *Course* and pivots on the choice of individuals within the social frame. A condition such as a highly infectious disease will clearly cause a major disruption to the social interactions of the person afflicted. However, other less obvious conditions can have an equally forceful impact. For example, someone who becomes mentally ill, is brain damaged, or begins to suffer from dementia may well cause themselves to alter their social interactions and also cause others to alter their usual social intercourse. However, we must be careful here not to suggest that it is the afflicted persons 'fault' but merely that it is the social interaction that is affected. There are many factors for this, but as examples it may be through embarrassment, lack of knowledge or merely because the condition incapacitates the social development.

Aesthetic qualities

This dimension refers to the extent to which there are signs and symbols of the condition that make the possessor repellent, ugly or upsetting in some way. Disfigurements which are obvious and are difficult to conceal can cause deep emotional pain to those who have them, but can also cause others to react instinctively by grimacing or recoiling. Such a reaction may be out of the person's conscious control, and they may deeply regret it; however, its impact on the disfigured person reinforces their condition as being aesthetically displeasing. Conditions such as facial burns and deformities of the face are difficult to conceal and are examples of this dimension. However, other conditions which may be hidden for part of the time, such as colostomy, may also be considered aesthetically displeasing and cause the person to become socially excluded.

Origin

This dimension refers to the aetiology of the circumstances that led to the condition and the perceived blame for its occurrence. Infectious diseases may be related, spuriously or otherwise, to the person's actual behaviour, and if there is a perceived relationship then responsibility and blame may follow. The early response to the number of gay men with AIDS was that it was retribution for their perceived aberrant sexuality. Previously, leprosy was conceived as divine retribution for past sins; and more recently smoking tobacco and alcohol consumption equate with personal responsibility, to the extent that medical interventions are questioned on the basis of dwindling resources and cost–benefit ratios.

Peril

This refers to whether the stigmatising condition poses any social danger and, if so, how imminent or serious it is. In this dimension there is a focus on the extent to which the social groups can be threatened by the condition. AIDS is one example, highlighting the extent to which sexual behaviour changed according to the perceived threat that the HIV virus caused. Earlier examples may include the numerous plagues that ravaged communities down the centuries with the result that perceived infected people were removed from their society. Furthermore, most readers will be familiar with the terms 'barrier nursing' or 'isolation nursing', in which an infected person is removed from the ward community and nursed alone in a room. In both these cases the exclusion is due to the perceived peril that the infection may cause, with the result that the 'appropriate' social precautions are taken. Although these may in reality be symbolic examples, we can see the structures of isolation, exclusion and marginalisation that are apparent throughout these reactions. As the infection causes a degree of peril to others, our social response is to remove the infected person and put up some form of protective 'barrier'.

Although Goffman, too, shows a deep concern with the relationship between deviance and stigmatisation, it should be acknowledged that some contemporary theorists are less happy with using the terms stigma and deviance interchangeably. While these latterday critics accept that both stigma and deviance are concepts from earlier writings in sociology, the term deviance has more recently acquired for them a sexual connotation tending towards perversion, while stigma focuses on the concept of the 'other' as a socially constructed normative outlier. Given that the use of linguistic terms continues to evolve, nevertheless many of the emotional and social reactions that people experience, in relation to such semantics, do not always change at the same pace.

The death of deviance?

For generations deviance has been taught as an integral part of undergraduate sociology programmes, as an academic subject in its own right. However, with the publication of Colin Sumner's book *The Sociology of Deviance: An Obituary* (1994), this perspective has shifted somewhat. Sumner's historical cultural analysis has resulted in his rejection of the concept of deviance as an academic subject and advocated that deviance should be replaced by a theory of censorship. An example of the rejection of the sociological issues associated with deviance is found in Sumner's demolition of Becker's contribution to labelling theory: 'My own theory of social censures suggests that it is rare that a stigmatisation or censure is anything other than an expression, sublimation or rationalisation of larger social divisions, such as those of social class' (Sumner, 1994: 225).

Both Goffman and Sumner argue that stigma is not a mutual experience shared by all societies: 'Killing is murder in some contexts and heroism in others. Sex in some contexts is a sign of deep love, and in others a sign of profound hate' (Sumner, 1994: 225). However, the question of the universality of stigma, rather than being rooted in individual issues across societies, is whether the concept of stigmatisation as a sociological process transcends all cultures. Thus, while accepting the possibility of the 'death of deviance as an academic subject', the object of deviance is all too alive and kicking.

Scambler and medical sociology

Graham Scambler has examined stigma and social exclusion within a framework of health and illness with his analysis (1993), bringing in the notion of the sick role as developed by Parsons, Gehardt and Freidson. The importance of these contributors lies particularly with Parsons, who observed a fundamental link between illness and deviance. Freidson's analysis of the sick role stretches beyond that of both Parsons and Gehardt, and is observed by Scambler: '... contrary to Parsons, Freidson sees the physicians' social control functions as extending far beyond the policing of the sick role and possessing negative as well as positive potential for society' (Scambler, 1993: 187). This latter point brings into focus a central theme of the current book, in that it attempts to deal with the role of healthcare professionals in the construction and maintenance of strategies that lead to stigma and social exclusion.

Both the medical and social nature of many conditions relate to Scambler's identification of certain medical structures that contribute to the process of exclusion through the force of a label. Scambler identifies a number of conditions as being stigmatising; these include AIDS, psoriasis, epilepsy and severe burns, and argues that these can be defined as conditions that set their possessors apart from 'normal' people, that mark them as socially unacceptable or as inferior beings (Scambler, 1993). Illness involves deviance and stigma on two levels. First, by individually deviating from the social 'norm' and being labelled as 'sick', and second, by having a condition which is socially uncomfortable for the rest of society. The deviance may involve appearance or behaviour, such as psoriasis or AIDS (as perceived). Again, this interplay of perceptions between individuals and society, and between the values of normality and prejudiced behaviour, is central to the concept of the current book.

Social Exclusion Unit

The Social Exclusion Unit was set up in 1998 by the government and comprises of a number of key personnel from both the civil service and people outside of government with front-line experience of tackling the problems of social exclusion. Their main remit is to concentrate on certain priorities within British society which are considered to lead to social exclusion. These are: (a) truancy and school exclusion; (b) sleeping rough; and (c) the most deprived housing estates. The unit is also required to report on improving mechanisms for integrating the work of departments, local authorities and other agencies, feeding into the Comprehensive Spending Reviews; and to draw up key indicators of social exclusion (SEU, 1998). The government hopes that the SEU will draw on its experience and identify key preventive interventions with children and young people; probe aspects of exclusion which disproportionately affect particular ethnic minorities; establish options for improving service access; and suggest ways to encourage individual and business involvement in addressing social exclusion (SEU, 1999).

Although this government initiative can be criticised as failing to address the wider social divisions in society that lead to the factors identified as precursors to social exclusion, it is an important development in recognising that the issues need to be seriously addressed. The fact that such a unit must itself be based on the identification of norms and values is stark testimony to the complexity and intransigence of the problems facing societies that at one level exclude aberrant behaviours, and at another level wish to be seen to include reformed characters. Again, this highlights the difficulty that healthcare professionals face in their identities, on the one hand, as socialised members of a particular society and, on the other, as members of the caring profession attempting to uphold those values.

Conclusion

The objective of this chapter has been to map out some of the more important historically based theoretical concepts of stigma and social exclusion. In doing this, the three central issues to emerge were, first, that to fully appreciate the concept of exclusion in its wide and varied forms requires its location in relation to particular scientific disciplines. For many sociologists the tracing back of stigma to deviance is a crucial starting point; for example, Durkheim's rules of deviance have been, and continue to be, a pivotal reference point for research that seeks to explore stigma and exclusion. Second, the fact that stigma and deviance do share this historical overlapping of the two concepts has made the changing dynamic difficult to pin down. Third, it is important to be aware of the psycho-social nature of the stigmatising process and the impact that it can have on the emotions. As we continue to observe and critique these historical developments it is this third issue, involving the profound emotional impact of stigma in relation to identification, anticipation, understanding and resolution, upon which we can have the most significant effect. As we look back, we will see how these historical landmarks have enabled us to progress from Durkheim's sociological phenomena of nineteenth-century Paris to the all-encompassing daily social interactions of the new twenty-first century.

References

Becker, H. (1963) *Perspectives on deviance: the other side*, Toronto: Macmillan.

Blumer, H. (1956) *Symbolic Interactionism – perspectives on method*, Englewood Cliffs, NJ: Prentice Hall.

Burns, T. (1992) *Goffman*, London: Routledge.

Freidson, E. (1961) *Patient views of medical practice*, New York: Russell Sage Foundation.

Gehardt, U. (1987) 'Parsons, role theory and health interaction', in G. Scambler (ed.), *Sociological theory and medical sociology*, London: Tavistock.

Goffman, E. (1990) *Stigma: notes on the management of spoiled identity*, London: Penguin.

Jones, E.E., Farina, A., Hastorf, A.H. *et al.* (1984) *Social stigma, the psychology of marked relationships*, New York: W.H. Freeman.

Parsons, T. (1951) *The social system*, New York: McGraw-Hill.

Scambler, G. (1993) *Sociology as applied to medicine*, London: Bailliere Tindall.

Social Exclusion Unit (1998) *So you'd like to know more?*, http://www.open.gov.uk/co/seu/more.html

—— (1999) *What's it all about?*, http://www.cabinet-office.gov.uk/seu/index/faqs.html

Sumner, C. (1994) *The sociology of deviance: an obituary*, Buckingham: Open University Press.

3 The changing dynamic of stigma

Elizabeth Whitehead, Tom Mason,
Caroline Carlisle and Caroline Watkins

Introduction

The experience of stigma has a profound effect both in its emotional impact for the individual concerned and in its social repercussions for the marginalised group as a whole. The stigmatising process is rooted deep within human nature and from earliest times to the present day there are examples that are gathered in stories, anthologies and historical accounts of one society or another stigmatising its neighbours (Parkin, 1993). The diversity and complexity of the human capacity to stigmatise is found in numerous symbolic expressive forms via a number of media, from litera-ture and film to news reports. The motives behind the stigmatising process are also extremely complex and often lie deep within individual psyches and culturalised prejudices. In modern times the most profound act of stigma revolves around what is now termed ethnic cleansing. From the mass slaughter of millions of innocent people, merely because they were of another race, creed or culture, or simply because they were different, is stark testimony to the darker side of human nature when the responses to the stigma are left unchecked. Therefore, understanding the cultural complexity of this marginalisation process is a vital step in changing the practice of exclusion (Social Exclusion Unit, 1999).

Stigma heightens our senses to the notion of difference and creates a tension within the self in relation to the context in which the stigmatised person is perceived. In healthcare settings these perceptions of difference may become professionalised, and thus to some degree legitimated, as they occur within a medical framework. That is, in this context treating someone differently becomes accepted because they are deemed to be in some way 'dis-ordered'. However, outside of the illness context the stig-mata are often viewed as blemishes, and for some this legitimates ridicule, avoidance, fear or disgust. For example, while the professional may accept the noise uttered by an autistic child in a residential home, some members of society are generally reluctant to accept such disturbance in the super-market. Outside of the life–death scenario the relationship between our health and the stigma representing the illness is relative to the context in which the sign symbolises the meaning. For example, our health is of central importance to most people, whether it is hidden dysfunctional muscles in muscular dystrophy or the visible imperfections of acne on the face of a teenager. Excepting the life-threatening and incapacitating nature of the former disorder, the context of stigma revolves around the presentation of self within the social status of the community (Goffman, 1972). Thus, the stigma of cancer equates with the stigma of acne depending on both the context in which society responds to it and its felt impact by the receiver of the stigma. This illustration of the stigmatising response to various conditions of 'disorder' serves to indicate the extent to which the concept of difference is confused with that of deviation.

Clarifying the meaning of difference in healthcare settings is crucial to developing our understanding of the stigmatising process, as most people wish to be considered different in some way but also wish to fall within the bounds of what is considered 'normal'. While being different may attract the response from society of being 'interesting', stigmatising conditions may attract responses that are governed by the degree to which they deviate from the 'norm'. This is often determined by their perceived origin. For example, a woman who contracts a sexually transmitted disease while being raped will receive a different response than if she had contracted the same disease through prostitution. And again, a person who has lost his sight in a bomb blast may well be responded to differently depending upon whether he was a victim or the bomber. In short, the origin of the stigma has some influence over the societal response to it.

The fluidity of stigma was reflected in the historical analysis of the concept presented in Chapter 2, and we can understand the cultural force of social exclusion if a community can establish an association between the perceived disorder and the behaviour of the person who is afflicted, even when the association is spurious. This was the case with such stigmatising diseases as, say, leprosy, when the causal relationship was perceived as referring to the person being considered to be possessed by the devil. In a similar, but contemporary, vein a relatively new stigmatising disorder is AIDS, which is socially associated with promiscuity, homosexuality and drug abuse. Thus, in establishing the changing dynamic of stigma in contemporary society, we must deconstruct the project into two main areas: (a) societal influences; and (b) cultural threats.

Societal influences

As we have already noted, there is a complex relationship between individuals and groups that stigmatise and those that become the stigmatised, and while on some occasions the process of exclusion is explicit, at other times it appears to operate at a subconscious level. In attempting to unravel this complexity it is important to understand some of the influences upon our attitudes and, ultimately, upon our behaviour.

Political influences

Whether politicians are leaders or followers of public opinion is open to debate and conjecture. However, what is central in either perspective is the extent to which they can impact on stigmatised groups. Political thought and action are only legitimate, in practical terms, when they can directly influence the behaviour of society (George and Wilding, 1985). As it is always a matter of power, we must be concerned as to the extent that political factors will determine the social response to socially excluded groups and, in terms of consequences, the effect that policy has on the quality of life of all concerned. This is a particularly thorny issue when the social members involved in decisions regarding marginalised groups also have a vicarious impact on 'innocent' others; for example, a pregnant teenager may well be socially excluded but this also has an impact on her unborn child, especially if an abortion is being considered (Worman, 1999). Furthermore, the enforcement of political policy may include calibrating state benefit payments or gatekeeping access to accommodation, with the corollary of added pressure in other aspects of people's lives that can, in turn, create further hardships and distress (Weeks, 1994).

Politicians also have freer access to media attention, although this can be negative as well as positive, and through this means they can wield further power to influence values and standards. Politicians who choose to attract media attention by championing a particular cause put themselves at risk to some degree; however, this is usually achieved by linking into lobby groups who represent a wider social membership. In contemporary times we can note the impact of political influences on socially excluded groups such as people with disability (the recent watering-down of legislation), teenage pregnancy (the development of the Social Exclusion Unit), and veterans of the Gulf War (the refusal to accept the existence of 'Gulf War syndrome'). Political views can clearly have a direct impact on which groups become marginalised and also on how members of society ought to respond to these groups (Social Exclusion Unit, 1998).

Media influences

Above and beyond the points mentioned in the foregoing section, the media have two further functions in relation to the changing dynamic of stigma. First, they are vehicles for the communication of values for those wishing to exercise their influence over others (Day and Page, 1986). This might be in the form of written views and commentaries stated in newspapers or on public platforms, or it might be via verbal statements made on radio and television. The important point here is that the method of delivery is central to the impact that the media can have on marginalised groups, and also in the process of marginalising them (Philo, 1996). For example, 'professional' broadcasting presenters, as well as some politicians, are often trained in public speaking and, through practice and experience, may be able to express their views more eloquently than their non-trained counterparts. Advertising companies know only too well the power of the means of communication rather than the content of the message (Campbell and Bonner, 1994).

Second, journalists who carry the mantle of reporting events, opinions and perspectives are also in a position of power to influence social values. In attempting to sensationalise a particular story, reporters and editors may emphasise a specific theme while omitting other information that might detract from the overall message. Editorial licence is a powerful means by which newspapers and other reporting sources can exercise their own ideological perspectives. A good example of this is the way in which a story can be re-worked to read from differing political viewpoints. It is worth remembering the comment of a former health minister, Edwina Curry, who in 1988 claimed that people from the North-West of England ate too much fried food. The political implication of her comment was that sufferers from heart disease in the North-West were responsible, and thus could be blamed, for their condition. This is similar to the argument that those who engage in cigarette smoking are also responsible for the diseases that may accompany this practice, or that those who drink too much alcohol are responsible for their diseased livers. In both cases there is already some debate concerning whether these latter two groups ought to receive healthcare, especially when they do not cease from smoking or drinking (Whitehead, 1992).

Campaigners' influences

Campaigners, lobby groups and voluntary organisations are driven by commitment to a particular cause, whatever that cause may represent. Many socially excluded groups have both supporters and critics from a number of fronts and are subject to a barrage of arguments, all of which are often claimed to be 'for their benefit'. Those who act as advocates may claim that we, as a society, have a shared responsibility for those who are marginalised, and that we ought to incorporate them into the body of society rather than expel them. However, some protagonists may claim that their plight is their own responsibility and they should be made accountable for their position. In any event, what is important is that all views strongly expressed tend to place upon those who are stigmatised a pressure to conform which can have deleterious effects on their physical, emotional and social health. Such campaigning influences are usually effective because the proponents tend to be specialists in their topic area and experienced in their lobbying. Furthermore, they also tend to express their views in a forceful and passionate manner. We cannot disentangle the interests that such stakeholders have in forming policy for excluded groups; as Williamson (1993) noted, 'interests are to do with advantage and detriment to individuals and to groups ... Everyone has interests in resources like influence, power, time, money, knowledge, the way situations involving themselves are defined'. Campaigners, like most others, have their own agenda to fulfil.

The influence of public opinion

In democratic societies the views of the masses are usually of central importance in affecting the social body. The weight of public opinion can affect changes in the law, government and social policy. It is well appreciated that such mass opinion can have both negative and positive reactions; for example, the public response to the development of AIDS in the 1980s was a case of the former and the public response to the outbreak of BSE in the 1990s was a case of the latter (although it is appreciated that other influences, such as economics, also had an impact). Public opinion can quickly switch to public outrage, with the result that groups and individuals can become further stigmatised. For example, people in general with mental health problems can become further ostracised and labelled as dangerous when a particular individual with a mental illness commits a serious crime.

There is a further complicating factor to this relationship which needs to be mentioned, and that concerns the role of the stigmatised person in response to the marginalisation process. If we take teenage pregnancy as an example, we can see that the public view of this condition is all-important in the case of a developing adolescent, as it is this weight of culturally determined opinion that will contribute to her feeling stigmatised. If she is unaware of the social perspective of her condition, then she is unlikely to feel the stigmatising force. On the other hand, if she misperceives that a social sanction has been applied, and in reality it is in fact not applied, then the perception alone is sufficient to create the feelings of stigma. With such stigmatised groups as pregnant teenagers, people who are HIV-positive, drug addicts, or 'glue sniffers', public concern leads into what is known as a moral panic. Recent moral panics have been fuelled and fanned by the 'new social policy' of both the current and the previous governments' focus on the family as a central tenet of contemporary society. Unfortunately, this focus has been less on the positive values of togetherness and the sharing of responsibility and more on the negative connotations of financial status and dependency. What is clear, however, is the interconnectedness of the relations between politics, media and the lay public in processing the influences of marginalisation.

Cultural threats

Threats to any culture are usually met with fierce resistance, and it is not surprising that there are numerous social structures that operate to safeguard members of a particular community. Marginalising others is a process that is employed to purify a given culture, at least by its own perceived views, and this lies as the basis of 'ethnic cleansing'. Some of these social processes will now be briefly outlined.

Values, norms and standards

When social groups are formed there are a number of strategic concepts that are employed to aid cohesion and strengthen the bonds of identity. Such concepts as values, norms and standards are well rehearsed in the sociological literature. *Values* are concerned with what members of a group consider to be good, valuable and important to them. They will vary between nations, cultures, groups, sub-groups and gangs. For example, one group of people may consider that polite manners are valued in their society, while members of a street gang might view them with distaste. However, it should be remembered that the gang culture will also have sets of shared values that other groups would view as without value. *Norms* are generally viewed as informal rules, which are often not written down but exist in tradition. Again, these vary across cultures, but each culture will have their own particular set of norms. In our culture it is a norm to eat with a knife and fork, in others with chopsticks, and in still others with the fingers. Interestingly, in our own culture eating with the fingers is a norm for certain foods and in certain contexts. *Standards* represent the expectation that certain levels of behavioural performance will be achieved by the accomplished, and aspired to by the trainee. 'Coming up to standard' is a socially accepted achievement in any group, no matter what the standard is, and 'falling below standard' is considered a failing.

For cultures, communities and gangs to exist, these norms, values and standards must be powerful enough to stir members to action in the face of their transgression. The society must be strong enough to reward conformists and to repel those who would attack the fabric of their community. The social structure of these groups provides a dynamic force that outlines their external boundaries, margins and internal structures. These are maintained through signs and symbols that often have a ritualistic quality. For example, Van Gennep (1909) showed how 'rites of passage' from one life-stage to the next was a common ritual found in many cultures (for example, from boyhood to manhood, and from being single to becoming married). The failure of this passage could often lead to exclusion, isolation and a devaluing of the person. What these 'rites of passage' highlight, of course, are the demarcation lines *between* one state and another which carry with them the status of inclusion, if successfully navigated. The lines are thresholds to be either crossed or not as the case may be, and they carry with them extensive rituals both in terms of their actual crossing and in defence of their boundaries. We could instance the ritual of 'carrying the bride over the threshold' as an example of the former and the 'ritual protection of bodily orifices as a symbol of social preoccupation about exits and entrances' (Douglas, 1996) as an example of the latter.

The internalised structures refer to the impact of those external social forces influencing the functioning of the individual member of the group. In this scenario, the transgression of socially legitimated behaviour may be seen to have an internal effect on the person. The obvious cultural example is witchcraft, in which the external force impacts upon the targeted individual (Evans-Pritchard, 1937). Irrespective of the type of belief system, there are few, if any, contemporary healthcare workers who do not believe that external conditions (home, work) can have an effect on the inner person (stress, burnout, depression). The important message here in understanding the forces of stigma, social exclusion and marginalisation is that these are social structures of demarcation which, if transgressed, may be considered as a form of 'pollution' (Douglas, 1996). This leads us to consider the central positions of demarcation in sociological terms: 'them' and 'us'.

Them and us

In the sociology of the outcast the distinction between 'them' and 'us' is often referred to as those in the in-group and those in the out-group. From this we can see that there is a clear relation between the two, in that one cannot exist without the other. As Bauman (1997) noted: 'the two members of the conceptual–behavioural opposition complement and condition each other; they acquire all their meaning from that opposition. "Them" are not "us", and "us" are not "them"; "me" and "they" can be understood only together, in their mutual conflict'. When individuals and groups sediment the opposition between 'them' and 'us' into value-laden social constructions, this can easily lead into prejudiced views and actions relating to the devaluation of the 'other'.

Other writers who have addressed this issue of marginalisation have produced differing terms for what in essence are similar social concepts. Norbert Elias (1965) highlighted the complexity of the prejudice-generating situation through his groupings of 'established' and 'outsiders'. He argued that a tension is always apparent between a set of newcomers and old-timers who exaggerate their differences in order to reaffirm their positions. Gregory Bateson (1980) employed the term 'schismogenesis' to identify the range of hostile feelings that, in turn, lead to hostile behaviour between conflicting parties. He distinguished between symmetrical schismogenesis, in which both sides attempt to become stronger and stronger against each other, and complementary schismogenesis where one side strengthens in the face of the other's weakness. What is important in these brief overviews is that this conflictual nature seems to reside as a natural phenomenon within social groups. It is as if we need, as members of a given society, an area in which we can establish a *difference*; a difference that makes them 'them' and us 'us'.

The threat of danger

The link between the cultural set-up of social communities and that of healthcare groups is very similar, with only one or two differences between them that need explaining. The similarities are not surprising given that we are socialised beings in our culture long before we enter the professional domain of healthcare. Although we would like to believe that we have the ability to bracket out our personal views in favour of professional ones, in reality there is a strong social and psychological link, and overlay, between the two (Billig *et al.*, 1988). The best that one can hope for is an open and challenging mind that can analyse and appreciate this relational position, and hopefully operate according to the professional standard if there is a discrepancy between the two. Before we focus more on the professional domain let us take a few moments to consider the lay, or public, response to the differences.

We can see that when groups of people are considered to be the same, that sameness becomes a form of familiar pattern, which in its familiarity feels safe and secure. Furthermore, we are all familiar with the concept of the stranger, and until we know that person, the stranger represents danger (Schutz, 1970). The person who is different disrupts the safety of the social patterning and draws attention from those who note the difference. This can be seen by the attention of children towards a person who is deformed or disfigured in some way. While adults may know the social etiquette of averting their eyes, children are not sensitive to such social requirements. Furthermore, children tend to have a 'natural' inclination to avoid physical contact with other children who are disfigured, if they consider that disfigurement to be unfamiliar (Hallas, Fraser and MacGillivray, 1974). In adulthood this inclination transcends into the physical avoidance strategies of adults and protective gestures towards their children when confronted with a person who is seen as different. Although, socially, this disorder impairs the patterning of society, its counterpart, order, re-establishes the limitations of what is considered 'normal'. 'So disorder by implication is unlimited, no pattern has been realised in it, but its potential for patterning is indefinite ... we recognise that it is destructive to existing patterns ... It symbolises both danger and power' (Douglas, 1996). In short, there is a discrepancy between the pure and the polluted.

Professionalisation

The role of the healthcare professional in the stigmatising process is not well understood, hence the need for this book. However, what is clear is the relationship between the professions, knowledge and power (Turner, 1987). High status, technical knowledge and increased power equate with lucrative incomes, while low status, low technical knowledge and reduced power equate with low pay. It should be an easy matter to see in this equation that doctors (medics) represent the former, and nurses the latter (Mumford, 1983). The relevance of this for the stigmatisation process, as a cultural artefact, rests on the notion of medicalised power. In all societies those who *apparently* have the power to alleviate pain and suffering or influence matters of life and death are viewed as high status and considered to have special powers. Clearly, with such influence, their role in society is held in high esteem, as is noted in Indian Ayurvedic spiritualists, Asian Shaman seers, Native American medicine-men and the medics of Westernised health belief models (Richman, 1987). With this esteem comes a technical wisdom (often fallacious) in which lay people have a deep-seated belief that medical knowledge is supernatural. This strength of feeling often blinds lay people, as well as some professionals, to the limitations of such medical knowledge (Illich, 1976) and may well contribute to the powerful–vulnerable relationship on which many health belief models are constructed.

As far as isolation and marginalisation are concerned we can see that, as medical science and technical sagacity march on to encompass ever-increasing areas of personal and social life, more and more individuals become identified as 'abnormal'. Under this 'medical gaze' (Foucault, 1973), those falling outside of particular parameters of normality may become stigmatised as, for example, too fat, too thin, too tall, too short, too ugly or too sick. Often unwittingly, under the guise of medicine, the technical scrutiny of individuals in our society is little more than the exercise of power with the corollary of an increasing mass of marginalised individuals.

Conclusion

We can see that there is a close interplay of psychosocial factors contributing to the changing dynamic of stigmatised groups and individuals in societies. Furthermore, we note that the stigma itself, i.e. the sign of the blemish, can change with the mores of the time. Although it is not surprising that as leprosy became less endemic it lost its potency as a stigma, and as witchcraft gave way to enlightenment so the fear diminished; none the less the social processes of exclusion remain as apparent in this epoch as in any other. There continues to be as much stigma surrounding AIDS as there is around teenage pregnancy and the eating disorders bulimia and anorexia. In our contemporary world, starvation and poverty stand beside beauty pageants and parades, and the focus on the excluded ranges from rickets to wrinkles. Although the focus is damningly different, the processes remain frighteningly similar.

In this chapter we have attempted to unravel some of the influences that contribute to having an impact on the marginalisation process in our society, highlighting some of the constructs to the cultural dynamic. In doing so there has been a strong suggestion that, as healthcare professionals, we are by the nature of our work closely involved with many individuals and groups who may well be part of the socially excluded. Through disease, deformity and disability, many persons turn to healthcare professionals for assistance and sympathy. However, we may be somewhat alarmed to realise that we might well become part of the stigmatising process ourselves, either deliberately or through ignorance and inattention. Unless we explore this relationship and begin to address the issues, we will be guilty of maintaining the status quo and contributing to the stigmatisation and exclusion of many individuals from or society. This is an unacceptable position.

References

Bateson, G. (1980) *Mind and nature: a necessary unity*, Glasgow: Fontana.

Bauman, Z. (1997) *Thinking sociologically*, Oxford: Blackwell.

Billig, M., Condor, S., Edwards, D. *et al.* (1988) *Ideological dilemmas: a social psychology of everyday thinking*, London: Sage.

Campbell, J. and Bonner, W. (1994) *Media, mania and the markets*, London: Fleet Street Publications.

Day, D. and Page, S. (1986) 'Portrayal of mental illness in Canadian newspapers', *Canadian Journal of Psychiatry*, 31: 813–17.

Douglas, M. (1996) *Purity and danger: an analysis of the concepts of pollution and taboo*, London: Routledge.

Elias, N. (1965) *The established and the outsiders: a sociological enquiry into community problems*, London: Frank Cass.

Evans-Pritchard, E.E. (1937) *Witchcraft, oracles and magic among the Azande*, Oxford: Oxford University Press.

Foucault, M. (1973) *The birth of the clinic*, London: Tavistock.

George, V. and Wilding, P. (1985) *Ideology and social welfare*, London: Routledge & Kegan Paul.

Goffman, E. (1972) *The presentation of self in everyday life*, London: Penguin.

Hallas, C.H., Fraser, W.I. and MacGillivray, R.C. (1974) *The care and training of the mentally handicapped: a manual for the caring professions*, Bristol: John Wright & Sons.

Illich, I. (1976) *Limits to medicine, medical nemesis: the expropriation of health*, London: Marion Boyers.

Mumford, E. (1983) *Medical sociology, patients providers and policies*, New York: London House.

Parkin, D. (1993) *The anthropology of evil*, Oxford: Basil Blackwell.

Philo, G. (ed.) (1996) *Media and mental illness*, London: Longman.

Richman, J. (1987) *Medicine and health*, London: Longman.

Schutz, A. (1970) *On phenomenology and social relations*, Chicago: University of Chicago Press.

Social Exclusion Unit (1998) *So you'd like to know more?*, http://www.open.gov.uk/co/seu/more.html

—— (1999) *What's it all about?*, http://www.cabinet-office.gov.uk/seu/index/faqs.html

Turner, B.S. (1987) *Medical power and social knowledge*, London: Sage.

Van Gennep, A. (1909) *Les rites de passage*, London: Doubleday.
Weeks, J. (1994) *Sex, politics and society*, London: New York Press.
Whitehead, M. (1992) *Inequalities in health: the health divide*, London: Penguin.
Williamson, C. (1993) *Whose standards?* Buckingham: Open University Press.
Worman, P. (1999) 'Pregnant women', *Sunday Times*, 24 January.

4 Relationship to practice

*Caroline Watkins, Caroline Carlisle,
Elizabeth Whitehead and Tom Mason*

Introduction

In the previous two chapters we focused on, first, the development of stigma as an academic topic which, by necessity, involved highlighting the various scientific disciplines that have traditionally addressed the issues of exclusion as central tenets of their paradigms. From sociology and social psychology to media studies and anthropology, many academic strands of study have been employed to develop our understanding of the social and psychological forces that contribute to the marginalisation of individuals and groups from various communities.

Second, we dealt with the changing dynamic of stigma across cultures, contexts and time, and, although we developed this theme in relation to the creation of stigma in healthcare settings, the main focus remained theoretical. The importance of theory cannot be denied as, largely through the evolution of conceptual frameworks, this influence has the potential to impact on practice. It can be argued that, if theory merely remains an esoteric exercise and does not affect the general well-being of the population, then its importance is greatly diminished. We are all probably well versed in the debate concerning the theory–practice divide, and this chasm exists merely because many theoreticians avoid pragmatical issues and many practitioners dismiss the importance of theory. We have attempted in this book to ensure that stigma, exclusion and marginalisation do not remain mere theoretical perspectives but are grounded in practice. Therefore, although Chapter 4 will briefly outline the macro perspectives of service policy, we will emphasise the more micro levels of practical impact that theory can have on individuals and groups. We will then explore the practical ramifications of personalised accounts by using vignettes from the two central areas of deviance and dilemmas. This will then set the scene for the remainder of the book in terms of relating theory to practice.

Service policy

The NHS, as outlined in the recent white paper 'The New NHS, Modern, Dependable' (DOH, 1998a), is charged with developing in a sustainable way a healthcare system which incorporates modernisation and new technologies. Not only must there be increased quality and efficiency, but attention must be paid to the needs of individuals.

In due recognition of the inequalities in healthcare provision and access to that care for some members of society, the government's green paper 'Our Healthier Nation' (Department of Health, 1998b) stressed the importance of improving the health of the worst off in society, in an effort to narrow the health gap. The government's resolve to tackle these issues has recently been reiterated, as evidenced in a press release by Alan Milburn, Secretary of State for Health (8 May 2000) in which he declared: 'I want the NHS to offer a first class service for all patients, no matter who they are or where they live'.

He was obviously speaking not personally but on behalf of the government, and acknowledged that 'This Government has done much to modernise the NHS, but there is still much more to do. ... NHS organisations must show what they can achieve, and for others to learn from them'.

The government aims not only to increase organisation in the NHS so that it is fast and efficient, but also:

- fair, by instituting mechanisms to ensure equity of access;
- shared, by introducing processes to identify examples of good practice (for example, Beacon sites);
- convenient, so that local health inequalities are addressed;
- in context, by being developed with due recognition of the wider health and social care system. That is, effective partnerships must be developed between formal (primary, acute and social services care) and informal services (voluntary organisations and carers).

Furthermore, services must be based on the best available evidence in order to ensure quality healthcare, which must be in line with the principles of Clinical Governance. This necessitates effective monitoring and evaluation mechanisms in place both locally and nationally. Locally, in the form, not only of Clinical Governance, but of:

- Primary Care Groups/Trusts;
- Explicit standards in service agreements;
- Health Improvement Programmes;
- Public healthcare Trust Boards;

... and nationally, in the form of:

- National Standards and Guidelines;
- the National Institute for Clinical Excellence, which will aim to promote evidence based practice, clinical and cost-effectiveness of provision;
- the Commission for Health Improvement, which will support and oversee these processes, intervening if requested by the Secretary of State.

The implementation of these changes requires improvements in education of all staff involved in healthcare provision. The educational emphasis must not just be on practical skills, but on developing and implementing mechanisms to ensure the acquisition of knowledge and to promote lifelong learning. Education must equip staff to reflect on current practice, to develop an insight into the strengths and limitations of the services that they are involved in providing, and to understand how services might be developed in a fast, fair and efficient manner. Although there will be an emphasis on cost-effectiveness with the consequent recognition of the importance of financial costs and sustainability, it is acknowledged that services must also be developed to meet the needs of all individuals and groups. Resources will be required to provide staff training in order to ensure effective leadership, effective dissemination, and innovative ideas for sharing learning. Educational establishments will be required to develop courses in line with current thinking and the needs on healthcare professionals, to allow these staff to work effectively in the new NHS. This will necessitate close collaboration between training providers, universities and colleges etc.

The NHS itself is promoting shared learning through its Beacon Service Programme (2000) which is seen as a key initiative in the government's agenda for modernising the NHS. The NHS is endeavouring to identify examples of good practice (Beacon sites) throughout the UK, so that these examples may be shared to allow improvements to be made to similar services elsewhere in the country. It is hoped that this will result in improvements in the quality of patient care, and result in standards being maintained and disseminated. Each Beacon site is expected to have services of demonstrable high quality that have already been evaluated, or have recently been introduced and have mechanisms in place which will allow them to demonstrate quality in the future. These Beacon sites will themselves be expected to offer interactive learning activities in order that they can share information and expertise.

These changes to the provision of healthcare must be structured and assessed to ensure that any improvements in health and health risks are demonstrable. Outcomes may include those relevant for public health, health services, patients and carers. In order to implement and evaluate such systems the emphasis on attitudes, which must also be modern, is important.

Individual impact

We have explored the importance of the policy context in ensuring fairness and equity in access to healthcare. A person's experience of discrimination, however, is most acutely felt at the individual level in their day-to-day interactions with others. It is at this individual level that healthcare professionals need to consider the ways that care delivery can acknowledge and address potential stigmatising attitudes.

The modern NHS aims to provide high-quality patient-centred care, and plans for reform to take place throughout the early twenty-first century emphasising the importance of patient empowerment and the strengthening of patient choice (Department of Health, 1998b). Stigmatising behaviour can result in a person being labelled and stereotyped and, as we shall see from the many examples included in the chapters of this book, the impact of this experience can have an adverse effect on self-esteem. The ability to take advantage of opportunities for self-empowerment is closely linked to a person's beliefs about their level of control and their self-esteem (Tones, 1998). Care planning which does not take account of ways in which a patient's self-esteem can be maintained, and which does not provide opportunities for involvement in decision making, can compromise the quality of healthcare. It is important, therefore, that healthcare professionals reflect on practice and identify any stigmatising attitudes and behaviour that could affect the care they provide.

When considering healthcare provision, it is important to remember that, in many cases, the identification of a stigmatising condition depends on a medical diagnosis. Later chapters of this book will deal with the complexities of living with a diagnosis of such conditions as epilepsy or schizophrenia, and the resultant effects of being labelled with a mental illness. Social meanings are attached to labels such as a medical diagnosis, and it is not only the effect of other's behaviour which is detrimental to the person so labelled. An individual's self-concept can also be affected by their own views which have developed from the social meanings they have previously ascribed to the condition. In this way, a person may well judge themselves to be unworthy and thus contribute further to their low self-esteem. Marris (1996) points out that illness or disability can help a person focus on their own essential and intrinsic value. People need support to do this, however, and unless their worth and value is reinforced by others, they will be unable to truly value themselves. Labelling and stereotyping that arises from the social meanings of illness will act as a powerful barrier to individuals with certain conditions developing their own sense of worth.

Clinical gaze and responsibilities

Within sociological circles the process of medicalisation is relatively well understood. The term 'medicalisation' refers to the way in which a particular aspect of human life, or the human condition, is brought within the professional medical domain of its scientific attention. From this perspective 'medicine' encompasses all those multi-professionals involved in all aspects of healthcare delivery and who base their assessment of the individual as differing in some way from the 'norm'. They usually refer to this difference as an illness, a standard (of size or weight), an imbalance, an abnormality, a disorder, a state, a condition, etc. In this manner many areas of human life may be subtly brought under what Michel Foucault called the 'medical gaze' (Foucault, 1973). This has now been popularised into the 'clinical gaze' which is concerned with how a state of human life may be brought within the frame of medical perception. An example may be useful here. At one time childbirth, and all its complications, was considered a traditional state of affairs that lay outside of medical focus. Each community would have its own village midwife whose authority was rooted in experience and whose knowledge would transcend the natural order of childbirth disasters and the divine cause and effect of apparent religious interventions. However, down the centuries medicine was able to gain control over the processes of childbirth through rationalisations based on the safety of 'science' and the natural fear of the mother for the unborn child.

There are said to be five stages within the medicalisation process which formulates the 'clinical gaze'. These are (a) identification, (b) classification, (c) diagnosis, (d) intervention and (e) prognosis. We will deal with these in a little more depth. First, *identification*, by this it is necessary for professionals to be able to establish a difference between the proposed condition and the normal state of affairs. Take, for example, a congenital abnormality that can be seen to differentiate between what is considered normal and what is an abnormality. This natural, but sad, event may then be seen as a medical condition. Second, *classification*, by which professional authority can locate the 'condition' into a nosological framework (that branch of medicine concerned with categorisation and classification of diseases). This classifying of conditions gives the impression of knowledge and provides a sense (often false) of medical interventive know-how. An example of this would be HIV and AIDS which are easily located within virological and immunological classificatory systems but which resist convincing interventive strategies to prevent their consequences. The third stage is *diagnosis*, which is often confused with classification since it appears to be closely related. However, the fundamental difference in diagnosis is that it carries a requirement to provide some degree of cause-and-effect relationship. In diagnosis there is a need to establish an aetiological explanation of the condition, i.e. where it has come from or how it has happened. Explaining a congenital abnormality in terms of genetic structures would be an example of this, although the important question of 'why?' could not be addressed. Fourth, *intervention*; for the medicalisation process to be convincing it must suggest some form of interventive strategy. This may or may not be effective; it may only be palliative;

but all medicalised conditions must be accompanied by medical 'science' to alleviate suffering which is real or perceived – even death. The final stage is *prognosis*, in which medicine must be able to form a prediction relating to the outcome of the condition. Often this is accompanied by a prediction relating to the set of medical interventions that is being applied under the previous stage; however, in reality it is the disease or the abnormal entity that lies at the centre of the prognosis in relation to the medical ability to correct it.

The medicalisation process, once completed, grounds the condition firmly within the scientific rationalism of contemporary society and makes any challenge to its authenticity, as a medicalised concept, extremely diffi-cult. However, it also has another feature and that is it locates the responsibility for succumbing to the process of correction on the individual concerned. As in a form of Parsonian sick-role adoption (Parsons, 1951) it is expected that the 'afflicted' person will wish to move towards a state of normality and will seek out medical help in order to achieve this. Should they not wish to do so, then this itself becomes another type of disorder, examples of which would include those in Western society who receive a diagnosis of cancer and decline medical interventions of surgery and chemotherapy only to allow nature to take its course; or those with anorexia who fight against medical intervention, preferring the conse-quences of their actions rather than to be force-fed. In these scenarios the person is either blamed for their actions or is given another medical label to account for their 'abnormal' decision; this additional label is usually a psychiatric one.

It is in this sense that we view healthcare professionals as part of the stigmatising process which can lead to the exclusion and marginalisation of patients. Furthermore, this is the central message that we hope to communicate in this book since, unless we begin to address the contribu-tion that we make, as caring professionals, on the stigmatising process, we are unlikely ever to change the negative impact that we may have on the patients themselves.

Users/competing agendas

For the most part we accept that we live in a society that is constructed of competing agendas. Rarely do we challenge the competition required to buy a house, win a place on a nursing course or, sadly, enter the market-place for healthcare. It is in this sphere that the vulnerable suffer the most. They have little or no voice to compete for limited resources. Without political acumen, influence, power and knowledge, the traditional 'Cinderella' groups are at risk of becoming sadly excluded. Such an example is the older lady who, after spending most of her life in a psychi-atric hospital, is discharged into the community. The support services are short-lived and, as she wanders the streets, unkempt and confused, this older lady is soon stigmatised by society, which feels uncomfortable in her presence. It is difficult to imagine how she can possibly stake her small claim for the most basic of services, but to compete with the city banker receiving state-of-the-art technological treatment that attracts global attention is an impossible task.

Case studies

We present two case examples, one from mental healthcare and one from acute general care, of the ways in which healthcare provision can contribute to stigma and marginalisation. We have noted that there may well be macro forces that converge to impinge on an individual's personal life, and that through the medicalisation process the 'clinical gaze' effects how 'conditions' arise to create pressure to succumb to medical rationality. Although there are many physical states that become the focus of this 'clinical gaze' it is in the realms of mental health that the boundaries between normal and abnormal, and between psychiatry and science, become most blurred. The following vignette, a real-life but anonymised account, highlights the relationship between the stigma of psychiatric labelling, the limitations of psychiatric theory to impact upon practice, and the devastating consequences for those involved in the clinical area.

Belinda: an example relating to deviance

Belinda was 21 years of age, came from a broken home, was from a poor housing estate in an inner city area, and had frequently been sexually abused by her father and brothers. She had run away from home many times and had eventually ended up in Social Service care facilities where she had again been abused by male workers. She learnt to self-injure by a variety of methods and did not dislike the notoriety of being a 'cutter'. She became pregnant on two occasions by different fathers and each child was taken from her to be fostered. She never saw either child again. Belinda gained her first admission to a psychiatric hospital at the age of 17 following the ingestion of illicit substances with a subsequent three-day fugue state. She was diagnosed as having a drug-induced psychosis and was eventually discharged back to care, having been settled on a depot injection. In her 17th year she had four more admissions to psychiatric hospitals in different catchment areas with incidents of violent outbursts, attacking other patients, setting minor fires and frequently absconding, only to return worse the wear for drink and drug abuse. She was variously labelled psychotic, schizo-affective, learning disabled and personality disordered. Belinda did not respond to treatment and frequently avoided the drugs that left her with unpleasant side-effects yet clamoured for those she enjoyed the effects of.

When she was 19 years of age she developed a relatively stable relationship with a male patient and was eventually discharged to private accommodation supported by Social Services. After a short period of cohabitation her partner seriously assaulted her and she was re-admitted to a psychiatric hospital from casualty as she was considered acutely psychotic. She set fire to the ward waste bin and began assaulting nursing staff. The numerous treatment programmes were eventually abandoned following frequent 'cutting' episodes. The mental health professionals were at a loss to know what to do and, following her refusal to speak or move for four days, a course of ECT was prescribed. She made a reasonable recovery and was discharged to new accommodation since her partner had disappeared with her few possessions.

Belinda became depressed and sought help at her out-patient appointment. She requested admission to hospital but this was refused. She turned up the following day at the admission ward and when asked to leave by the attending doctor she scratched her wrists in the toilet with a piece of glass hidden for that purpose. The superficial wounds were dressed and she was advised to see her GP after the weekend. She demanded to stay; staff demanded that she go. She was informed that she was 'black-listed' from the hospital and was trespassing. She was escorted by nursing staff to the main hospital gates. She walked out of sight of the nurses, climbed onto a railway bridge, and jumped. She was 'lucky': a train was coming. At the inquest she was described as a deviant and untreatable. At the funeral she was considered a tragedy and a victim.

In this vignette we see, first, the stigma of the labelling processes that were employed to exclude Belinda from society and to marginalise her in a psychiatric hospital. Second, when she did not respond to the many and varied psychiatric attempts to help her, similar derogatory labels were used to exclude her from the psychiatric system. The mental health professionals clearly played their part in this, as did Belinda, and the end result was a negative experience for all concerned.

The newly qualified nurse: an example relating to dilemma

Professional caring relationships to some extent will always present conflicts and dilemmas, particularly in circumstances where the patient or client requires psychological support. Many dilemmas which nurses face are the result of the conflicting value systems between the patient and the nurse (Kagan and Evans, 1995). The values which nurses hold about the family, health, politics, sexuality and so on may be very different from those of the people they help as part of their professional role. It can be a challenge to maintain a balance in which the patient's values are respected, the nurse's values are upheld and no labelling or judgemental attitudes are conveyed during the delivery of healthcare.

Consider, for example, that you are a newly qualified staff nurse on a busy medical ward. You are the primary nurse for a middle-aged man who has an exacerbation of a severe gastric condition brought on by drinking excessive quantities of alcohol. You know that if he continues to drink his physical health will deteriorate rapidly, but he has told you that he doesn't care any more as his wife and children have left him and he has lost his job. At handover during your first week on the ward you hear the leader of the early shift refer to him as the 'alcoholic in bay 3' who has been admitted 'yet again' because of his 'drinking'. You are anxious to fit in and be accepted by your colleagues, and are finding it difficult to challenge such stigmatising behaviour. Your anxiety is increasing as you cannot come to terms with the conflicting values which are expressed through the behaviour of both the patient and some of your nursing colleagues.

The example illustrates a number of important things about the nature of professional dilemmas. Stigmatising attitudes conveyed by staff can reduce any opportunities a patient may have to increase their self-esteem to a point where they can begin to value themselves and play an active part in decision making about positive health outcomes. Even in situations where an individual nurse has the ability to deliver non-judgemental care, conflicting value systems between staff can pose an additional dilemma for a nurse who feels they, too, may be judged for being 'different' in their approach to certain patient groups. A nurse who has no access to clinical supervision, and is not facilitated to reflect on challenges such as this, can find it difficult to uphold their own value system and may well suffer a great deal of anxiety, stress and burnout if continually confronting such situations.

This chapter has explored both policy and practice issues in relation to stigma and marginalisation. The next section of the book highlights specific clinical situations in more detail and provides explicit examples of the challenges facing both patients and practitioners.

References

Department of Health (1998a) *The new NHS, modern, dependable: a national framework for assessing performance*, London: Department of Health.
—— (1998b) *Our healthier nation*, London: The Stationery Office.
Foucault, M. (1973) *Birth of the clinic: an archaeology of medical perception*, New York: Vintage.
Kagan, C. and Evans, J. (1995) *Professional interpersonal skills for nurses*, London: Chapman & Hall.
Marris, V. (1996) *Lives worth living*, London: Pandora.
Parsons, T. (1951) *The social system*, London: Routledge & Kegan Paul.
Tones, K. (1998) 'Empowerment for health: the challenge', in S. Kendall, *Health and empowerment*, London: Arnold.

Part II

Applications to practice

Section I: Difference

5   The stigma of congenital abnormalities

Mike Farrell and Kathy Corrin

'What did I do to deserve this fate?'

(Desperate, *Miss Lonely Hearts*, quoted in Goffman, 1963)

Introduction

Goffman's classic book *Stigma, Notes on the Management of Spoiled Identity* opens with a poignant letter written by a 16-year-old girl born with a congenital defect (Goffman, 1963). The letter, which had been sent to an 'agony aunt', expresses the writer's sense of sadness, loneliness and personal hurt for herself and her family due to an abnormality causing a serious facial disfigurement. The letter ends in the young writer's anguished plea, 'Ought I to commit suicide?'

This letter reflects the real, sustained and profound stigmatising impact of congenital disfigurement, and although written over thirty-five years ago, captures a sense of stigma which still has relevance today. Despite an increased understanding of the social and psychological impact of congenital abnormality lowering the intensity of feelings of desolation and stigma, the stigmatising potential is retained. There is a challenge for society in how best to support those distinguished by congenital abnormality, to enable inclusion and participation in a society that claims to accept, value and celebrate human diversity.

This chapter will consider the potential stigmatisation provoked by congenital abnormalities. Factors that influence the development of a stigmatised response will be explored from historical and contemporary perspectives. The role that health professionals have in lessening stigma response, when involved in caring for children with congenital abnormalities and their families, will be discussed. Health professionals have a critical role in promoting a positive adaptation to the impact of any disability and can model a professional and social response that has benefits for both child and family.

Congenital abnormalities: course and outcome

Congenital abnormalities are structural defects present at birth. Major life-threatening congenital abnormality is seen in 16 per 1000 live births, while minor abnormalities are seen in 33 per 1000 (Forfar, 1998). Many congenital abnormalities are amenable to treatment, often with positive treatment outcomes.

The historical impact of congenital abnormalities

Children with congenital abnormalities, and their families, face at best an uncertain social response and at worst a response which exemplifies the essence of stigma. Congenital abnormalities can delineate a stigma response with features which are not evident in other stigmatising conditions.

Historically, children born with abnormalities and their families have been viewed in a stigmatised manner. In Greek society congenital deformity was seen as a sign of divine retribution, as a means of atonement for transgressions in an earlier life (Garland, 1995). Likewise, in Roman civilisation there is evidence that statutes were decreed which instructed the head of a family to kill a child with a congenital deformity (Garland, 1995). Garland in his exposition writes that, in some sections of Roman society, most notably the higher social classes, this law was not always followed, suggesting an increasing sympathetic and compassionate response. It seems that important factors influencing reactions to the disabled in these early civilisations included concerns about the functional economic ability of the individual. A broader concern was related to contamination of society by the 'tainted', with the fear that deformity resulted in weakness of the race, a fear that is sadly mirrored in the orientation of Hitler's Third Reich (Meyer, 1988).

In medieval times and the Tudor age, children with deformities were viewed as *changelings*, the devil's substitutes for human children, with the perception that deformed children represented the parents' involvement with black magic. Even the great protestant reformer, Martin Luther, considered the disabled child as the *devil incarnate* and recommended killing it. It is probable that the prevalence of such beliefs could be attributed to the perception that the person and their impairment were one. In other words, that the person was defective.

Superstitions and attitudes towards children born with congenital abnormalities began to shift in the nineteenth century due to increased awareness of the association of abnormality and environmental conditions (Fletcher, 1977). Nevertheless, the perception and belief that deformity was a sign of divine retribution for sins committed in a previous life continued and remained widespread even until Victorian times (Buhler, 1886, cited in Miles, 1995).

Miles (1995) states that from East to West, from one civilisation to the next, congenital deformity has the capacity to mark out 'differentness' and provoke a powerful discriminating, stigmatising response. While there has been an apparent societal change in the way that those affected by abnormalities and disability are viewed, others worry that all that has happened has been transformation of discrimination to more subtle and less obvious forms (Barnes, 1991).

Great expectations – impending birth of the child

There is usually a great sense of anticipation at the impending birth of a child. While some of this anticipation might relate to the demands of parenthood there is also a great sense of expectation about the baby itself. What sex will it be? Who will the baby look like? Will the baby be alright? There is a common expectation of the 'perfect baby' (Lynch, 1989). These expectations are raised further when, during social interactions and discourse, expectations of perfection are perpetuated and validated by others. In this way the impending birth of a child becomes a social event, generating a sense of anticipation, oriented around positive expectations that this will be a time for great celebration and hope.

However, these expectations can be soon shattered when it becomes evident that the baby has a congenital abnormality. The vision of the baby as perfect and unspoilt is damaged in a most significant way. This then triggers a series of reactions and feelings, ultimately requiring a process of adjustment where personal and social expectations must be re-aligned and re-evaluated.

Parental reaction

Of critical importance is the loss of the image of the 'perfect child'. This can be such a powerful reaction because children are often seen as an extension and embodiment of their parents (Lemons, 1986; Pate, 1987). Thus any congenital abnormality can be perceived as 'genetic corruption' caused by the parents, leading to feelings of shame, embarrassment and guilt (Niven, 1992). The prime expectation for a 'healthy baby' is lost and is replaced with the reality of abnormality, giving rise to a perception of weakness, vulnerability and pity.

Linde (1982) suggests that the parents' narcissistic self-image as 'good parents' is assaulted by the birth of a child born with abnormalities, and can lead to intense parental psychological reaction. Linde (1982) further suggests that the impact upon fathers can be particularly strong, perhaps reflecting a primeval feeling of failure. Taylor (1992) notes that no parents would wish for 'a child burdened with imperfections'. In a particularly powerful comment, Taylor (1992) captures what he considers to be the parents' perception of the futility of this tragic event when he writes (about the child):

He will not represent their happy synthesis nor offer continuity of their biological substance: not an adornment, no achievement, but a stigma; not even a useful chattel, but a burden.

(Taylor, 1992: 54)

Naturally parents often seek to identify the cause and reason for any abnormality. This might stimulate reflection and enquiry around the progress and management of the pregnancy. From this process, feelings of blame and recrimination might be provoked if parents attribute past undesirable behaviours as a possible cause for the defect.

As Miller and Gwynne (1972) affirm, a particular test for parents is that their internal values about abnormality and disability are awakened and challenged by the birth of the disabled child. Douglas (1966, cited in Barnes, 1991) notes that perceptions of impairment and disability are influenced by a deep-rooted psychological fear of the unknown, the anomalous and abnormal. Accordingly these fears and internal values will then be exposed and will manifest themselves through the strategies and responses of parents. Parents might respond by denying, diminishing or concealing the impact of the abnormality; for example, by avoiding social contact or, conversely, by seeking as much information as they can so as to explain and 'legitimise' the existence of the defect. Frequently, as a means of coping, parents react by using protective strategies of over-compensation. However, for parents ultimately to respond they first have to experience and acknowledge the loss of the perfect child (Garth, 1985; Ludder Jackson, 1985; Cheetham, 1987; Lynch, 1989; Taylor, 1992; Hall and Hill, 1996). This resembles a grief reaction and results in a burden of chronic sorrow (Lemons, 1986).

Parental feelings can range from ambivalence to revulsion, leading to stigma through what Goffman (1963) believes is the social response to the 'undesired differentness from what had been expected'. This sense of differentness is perhaps even more accentuated given the representation of children in the media. Images of the 'perfect child' are frequently offered as being healthy, and with signs of physical beauty; children with disabilities are frequently portrayed as being brave, tragic and deserving of our sympathy. Such images perpetuate the expectation of the ideal while promoting attitudes of sympathetic benevolence when this ideal is not achieved. This in itself can be stigmatising, given that this type of response suggests a sense of devaluing. This is perfectly captured in Brearley (1997) by the comments of a boy with disabilities who reflects that he is expected 'to be either a PBC (poor bloody cripple) or a Supercrip', capable of undertaking heroic feats such as scaling Mount Everest!

Social reaction

Given that the majority of congenital abnormalities are present at birth, the process and success of social acceptance is challenged from birth. Moreover, it could be argued that the advances of perinatology, offering the increased ability to detect foetal abnormality, could begin this process even sooner.

Many families with children who have abnormalities can experience isolation (Cheetham, 1987). Cheetham suggests that 'people are hesitant about becoming close to a family who have an abnormal or handicapped child fearing that they too may become stigmatised'. One explanation for this social isolation may be that people involved in the social world of those affected by congenital abnormality (for example, friends and relatives) are unable to provide an effective and supportive response at a difficult time. Having been part of the social world that eagerly awaited and anticipated the birth of the normal child they, too, experience a sense of loss of the perfect child. Aware of the sense of disappointment felt by the parents they become uncertain of how to respond, and distance themselves until more confident in the approach to take. This process of social distancing reinforces parental feelings of isolation and stigma.

Those affected by congenital abnormality often seek contact with others who are in a similar situation to themselves, in the hope that they will be able to offer support to others and to understand the situation in which they find themselves. This is evident when parents join a support or action group, formed to give and share information about specific abnormalities, or to advance the awareness of the child's and affected families' specific needs. There are a number of benefits to joining support groups, including the psychological benefits promoted by gaining information about coping with daily living. The other major benefit is the sense of social acceptance afforded by joining such groups. Individuals can develop increased coping responses and strengths when they become part of an organisation representative of their position (Whitehead, 1995). Thus membership of such groups offers the opportunity to be part of a social community that shares a common identity and which tolerates and accepts the 'differentness' that the wider social community perhaps cannot.

Recently it has been suggested that other social settings can have a valuable social function for those affected by abnormality. For example, the Internet increasingly offers an additional, albeit electronic, source of social support which can be valuable for those marginalised in 'real life', and is a social setting in which strangers can exchange useful information (Mickelson, 1997).

Congenital abnormalities, healthcare professionals and stigma

Medical advances primarily aim to relieve the health deficit or complications caused by a congenital abnormality. So, for example, the advances in paediatric cardiac surgery have afforded real benefit in lessening the mortality associated with congenital heart defects. Similarly, developments in orthopaedic limb surgery have given children greater independent mobility and facilitated a reduction in the pain and discomfort associated with congenital skeletal abnormalities.

However, in treatments of some congenital abnormalities it could be argued that the focus is less about cure and directed more to 'concealing' the defect, responding to the anticipated fear and impact of stigma. An example of this may be found in the surgical elimination of the facial features of Down's syndrome.

A prime reason for undertaking this type of cosmetic surgery, which gained popularity in the 1980s, was to enhance the social functioning of the individual by removing the visible barriers which negatively impacted upon their social interactions. Such surgery has been suggested as having a positive influence upon social functioning in children with Down's syndrome (Lewandowicz and Kruk-Jeromin, 1995), although this type of treatment has significant ethical and social implications (Aylott, 1999). A key ethical challenge relates to the issue of consent, given the child's inability to articulate their own decision due to the cognitive effects of the condition. This is further compromised because, typically, the surgery has to be conducted in the pre-school years, at a time when the child is cognitively immature. The social implication of this type of medical intervention is that difference need not be tolerated but can be repaired. A change in social attitudes has mainly been promoted through exposure to children with disabilities rather than in trying to hide the deformity through cosmetic surgery (Aylott, 1999).

It is interesting to note that, while the social benefits of cosmetic surgery for children with Down's syndrome are apparent, and would therefore be clearly attractive, the research evidence supporting the benefits is not conclusive (Serafica, 1990). Indeed, the arguments that the child's social functioning would be improved through surgery have been disputed (Cunningham *et al.*, 1991; Kravetz *et al.*, 1992). It has been suggested that the acceptance of congenital features can be influenced by the values of healthcare professionals. For example, in a study investigating both parents' and physicians' attitudes and perceptions concerning facial plastic surgery in children with Down's syndrome, more physicians (63 per cent) than parents (28 per cent) felt that that the children's facial features negatively affected their social development and interaction (Pueschel *et al.*, 1986). While most parents (85 per cent) felt that their children were well accepted by society as compared to 4 per cent of physicians, 44 per cent of physicians supported the use of facial plastic surgery in children with Down's syndrome, as compared to 13 per cent of parents. At a time when parents are struggling to adapt and respond to this challenging situation, they can be influenced by the beliefs and attitudes of healthcare professionals, and a health system that seeks and values only cure (or at the very least some amelioration of the signs of the presenting abnormality).

It is of great concern that the parents of children born with congenital abnormalities (and indeed the children themselves) are still exposed to remarks made by healthcare professionals which can only be described as offensive, judgemental and stigmatising.

In a recent survey conducted by the Down's Syndrome Association (1999) there is a catalogue of offensive remarks made by healthcare professionals which portray stigmatising attitudes and a sinister lack of regard. One mother recalls how an ophthalmologist treating her young son said, 'We won't bother with glasses as he's not what you would call university material'. The parents of a 2-year-old child were told by a paediatrician 'He'll never be a brain surgeon'. These comments not only reflect a complete lack of respect but gives some indication of the attitudes and values of professionals in terms of what is considered as a desirable level of achievement. There is a significant chasm between the expectations and attitudes of some healthcare professionals and parents in relation to caring for a child with a congenital abnormality (Cooley *et al.*, 1990). It is essential that healthcare professionals have balanced attitudes if they are to be effective in their interactions with affected children and families.

Hall and Hill (1996) rightly caution that medical terminology such as diagnostic labels, and participation in certain types of therapy, have the potential to stigmatise the child as much as any disability. Both the labelling process and the label itself have enduring consequences for the child and can limit the life-achieving potential of the child. A real tension, perhaps encouraged by the labelling process, is that it shapes the responses of the healthcare professionals which can become technical and condition-focused, clouding recognition of the specific and individual needs of the child and of the family (Holmes, 2000). The family will also have to learn a new technical language related to the management of the congenital defect, and to make decisions about treatment options which can often mean an extensive programme of care. Given the 'valued status' of healthcare professionals, the child and family will be expected to engage with these professionals in a way that appreciates, and is respectful of, this valued status. This can mean 'doing what the doctor or the health professional thinks is good for them' even where this might diminish their own instinct, sense and right to self-determination.

Congenital abnormalities – lessening the stigma

Healthcare professionals are in a strong position to lessen the stigma of congenital abnormalities. A range of strategies can be used which can be supportive to both the child and the family. These will now be explored.

The importance of reflection

All healthcare professionals involved in the care of children with congenital abnormalities and their families should consider and appreciate their potential for creating and maintaining stigma. Using a reflective approach, healthcare professionals could explore their own personal values and beliefs and the impact of these when caring for children and families.

Recognising the individuality of the child and family

Healthcare professionals in frequent contact with families affected by congenital abnormalities become desensitised to the impact of the experience for family members. Remaining sensitive, critically aware and attuned to the individuality of the experience demonstrates high regard for both the child and the family. It affirms a sense of personal worth and value for those affected.

Personal attributes of the child

A positive strategy that can be used to support families of children born with a congenital abnormality is to highlight the personal and unique attributes of the child. This can be promoted in several ways.

- Making specific and repeated references to the name of the child during any discussions or care activities. Reference to the child's name should not just occur in the presence of family members. It should be a feature of any interaction in which the child's needs are being discussed. References which represent the child just within the context of their diagnostic label, for example, 'the child with the cleft', should be considered inappropriate and be condemned.
- Supporting family members to focus on the individual characteristics of the child. This can be achieved by noting simple observations such as the colour of hair and eyes, or comments on how the child seems to respond to the parent's interactions. However, caution is needed to ensure that, when highlighting any personal attributes, this is done with a sense of balance. There is a danger that over-emphasis could be seen as misdirected and facile, engendering negative feelings which would leave the child and family feeling patronised and diminished.

These actions confirm the personal identity of the child. In celebrating with families the uniqueness of their child there is an acceptance of the child in its own right. This is a critical first step in encouraging inclusion and preventing potential adverse stigma response.

Active listening and response

On the birth of a child with an abnormality, families can experience a range of powerful reactions. Responding to and supporting family members requires an active response. This is essential to demonstrate acknowledgement of the feelings and reactions experienced. Through a process of active listening, healthcare professionals validate parental reactions. This encourages an atmosphere of openness, which in turn facilitates expression of negative feelings. In enabling the expression of such feelings, parents have an opportunity to release and reorganise negative emotions which, if not expressed, might thwart their adaptation response. Moreover, an active listening response gives the parents and family members a voice, demonstrating respect and offering them the dignity of being noticed and heard. These conditions are crucial to promoting an anti-stigma response.

Therapeutic relations framework

The development of specific therapeutic relation guidelines, relevant to the field of professional and clinical practice, can be a useful way to promote an equitable and sensitive approach to care. Such guidelines should reflect the caring ethos and endorse the values and beliefs considered fundamental for the promotion and demonstration of non-discriminatory practice. Guidelines produced by the American Association of Rehabilitation Nurses to guide ethical practice offer an example which could be adapted for other settings (American Association of Rehabilitation Nurses, 1994). The development of these guidelines can have several advantages: they are a tangible statement and commitment to care; they can be used as a tool in the education of practitioners, new to a particular clinical setting; they can be used as a benchmark to compare and evaluate quality of care; finally, such guidelines can be advantageous for individual practitioners to use as prompts to encourage reflection and the development of individual practice.

The need for education and support

Fradd (1994) identifies the importance of education and access to support systems to ensure care commensurate to the expectations and scope of professional practice. Research has shown that focused education programmes can have a measurable benefit in promoting positive attitudes and therapeutic engagement with those perceived in a position of disadvantage (Oermann and Lindgren, 1995). Pre-registration nurse education pro-grammes often include an exploration of issues of discrimination within a healthcare context. However, as Slevin and Sines (1996) assert, there remains a considerable need to educate the many thousands of nurses in practice that have had little opportunity to explore such key issues. Given the constraints and demands upon practitioners, a range of creative educational approaches and the effective use of a diverse range of media will be required to address this significant educational need.

Conclusion

A congenital abnormality is a burden in itself without the additional stress of a stigma response. Central to the ethos of care is the recognition of individual worth, and this is powerfully demonstrated when, in caring for children afflicted with congenital abnormality, we recognise this value by ensuring rigorous non-discriminatory practice. The challenge for practitioners involved in the care and support of children and families affected by congenital abnormalities is to remain critically aware of their own attitude and potential capacity in conveying a stigmatising response. Accordingly, it must be a challenge which we do not fail.

References

American Association of Rehabilitation Nurses (1994) *Standards and scope of rehabilitation nursing practice* (third edn), American Association of Rehabilitation Nurses.

Aylott, J. (1999) 'Should children with Down's syndrome have cosmetic surgery?', *British Journal of Nursing*, 8, 1: 33–8.

Barnes, C. (1991) *Disabled people in Britain and discrimination – a case for anti-discrimination legislation*, London: Hurst and Company.

Brearley, G. (1997) *Counselling children with special needs*, Oxford: Blackwell Science.

Buhler, G. (1886) 'The Law of Manu, in SBE 25', in M. Miles (1995), 'Disability in an Eastern religious context: historical perspectives', *Disability and Society*, 10, 1: 49–69.

Cheetham, C. (1987) 'Congenital abnormalities', *Nursing*, 13: 487–90.

Cooley, W.C., Graham, E.S., Moeschler, J.B. and Graham, J.M. Jr. (1990) 'Reactions of mothers and medical professionals to a film about Down syndrome', *American Journal of Diseases in Children*, 144, 10: 1112–16.

Cunningham, C., Turner, S., Sloper, P. and Knussen, C. (1991) 'Is the appearance of children with Down's syndrome associated with their development and social functioning?', *Development Medicine and Child Neurology*, 33, 4: 285–95.

Douglas, M. (1966) 'Purity and danger', in C. Barnes, *Disabled people in Britain and discrimination – a case for anti-discrimination legislation*, London: Hurst and Company.

Down's Syndrome Association (1999) *He'll never join the army*, London: Down's Syndrome Association.

Fletcher, J. (1977) 'Attitudes towards defective new-borns', in T.V.N. Persaud, *Problems of birth defects. From Hippocrates to Thalidomide and after*, Lancaster: MTP.

Forfar, J. (1998) 'Demography, vital statistics and the pattern of disease in childhood', in A.G.M. Campbell and N. McIntosh (eds), *Forfar and Arneil's textbook of pediatrics*, Edinburgh: Churchill Livingstone.

Fradd, E. (1994) 'A broader scope to practice', *Child Health*, April/May, 233–8.

Garland, R. (1995) *The eye of the beholder: deformity and disability in the Graeco-Roman world*, London: Duckworth.

Garth, A. (1985) 'Parental reactions to loss and disappointment; the diagnosis of Down's syndrome', *Developmental Medicine and Child Neurology*, 27, 3: 392–400.

Goffman, E. (1963) *Stigma, notes on the management of spoiled identity*, Harmondsworth: Penguin.

Hall, D.M.B. and Hill, P.D. (1996) *The child with disability* (second edn), Oxford: Blackwell Science.

Holmes, L. (2000) 'Nurses' attitudes to disability', *Paediatric Nursing*, 11, 10: 18–20.

Kravetz, S., Weller, A., Tennenbaum, R. *et al.* (1992) 'Plastic surgery on children with Down syndrome: parents' perceptions of physical, personal, and social functioning', *Research In Developmental Disabilities*, 13, 2: 145–56.

Lemons, P.M. (1986) 'Beyond the birth of a defective child', *Neonatal Network*, Dec., 13–20.

Lewandowicz, E. and Kruk-Jeromin, J. (1995) 'The indications and the plan of plastic operations in children with Down's syndrome', *Acta Chirurgiae Plasticae*, 37, 2: 40–44.

Linde, L.L. (1982) 'Psychiatric aspects of congenital heart disease', *Psychiatric Clinics of North America*, 5, 2: 399–406.

Ludder Jackson, P. (1985) 'When the baby isn't "perfect"', *American Journal of Nursing*, April, 396–9.

Lynch, M.E. (1989) 'Congenital defects: parental issues and nursing supports', *Journal of Perinatology Neonatal Nursing*, 2, 4: 53–9.

Meyer, J.E. (1988) 'The fate of the mentally ill in Germany during the Third Reich', *Psychological Medicine*, 18: 575–81.

Mickelson, K.D. (1997) 'Seeking social support: parents in electronic support groups', in S. Kiesler *et al.*, *Culture of the Internet*, Mahwah, N.J.: Lawrence Erlbaum Assocs.

Miles, M. (1995) 'Disability in an Eastern religious context: historical perspectives', *Disability and Society*, 10, 1: 49–69.

Miller, E.J. and Gwynne, G.V. (1972) *A life apart. A pilot study of residential institutions for the physically handicapped and the young chronic sick*, London: Tavistock.

Niven, C.A. (1992) *Psychological care for families: before, during and after birth*, Oxford: Butterworth Heinemann.

Oermann, M.H. and Lindgren, C.L. (1995) 'An educational program's effect on students' attitudes towards people with disabilities: a one-year follow up', *Rehabilitation Nursing*, 20, 1: 6–10.

Pate, C.M.H. (1987) 'Care of the family following the birth of a child with a cleft lip and/or palate', *Neonatal Network*, June, 30–37.

Pueschel, S.M., Monteiro, L.A. and Erickson, M. (1986) 'Parents' and physicians' perceptions of facial plastic surgery in children with Down's syndrome', *Journal of Mental Deficiency Research*, March, 30 (1), 71–9.

Serafica, F.C. (1990) 'Peer relations of children with Down's syndrome', in D. Cicchetti and M. Beeghly, *Children with Down's syndrome: a developmental perspective*, New York: Cambridge University Press.

Slevin, E. and Sines, D. (1996) 'Attitudes of nurses in a general hospital towards people with learning disabilities: influences of contact, and graduate–non-graduate status, a comparative study', *Journal of Advanced Nursing*, 24: 1116–26.

Taylor, D.C. (1992) 'Mechanisms of coping with handicap', in G.T. McCarthy, *Physical disability in childhood. An interdisciplinary approach to management*, Edinburgh: Churchill Livingstone.

Whitehead, E. (1995) 'Prejudice in practice', *Nursing Times*, 91, 21: 40–41.

6 Aspects of stigma associated with genetic conditions

Caroline Benjamin

Introduction

This chapter aims to inform healthcare professionals in order that they can understand and work towards minimising the potential for stigma associated with genetic conditions. The personal narratives illustrate the emotional issues faced by individuals and families affected by genetic disease. Strategies are suggested which could serve to identify the difficulties surrounding the diagnosis of a genetic condition in the family.

All individuals and families manifest genetic differences and this genetic variation is part of the diversity of the human race. How genetic differences are viewed by and shaped by society is ambiguous, transient and changeable. The terminology used by healthcare professionals such as genetic 'disease' seem to accentuate the 'medical model' in defining disability or difference in terms of impairment. It is argued that social barriers create disability out of difference, and that the difficulties of living as a disabled person are due to discrimination and prejudice, rather than impairment (Shakespeare, 1998). This social model of disability, to which I subscribe (Oliver, 1990), distinguishes impairment (the medical condition of the body) and disability (discrimination, prejudice and physical barriers in society).

Genetic knowledge and molecular genetic technology

Inheritance

Genetics can be defined in a number of ways; within the context of human genetics it can be defined as the study of the ways in which heritable characteristics and conditions are passed from parents to children through generations. Research into the lay understanding of genetics and the concept of culture, kinship and genes shows that the biomedical model of Mendelian genetics described below is often not simply received and understood without modification. Individuals often try to create a personal meaning for the origin of their particular genetic condition (Richards, 1996).

The science of inheritance is important for understanding the differences between genetic conditions and is fundamental to the meanings and consequences the condition has for an individual or family. Some genetic conditions result in carrier status, where the individual is not affected but may 'silently' carry the disease. Others result in the presence of a genetic illness, the onset of which can be variable and can show a great range in disease symptoms between affected individuals. A more detailed explanation of the biological mechanisms of inheritance can be found in most biology textbooks (for example Strachan and Read, 1999).

Molecular genetic technology

There are now over 4,000 distinct conditions and characteristics which are recognised to be genetic in nature, and the Human Genome Project (HGP) is expected to achieve the complete sequence of human DNA by the year 2005 (National Human Genome Research Institute, 2000). The societal acquisition of genome information, the prevention of stigmatisation and discrimination of individuals and groups and the maintenance of respect for the priceless diversity of the world's cultures is the responsibility of the Human Genome Organisation (HUGO) (Human Genome Organisation, 2000; Cassel, 1997). There is difficulty in providing healthcare professionals with information in this rapidly changing field.

Societal influences on genetic stigma

An important distinction has to be made between the application of certain genetic technologies at a personal level (individual genetic tests) as opposed to that at a societal level (population targeted screening programmes). Often people would support the personal choice of a woman to choose to have a screening test and perhaps a termination of a child with Down's syndrome, but would be much more likely to be against a compulsory screening and termination policy. Individual genetic testing as distinct from population screening provides diagnostic information about an at-risk individual for whom there is prior indication of a genetic condition or defect being present (Nuffield Council on Bioethics, 1993).

Societal issues

It has been suggested that the recent advances in genetic knowledge, which bring with them new choices for the management, avoidance or prevention of genetic disease, will result in a paradigm shift in healthcare towards a genetic explanation of health (Baird, 1990). This knowledge could be used to make reproductive choices, identify individuals with faulty genes, give advanced warning to those at risk and also plan possible preventative strategies and therapies. The term 'geneticisation' has been used to describe the dominance of genetic modes of thought and explanations for disability in purely genetic terms, as opposed to social and environmental explanations and the overemphasis of genetic factors in the planning and provision of healthcare (Lippman, 1992; Ramsay, 1994; Baird, 1990).

The boundaries between what is genetically desirable and what is undesirable will change in accordance with the values of those who select the criteria for what is a genetic defect or handicap. This classification may depend on the costs or benefits to society, and the value or availability of certain characteristics or qualities (Thomas, 1982). Unfortunately, the term genetic disease is often misused to describe a healthy individual potentially at risk of ill health or having a child with ill health. The term genetic condition, which I prefer, acknowledges that many individuals have genetic differences.

Knowledge of the historical context of population screening programmes and some past and present abuses of genetic information is important in appreciating the present concept of stigma associated with genetic conditions. In the early twentieth century the eugenics movement (Davenport and Muncey, 1916; Panse, 1942) resulted in the science of improving the human population by controlled breeding for desirable inherited characteristics. The abuses of genetics in Nazi Germany, and the compulsory Sterilisation Act of 1933, not only targeted individuals with genetic diseases but also those with racial differences. These individuals were not only stigmatised by the fact that they had poor mental or physical health but that the condition was hereditary and therefore was a perceived threat to the future of society.

As recently as 1995 the People's Republic of China passed the legislation, 'Maternal and Infant Health Care'.

> Physicians shall, after performing the pre-marital physical check-up, explain and give medical advice to both the male and female who have been diagnosed with certain genetic disease of a serious nature which is considered to be inappropriate for child-bearing from a medical point of view; the two may be married only if both sides agree to take long-term contraceptive measures or to take ligation operation for sterility. Genetic diseases of a serious nature refer to diseases that are caused by genetic factors congenitally, that may totally or partially deprive the victim of the ability to live independently, that are highly possible to recur in generations to come, and that are medically considered inappropriate for reproduction ... relevant mental diseases include, schizophrenia, manic depressive psychosis and other mental diseases of a serious nature.
>
> (Harper, 1997a)

At present, UK newborn and targeted population screening programmes exist for phenylketonuria, Duchenne muscular dystrophy, Tay-Sachs disease, cystic fibrosis, sickle cell disease and the thalassaemias. There are also many prenatal screening tests that identify genetic conditions, routinely offered in pregnancy, including maternal blood tests (spina bifida and chromosome abnormalities) and screening for ultrasound markers of abnormality.

Stigma associated with the concealability of the condition

Concealability, as described by Jones *et al.*, (1984) is a dimension of stigma that focuses on those characteristics of marks that make some irrevocably obvious to others, while some remain undetected (Jones *et al.*, 1984). Conditions such as physical birth defects, blindness, deafness and severe neurological conditions are obvious to the observer, whereas others such as mental health problems or carrier status may be completely undetected by others and may or may not be known to the individual themselves. More recently the concept of the 'worried well', first described in the HIV positive community (Sherr, 1995), has been used to describe individuals who are at risk of developing disease or have had a predictive genetic test to show that they will develop a disease in the future.

Visibility plays a central role in producing a negative social reaction from others. Individuals with genetic conditions have avoided making claims on their health insurance for fear that they will be labelled as different. Individuals at risk of developing a late onset condition such as Huntingdon's disease, a severe neurological disorder, often describe difficulties planning long-term relationships and conceal their genetic status from their partner or their close family. This places strain on interpersonal relationships, and feelings of guilt, shame and fear of discovery have been described (Kessler, 1993). The concept of 'survivor guilt' has been described when, within a group of siblings, one individual may not have inherited the condition and they describe feelings of responsibility or guilt towards the affected siblings. Family members, formerly united by a bond of risk, may suddenly find themselves separated by the outcome of a predictive test. The following poem was written by a 13 year old whose father was affected by Huntingdon's disease and who herself is at risk of developing the disease.

HD and me

Huntingdon's disease means a lot of things to me.
It means pain and suffering. I watch my dad disappear and become someone else, I shouldn't have to do that.
It means fear. It terrifies me, scares me to death. I watch my dad knowing that one day it may be me. Everything that I enjoy slowly being taken away. I confront that every day – it scares me.

It means embarrassment. When dad collected me from school you could see the teachers gossiping, making judgements – deciding he was drunk.

It means stigma – being from the 'HD' family, the funny or nutty family.

It means discrimination – who will employ, loan money, insure?

It means strength – I am a much stronger and courageous person.

It means friendship – I have met and made friends with many lovely people.

It means fun – you learn to keep life's problems in proportion.

It means hope – there is so much hope for the future.

(Sarah, aged 13)

Carrier status

Identifying an individual as a carrier of a genetic condition can have both psychological and social risks, such as stigmatisation, discrimination and a negative effect on self-image (Childs *et al.*, 1976; Haan, 1994). There is evidence that knowledge of carrier status is related to a less optimistic perception of future health (Marteau *et al.*, 1992) and that siblings of children with cystic fibrosis have a fear of intimacy and of interpersonal relationships (Fanos and Johnson, 1995). Children affected by cystic fibrosis described being teased and picked on at school and the central phenomenon of 'discovering a feeling of difference' emerged from the interviews of twenty children (D'Auria *et al.*, 1997).

The history of mass screening for carrier status has been interesting. In 1966 a programme was introduced in Greece, aimed at reducing the number of children born with haemoglobinopathies (Stamato-yannopoullos, 1974). In a study prior to the introduction of the programme, 7 per cent of the population stated that they would avoid relationships with known carriers. This stigmatisation of known healthy carriers caused young people to hide their carrier status, for fear of rejection. Carrier testing can also produce feelings of a less positive self-image, and projected negative feelings towards other carriers (Evers Kiebooms *et al.*, 1994).

The study by Jolly *et al.* (1998) suggests that, when individuals were told of their carrier status for a chromosome condition, they experienced similar reactions to those described by Falek (1977), i.e. shock and denial, anxiety, anger/guilt, depression and eventually psychological homeostasis (Falek, 1977; Lazarous and Folkman, 1984). Participants were selective about with whom they shared information, suggesting that it seemed easier for participants to share the information of their carrier status within the family than with friends or healthcare professionals.

Discrimination

Genetic discrimination refers to discrimination directed against an individual or family based solely on an apparent or perceived genetic variation from 'normality'. In 1972 the United States passed legislation to screen Afro-Americans for the sickle cell trait; this was a mandatory targeted population screening of a minority group. This lead to discrimination by employers such as airlines against healthy workers, in the mistaken belief that carriers would pass out at high altitude (Reilly, 1976).

There is now evidence of discrimination in health and life insurance in the United States as well as life insurance in the UK (Billings *et al.*, 1992; Harper, 1997b; Low *et al.*, 1998). It is therefore important to consider the confidentiality of genetic information within the healthcare system and the potential for harm to an individual or their extended family members which could occur if used inappropriately. Workplace screening, in which job applicants and employees are tested for inherited traits that may predispose them to industrial disease, has led to exclusionary practices at work (Drapper, 1991). It is a concern that policies may bring about the exclusion of certain workers rather than the removal of hazards or the introduction of safeguards to provide a safer workplace for all. If a genetic approach to health is undertaken, then this individualises and privatises health problems without challenging the systems that create ill health.

Stigma associated with the course of the condition

An important aspect to consider is whether the marker, to use the term applied by Jones *et al.* (1984) to indicate the person who is inflicting the stigmatisation, is aware of the genetic nature of the disorder. Different reactions are observed if the origin of the stigma was the result of a personal choice or a societal influence, such as an approved screening programme. Being personally responsible for causing one's own blemish or the extent that someone or something else (nature/God) can be blamed changes the extent of the stigmatisation, being stronger when the marker perceives the individual to be personally responsible. Individuals who choose not to have prenatal screening tests or have children in the knowledge of a known genetic risk may be perceived as being personally responsible for the outcome (Hubbard, 1984).

The dimension of 'the course of the mark' can be described by the example of Huntington's disease. Huntington's disease shows three of the features described by Jones *et al.* (1984) as contributing to the stigmatisation process. The disease is progressively crippling and deforming, it is non-fatal and chronic, running a long course, and it appears to be incurable. If people believe that the mark can be cured, then they are more likely to present a favourable attitude to the affected individual. One issue is that most genetic conditions can not be cured or repaired; this can be less acceptable and more open to stigmatisation. There is great variation within genetic conditions. The multifactorial nature of disease, the variations in class, culture, education levels and socio-economic circumstances, make it impossible to predict with any accuracy the impact of some genetic conditions on any one individual and their family (Ramsay, 1994).

New developments in prenatal diagnosis have altered the experience of pregnancy in Western society. Rothman describes the 'feeling that a pregnancy is only provisional until the foetal quality control investigations have been reported as satisfactory. Until then a women may find it difficult to let herself feel unconditionally positive about her pregnancy' (Rothman, 1988).

Altering the course

As with many conditions, the course of some can be altered. Surgery is now more readily available for many physical birth defects, such as birthmarks and malformations. The early repair of a child's cleft lip has resulted in a far different outcome for children born in families in which 50 per cent of the children in the past have been affected. Often society will expect that efforts are made by the individual or family to remove the marks, or to reduce their salience, by such means as surgical cosmetic surgery and prosthetic limbs, and concurrence with these social demands brings approval and better acceptance.

Issues of shame and guilt

Genetic conditions have been linked to feelings of shame and guilt in a number of studies (Kessler *et al.*, 1984; Chapple *et al.*, 1995). Shame has a number of elements, including embarrassment and stigma, and it is thought to arise from diminished self-esteem, feelings of loss of control, and deficiency. Parents of children with disfigurements have become socially isolated as they find others' expressions of sympathy to be painful, implying they are pitiful or deviant. The issue of guilt arises when someone believes he or she has done something or failed to do something, which might have averted the occurrence of a genetic problem. Questions such as 'what did I do wrong to cause this to happen?' are frequently raised in counselling sessions.

The influence of healthcare professionals and health policy

It is acknowledged that nurses should deliver healthcare to all and should not allow negative attitudes to adversely affect the delivery of healthcare (UKCC, 1992). A review of nursing research demonstrated that nurses' attitudes towards children with learning disabilities resulted in the stigmatisation of certain patients and acted as a barrier to providing care of an appropriate quality (Kelly and May, 1982; Goodyear, 1983). It has been stated that virtually all diseases have a genetic component and the contribution of genetic conditions to ill health is considerable (Welsh Health Planning Forum, 1995). Many healthcare professionals, from laboratory scientists to speech therapists, will care for families and individuals with a genetic diagnosis. The preceding sections have described some of the potential for discrimination and stigmatisation, which have been inflicted by healthcare professionals or maybe felt by the families themselves. A sense of insecurity and lack of knowledge when caring for children with learning disabilities has been found to adversely affect nursing care, leading to stigmatisation (Ryan, 1983; Shanley and Guest, 1995). As many genetic conditions are individually rare but collectively common, it is probable that most non-specialist healthcare professionals will be confronted with a situation they have not previously encountered.

Ethical framework

This section describes a framework of practical and ethical boundaries which many specialist nurses in genetics use to define their own practice (Williams, 1994). The code of conduct of the National Society of Genetic Counsellors is also very helpful in exploring difficult issues relating to the care of families at genetic risk (National Society of Genetic Counsellors, 1992). In many situations the care of the individual will also have an impact on the extended family in genetic conditions. There is a duty of care to avoid misusing your relationship with the family, which could lead to the disruption of established family structures. Healthcare professionals may work with families in a number of circumstances, such as seeking to understand the birth of a handicapped child, undergoing prenatal diagnosis and considering termination of pregnancy, or coping with the threat of chronic illness such as cancer or muscular dystrophy. The ability to provide a caring environment for the giving of bad news or the discussion of distressing subjects is important. Families need time to seek advice and information, both from specialists and from their own trusted sources of support. Healthcare professionals need to work with the family to promote benefits and minimise harm. For individuals to exercise autonomy they need sufficient information to enable them to understand and evaluate their options. Individuals facing new genetic information need support not only to comprehend the risk information they have been given in an intellectual sense, but also to incorporate an emotional element of understanding and belief. This way the information given is experienced as relevant to themselves in a meaningful way (Williams, 1994; Richards and Ponder, 1996).

Support and non-directiveness

It is important to help patients express their grief, often related to the loss of normality or their image of themselves as normal, and support them in their search to re-evaluate themselves, their role and place in society (Resta, 1997). Families affected by genetic disease need supportive care when decisions need to be made: whether to 'have a prenatal test', to 'have a termination' or to 'have corrective or prophylactic surgery'. The desire to respect autonomy and support patient choice can be a difficult one, especially if the choice is contrary to the healthcare professional's own or society's view of what is right or healthy. Clarke (1991) has argued strongly that the non-directive aim of genetic counselling is not possible and therefore, within the limits of acknowledging our possible directiveness, we have an obligation to offer most support at a time when patients are making difficult decisions (Clarke, 1991). Caring for a family with a genetic condition starkly demonstrates that the provision of health-care takes place against a background of social, political and commercial interests, and that these interests change with the rapid discovery of new knowledge in this field. Also it is important to acknowledge that the process and content of genetic counselling differs between professional groups and cultures. Research has shown that, when providing genetic counselling for foetal abnormality, obstetricians were most likely to be directive, with clinical geneticists and genetic nurses being more non-directive (Marteau *et al.*, 1994). Internationally there are wide cultural differences in how genetic counselling is practised and in the attitudes of genetics professionals to contentious issues (Wertz, 1998). This emphasises the importance for healthcare workers to examine their own cultural background and moral values when providing support and information for families from their own or different communities.

A problem encountered by healthcare professionals caring for families is the lack of education about genetic healthcare available through formal routes of training. A review of genetic education in nursing in the UK and the United States showed very few, if any, formal lectures on genetics (Anderson, 1996; Kirk, 1999). A number of resources exist to provide information for healthcare professionals, two of which are the public health genetic website (Public Health Genetics Unit, 2000) and the national coalition of health professional education in genetics (National Coalition of Health Professional Education in Genetics, 2000). A recent text written specifically for nurses helps to highlight some of the nursing approaches to the care of families affected by genetic disease (Lea *et al.*, 1998). The resources available to most healthcare professionals are their local Regional Genetic Centres. These are organised around the NHS Regions and will discuss and inform on most genetic issues, from laboratory services to patient care. These centres are staffed by consultant clinical geneticists and non-medical genetic counsellors/nurse specialists in genetics (Skirton *et al.*, 1997, 1998).

Nurses need to be aware that the public has a poor understanding of how genetics relates to illness and therefore need to inform and be aware of the potential for stigmatisation by other colleagues and also other patients (Durant *et al.*, 1996). Table 6.1 lists ways in which stigma can be overcome in relation to genetic conditions.

Families affected or at risk of genetic conditions not only have to cope with the physical, psychological and social problems associated with their condition, but have to contend with the genetic aetiology and future decisions relating to reproduction and their own health. These issues are complex, and healthcare workers can cause great harm by not realising the importance of the issues described here, which are common to many genetic conditions. By having the knowledge, awareness and skills to offer sensitive care, the potential for stigmatisation can be reduced.

Table 6.1   **What can be done to overcome stigma**

Be informed

Be aware of the basic genetic principles – the difference between carrier status and disease.
Obtain knowledge about the impact of specific genetic conditions upon the family.
Obtain up-to-date knowledge about the origin, course and prognosis of the specific condition affecting the family.
Be aware of the implications for other family members, such as at-risk status and risk to children.

Examine your own ethical boundaries and cultural differences

Give support and provide an environment where difficult issues can be discussed and questions asked.
Be honest when you are not personally comfortable with a decision made by a family (for example, termination of pregnancy) and perhaps refer them to another professional who will feel able to support the family's decision.

Multidisciplinary practice

Providing healthcare to individuals and families affected or at risk of genetic disease is by necessity a multidisciplinary task. It is important that the carer be comfortable moving between the fields of biological science, counselling/support, new technologies and ethics.

References

Anderson, G.W. (1996) 'The evolution and status of genetics education in nursing in the United States 1983–1995', *IMAGE Journal of Nursing Scholarship*, 28: 101–6.

Baird, P. (1990) 'Genetics and health care', *Persp Biol Med*, 33: 203–13.

Billings, P., Kohn, M. and de Cuevas, M. (1992) 'Discrimination as a consequence of genetic testing', *American Journal of Human Genetics*, 50: 476–82.

Cassel, C. (1997) 'Policy implications of the human genome project', *Woman's Health Issues*, 7: 225–9.

Chapple, A., May C. and Campion, P. (1995) 'Lay understanding of genetic disease: a British study of families attending a genetic counselling service', *Journal of Genetic Counselling*, 4: 281–300.

Childs, B., Gordils, L., Kayback, M. and Kazazain, H. (1976) 'Tay Sachs screening: social and psychological impact', *American Journal of Human Genetics*, 28: 550–8.

Clarke, A. (1991) 'Is non directive counselling possible?', *Lancet*, 338: 998–1001.

D'Auria, J.P., Christian, B.J. and Richardson, L.F. (1997) 'Through the looking glass: children's perceptions of growing up with cystic fibrosis', *Canadian Journal of Nursing Research*, 29: 99–112.

Davenport, C. and Muncey, D. (1916) 'Huntington's chorea in relation to hereditary and insanity', *American Human Insanity*, 73: 195–222.

Drapper, E. (1991) *Risky business*, Cambridge: Cambridge University Press.

Durant, J., Hansen, A. and Bauer, M. (1996) 'Public understanding of the new genetics', in T. Marteau and M. Richards (eds), *The troubled helix*, Cambridge: Cambridge University Press.

Evers Kiebooms, G., Denayer, L., Welkenhuysen, M. *et al.* (1994) 'A stigmatizing effect of carrier status for cystic fibrosis', *Clinical Genetics*, 46: 336–43.

Falek, A. (1977) 'Use of the coping process to achieve psychological homeostasis in genetic counselling', in H. Lubs and F. de la Cruz (eds), *Genetic counselling*, New York: Raven Press.

Fanos, J. and Johnson, J. (1995) 'Perception of carrier status by cystic fibrosis siblings', *American Journal of Human Genetics*, 57: 431–8.

Goodyear, R. (1983) 'Patterns of counsellors' attitudes towards disability groups', *Rehabilitation Counselling Bulletin*, 26: 181–4.

Haan, E. (1994) ' Screening for carriers of genetic disease: points to consider', *Medical Journal of Australia*, 158: 419–21.

Harper, P. (1997a) 'China's genetic law', in P. Harper and P. Clarke (eds), *Genetics society and clinical practice*, Oxford: BIOS Scientific Publishers.

—— (1997b) 'Genetic testing and insurance', in P. Harper and P. Clarke (eds), *Genetics society and clinical practice*, Oxford: BIOS Scientific Publishers.

Hubbard, R. (1984) 'Personal courage is not enough: some hazards of childbearing in the 1980s', in A. Arditti, R. Klein and S. Minden (eds), *Test tube women: what future for motherhood?*, London: Pandora Press.

Human Genome Organisation (2000) *Human Genome Organisation*, vol. 2000, http://www.hugo-international.org/hugo.

Jolly, A., Parsons, E. and Clarke, A.J. (1998) 'Carriers of balanced chromosomal translocations', in A. Clarke (ed.), *The genetic testing of children*, Oxford: BIOS Scientific Publications.

Jones, E., Farina, A., Hastorf, A. *et al.* (1984) 'The dimensions of stigma', in R. Atkinson, G. Lindzey and R. Thompson (eds), *Social stigma: the psychology of marked relationships*, New York: W.H. Freeman and Company.

Kelly, M. and May, D. (1982) 'Good and bad patients: a review of the literature and a theoretical critique', *Journal of Advanced Nursing*, 7: 147–56.

Kessler, S. (1993) 'The spouse in the Huntington disease family', *Family Systems Medicine*, 11: 191–9.

Kessler, S., Kessler, H. and Ward, P. (1984) 'Psychological aspects of genetic counselling. III: Management of guilt and shame', *American Journal of Medical Genetics*, 17: 673–97.

Kirk, M. (1999) 'Preparing for the future: the status of genetics education in diploma-level training courses for nurses in the United Kingdom', *Nurse Education Today*, 19: 107–15.

Lazarous, R. and Folkman, S. (1984) *Stress, appraisal and coping*, New York: Springer-Verlag.

Lea, D.H., Jenkins, J.F. and Francomano, C.A. (1998) *Genetics in clinical practice: new directions for nursing and healthcare*, Boston: Jones & Bartlett.

Lippman, A. (1992) 'Mother matters: a fresh look at prenatal genetic testing', *Issues in reproductive and genetic engineering*, 5: 141–54.

Low, L., King, S. and Wilkie, T. (1998) 'Genetic discrimination in life insurance: empirical evidence from a cross sectional survey of genetic support groups in the UK', *BMJ*, 317: 1632–5.

Marteau, T., Drake, H. and Bobrow, M. (1994) 'Counselling following diagnosis of a fetal abnormality: the differing approaches of obstetricians, clinical geneticists and genetic nurses', *Journal of Medical Genetics*, 31: 864–7.

Marteau, T., van Duijn, M. and Ellis, I. (1992) 'Effects of genetic screening on perceptions of health: a pilot study', *Journal of Medical Genetics*, 29: 24–26.

National Coalition of Health Professional Education in Genetics (2000) *National Coalition of Health Professional Education in Genetics*, vol. 2000, http://www.nchpeg.org.

National Human Genome Research Institute (2000) *National Human Genome Research Institute*, vol. 2000, http://www.nchgr.nih.gov.

National Society of Genetic Counsellors (1992) *Code of Ethics*, Wallingford: NSGC.

—— (2000) http://www.nsgc.org, NSGC.

Nuffield Council on Bioethics (1993) *Genetic screening – ethical issues*, London: Nuffield Council on Bioethics.

Oliver, M. (1990) *The politics of disablement*, Basingstoke: Macmillan.

Panse, F. (1942) *Die Erbchorea, eine Klinische-genetice Studie*, Leipzig: Thieme.

Public Health Genetics Unit (2000) *Public Health Genetics Unit*, vol. 2000, http://www.medinfo.cam.uk/phgu/info, Cambridge: University of Cambridge.

Ramsay, M. (1994) 'Genetic reductionism and medical genetic practice', in A. Clarke (ed.), *Genetic counselling practice and principles*, London: Routledge.

Reilly, P. (1976) 'State supported mass genetic screening programs', in A. Milunsky and G. Annas (eds), *Genetics and the law*, New York: Plenum Press.

Resta, R. (1997) 'Carolyn's feet', *American Journal of Medical Genetics*, 72: 1–2.

Richards, M. (1996) 'Families', in T. Marteau and M. Richards (eds), *The troubled helix*, Cambridge: Cambridge University Press.

Richards, M. and Ponder, M. (1996) 'Lay understanding of genetics: a test of a hypothesis', *Journal of Medical Genetics*, 33: 1032–6.

Rothman, B. (1988) *The tentative pregnancy: prenatal diagnosis and the future of motherhood*, London: Pandora.

Ryan, L. (1983) 'Discrimination in nursing care, reality or fallacy?', *Australian Nurses Journal*, 12: 35.

Shakespeare, T. (1998) 'Choices and rights: eugenics, genetics and disability equality', *Disability and Society*, 13: 665–81.

Shanley, E. and Guest, C. (1995) 'Stigmatisation of people with learning disabilities in general hospitals', *British Journal of Nursing*, 4: 759–61.

Sherr, L. (1995) *Grief and AIDS*, Chichester: John Wiley and Sons.

Skirton, H., Barnes, C., Curtis, G. and Walford-Moore, J. (1997) 'The role and practice of the genetic nurse: report of the AGNC working party', *Journal of Medical Genetics*, 34: 141–7.

Skirton, H., Barnes, C., Guilbert, P. *et al.* (1998) 'Recommendations for education and training of genetic nurses and counsellors in the UK', *Journal of Medical Genetics*, 35: 410–12.

Stamatoyannopoullos, G. (1974) 'Problems of screening and counselling in the haemoglobinopathies', in A. Motulsky and F. Ebling (eds), *Birth defects. Proceedings of the Fourth International Conference*, Amsterdam: Excerpta Medica.

Strachan, T. and Read, A.P. (1999) *Human molecular genetics 2*, Oxford: BIOS.

Thomas, D. (1982) *The experience of handicap*, London: Methuen.

United Kingdom Central Council (1992) *Code of professional conduct for nurses, midwives and health visitors*, London: UKCC.

Welsh Health Planning Forum (1995) *Genomics: the impact of the new genetics on the NHS. The Cardiff Debate*, Cardiff: Welsh HPF.

Wertz, D.C. (1998) *International perspectives*, Oxford: BIOS.

Williams, A. (1994) 'Genetic counselling: a nurse's perspective', in A. Clarke (ed.), *Genetic counselling practice and principles*, London: Routledge.

7 Hearing loss

Scope for concealment

Janet Heyes

Introduction

Having spent considerable time, thought and energy while working on a clinical account of stigma and deafness, I now realise that anything useful that I may have to say is based on my personal experience of forty years of varying severity of hearing loss, due to otosclerosis.

Otosclerosis is a familial disorder, previously unknown in our family, in which the stapes, one of the chain of small interlinked bones in the middle ear, becomes immobilised by fibrous tissue and no longer transmits the vibration which is converted to sound.

My ears had been troublefree in childhood, and I was a fifth-year medical student when the first hint of trouble arose. I was unable to hear foetal hearts with my right ear, was referred to the student health service, saw an Ear, Nose and Throat consultant (ENT), was reassured and forgot all about it.

Four years later, working as a senior house officer in London, I was startled and rather offended when the consultant for whom I was working suggested that I should see another ENT specialist, as he had noticed that I possibly had hearing problems. I certainly had not noticed it myself, as far as I remember. The outcome of the ENT consultation was distressing. From the audiogram I was diagnosed as having bilateral otosclerosis, with significant loss of hearing in both ears. I was fortunate in having seen a consultant who was at the forefront of treatment for otosclerosis, and he described the new surgical treatments of mobilising the stapes, or more radically replacing the stapes with a Teflon piston, which had been developed by Shea in the United States about five years previously. This was available to me if I wished it later. But I was managing well and, despite the fear of what lay ahead, carried on working, became married, had a baby and put the matter to the back of my mind.

I had no idea how impaired my hearing was. I was enjoying life, and it was only after accepting with enthusiasm an unissued invitation that I realised that my hearing should be reviewed. In retrospect it is interesting how the period of self-deception lasted so long. I had moved to a new city and had stopped work for a period to bring up two children, so there were few familiar people around me and I was moderately isolated. I was not aware of any need either to reveal or conceal my hearing loss. The process of withdrawal was very slow and insidious. It was only the sudden improvement following stapes mobilisation, when I began to initiate conversations with strangers and laugh at jokes, puns and innuendo, that I realised what deep and subtle changes had crept up on the person I had been before this all began.

The fact that I had not noticed what was happening, despite the knowledge, shows how difficult it can be for others to help. Everyone knows at some time what it is like not to hear something. There is perhaps the irritation that the speaker did not speak clearly, and the hope that the essential part of the message will be appreciated a little later when the context is clear; and there is the self-confidence needed to ask to have something repeated which may interfere with the flow of the speaker's thoughts. We will all have been attendees at talks and lectures when we are absolutely certain that half of the audience cannot hear, and yet no one takes action. It is very difficult to tell whether words are being heard by another, and there is likely to be unintentional concealment, waiting for the penny to drop or to catch a clue about topic change, to place the missed words in context and make them comprehensible.

Sound, and its higher development speech, have many functions. Among them, the essential one is the provision of information, and this makes the early stage of learning to use a hearing aid bearable. But a much more subtle and far-reaching form of verbal intercourse is presented by the trivia with which we build bridges before deciding whether to become closer, more intimate and more open with another. The well-known British obsession with the weather is really a dipstick. Is the recipient amiable, cordial, irritable, interested? Is it worthwhile talking about the cost of fuel, a family holiday or a recent bereavement? It is impossible to repeat the trivia without seeming ridiculous (instead of repeating, we usually say 'Never mind, it doesn't matter'). But it does matter to the recipient, because without these bridges very many opportunities to draw close to another person are lost. Humour, too, depends greatly upon speech. Without being able to hear speech, tone of voice, innuendo, pun and punch line are lost.

Laughter is often the first area in which people with hearing loss deliberately practice deception. There is unease in a group if each member except one laughs together. The joke will probably be killed by explanation. It is easier for the deaf person to laugh, but there is always the risk of laughing at the wrong moment or inappropriately. My dishonesty is compounded by a helpful friend who asks after I have laughed, 'Did you get that?' That question can only ever have an affirmative reply! There may also be practical reasons for concealment. One of my worst experiences was spending an evening as a guest of a group of relative strangers in a dimly lit room shortly before I was to have further surgery. I was managing one-to-one with a hearing aid which failed that evening. The attempted concealment was deliberate, although whether it was successful I do not know; I was never invited there again.

What causes us to conceal our hearing loss? There are many factors. It is significant that, whereas blind people are portrayed in tragedy, deaf people are seen in comedy. Mishearing can lead to many jokes, usually at the expense of the hearing impaired person. There is the common and understandable irritation of those with normal hearing at the need to repeat, to attract attention, to communicate face-to-face – and the often-voiced suspicion that the deaf one could hear if they wanted to. This is often accompanied by exasperation that the hearing impaired one will not obtain or use a hearing aid, or will discard one after it has been seldom used. Usually when communication is difficult the first remedy is to shout. Shouting is almost never helpful, and the facial changes and apparent attack of the attempt evoke in the recipient feelings of threat, confusion and a wish to escape. Listening intently is very tiring, and attempting to conceal the impairment imposes a watchfulness and guardedness which is quite alienating of others. Tied up in all of this is one's sense of worth. While engaged to work as an audit facilitator by a committee of doctors who knew that I had severe hearing impairment, sometimes it seemed to me that they made no attempt to ensure that I was able to hear. They covered their mouths as they spoke, muttered, spoke in duets and were generally unhelpful. On these occasions I became silently angry with the group, then usually felt that it was unreasonable to expect them to remember to make special allowances for me, eventually feeling very sad, unworthy and near to tears. By this time my concentration was so fragmented that little was heard.

However, hearing loss does not only involve difficulty with speech (Lysons, 1996). Underlying speech there is a more primitive use of sound which is also lost. The background noises which in normal circumstances are ignored are essential monitors of our environment and safety. Birdsong may be ignored until the panic messages to warn of a predatory cat are heard; footsteps in a dark road will only be heard if there is an approach, or a change of pace; and traffic noise will only impinge when brakes squeal. All these unconscious clues are no longer available to a person with significant hearing loss, making them much more vulnerable and anxious, probably without realising why. It is generally assumed that we live in a hearing world, and that normal people are hearing people who will get out of the way of approaching cars, answer the doorbell if it rings, and respond if spoken to. If the person does not respond in the expected way they are seen as 'deviant'; in other words, they do not follow the generally accepted norms of society. When a hearing impaired person deviates from the expected norm, it is seen as something discreditable and experienced as 'stigma'.

As Goffman (1963) says, the rewards of appearing normal are so great that most people with a disability will pretend to be normal, and as hearing impairment usually has no outward mark, pretence is very common in hearing loss. Because of this, many will not wear a hearing aid, and this is reinforced by manufacturers of hearing aids who emphasise the invisibility of their devices, even at the cost of loss of efficiency. This contrasts markedly with the response to visual impairment, where spectacles are accepted without comment as part of the ageing process. A common reason given by people who hide hearing loss is that they do not want other people to need to make a special effort to communicate with them. There are several components in this statement. One is that it is even more painful if the other realises that extra help is needed, but does not attempt to provide it. Another is that because of the stage of life at which hearing loss is usually experienced, most people will have uncomfortable memories of occasions in the past when they have been less than helpful to others with hearing loss, and may in fact have deliberately excluded them.

Hearing loss almost invariably produces personality and life changes in those affected. The recognition that hearing loss tends to be progressive, and that an unpredictable worsening of the situation has to be faced in the future, leads almost always to feelings of depression and fear. There is also a general constriction of life, which has been described by McCall (1981) as including:

- diminished opportunities for conversation and the embarrassment of misunderstandings;
- missing the tone of voice, which conveys so much;
- the humiliation of being thought stupid;
- the impossibility of easy participation in discussions, groups, etc.;
- fatigue caused by constant alertness;
- the diminution of social information from which to assess the social mood;
- the reasons for decisions not being clearly understood;
- lack of stimulation of discussion and debate;
- the uncertainty caused when people act suddenly without explanation;
- the enormous difficulty of simple encounters; even asking a shop assistant to repeat something twice may cause embarrassment;
- the reality of being left out.

The feelings of depression tend to last longer and can be reactivated in many situations. Eventually it may become easier to avoid social situations which are likely to be difficult, which may well lead to even further constriction of life.

Many of the effects can be reduced by being honest and open about the hearing loss. Despite the problems that people have in coping with another's hearing loss, the outcome of openness is nearly always a great improvement. A clear example of this is given by the case of a colleague who has severe impairment, and who always seemed to be a rather austere and aloof person. His acquisition of a 'hearing dog', a sociable mongrel that wears a coat with the large, clear message, 'I am a hearing dog', has transformed the attitude of others who, knowing what the problem is, now approach him with confidence and make determined attempts to overcome it. In my own case, now that I always tell people at the outset that I have hearing loss, communication is much easier and I feel less isolated.

Measurement of hearing

Sound is created by vibration which reaches the ear and is perceived as hearing. The sound is registered as having both pitch, which depends on the frequency of the vibration, and volume, which depends on the force of the vibration. Sound is measured in decibels, one decibel being a measure of sound energy based on the relation to the sound which is just audible to a person with normal hearing. Ten decibels is sound which has twice the impact of zero decibels, and sixty decibels is a sound which has a million times the impact of the sound which is just audible to a normal ear. Ninety decibels has one thousand million times the impact, and at that level of loss, when such a powerful stimulus is needed, it is not possible to hear speech without a powerful hearing aid.

The pitch, or frequency of vibration, is also measured as part of the common method of hearing assessment, the audiogram, a chart on which is plotted the intensity of sounds at different pitches that are just audible to the person being examined. The pattern of the graph can help with the diagnosis of the cause of deafness. But it tells little about discrimination, the ability to decipher the sound into useful speech which is also commonly damaged and which can only be helped to a very limited extent by adjusting a hearing aid to emphasise higher or lower pitches. This is one of the most difficult aspects of hearing loss, partly because other people expect an aid to correct hearing in the way that spectacles often correct sight, when in fact it may only amplify noise. Understanding hearing loss is compounded by the fact that different groups of experts use different systems of classification. Any loss of hearing causes different loss of high or low pitched sound. Particularly in older people, it is common for the loss to be in frequencies of higher pitch, making it difficult to hear the consonants which define speech clarity, and often causing increased sensitivity to lower pitches, which causes discomfort if the aid is effective enough to amplify the consonants. The aid also amplifies any background noise such as traffic, noise of cutlery on plates, wind, or music. These difficulties often make older people unwilling to use an aid and lead to mutual irritation between the hearing impaired person and their family. Irritation does not help communication, nor does mutual blaming; instead it tends to lead to exclusion, or to shouting. It is important when a hearing aid is first provided that, to become accustomed to it, the wearer uses it regularly for short periods in a quiet environment. (For further reading about hearing loss, Lysons' book *Understanding Hearing Loss* (Lysons 1996) is strongly recommended.)

Table 7.1 Estimates of the number of adults in Britain in different hearing categories

Description of hearing loss	dBHL better ear average	Number of adults	Total adult population (%)
Mild hearing loss	25–40	5 million	11.33
Moderate hearing loss	41–70	2.2 million	4.99
Severe hearing loss	71–95	0.24 million	0.54
Profound hearing loss	95	0.06 million	0.14
	Total	7.5 million	17

Source: Ballantyne, 2000.
Note: dBHL = hearing loss in decibels.

Table 7.2 Rough relationship between hearing loss and social difficulty

Loss	Effect
25–40dB	Impairment in church or theatre
40–50dB	Difficulty in direct conversation
55dB	Difficulty with telephones
90dB	Total deafness for speech

Source: Lysons, 1996 (with permission of Jessica Kingsley Publishers).

Hearing impairment and healthcare

Given the prevalence of hearing impairment and the frequency of conceal-ment, it is reasonable to assume that everyone might be deaf, and to make allowances accordingly. In any six-bedded hospital ward, one person is likely to have a significant hearing loss, and at any general practice surgery at least three or four people will be affected. The organisation of health-care certainly traps the concealers. The patient call systems of out-patient clinics and GP surgeries depend almost entirely on spoken names, often spoken by a receptionist or nurse perhaps with a light and quiet voice. This causes much unwarranted anxiety and a fair degree of muddle. It is very rare to have hearing impairment noted on a file, and it is rare for a surgery or hospital reception area to have an induction loop installed or to publicise that they participate in a sympathetic hearing scheme, with the appropriate symbol.

A recent study commissioned by the Royal National Institute for Deaf People (RNID, 2000) found that more than a fifth of deaf and hard of hearing patients leave a doctor's appointment unsure of what is wrong with them. A fifth felt upset by the way they had been treated and more than one in ten put their health at risk by avoiding doctors because of communication difficulties (Beecham, 2000). The RNID have produced an information pack for GPs, which includes simple advice for care of people with hearing loss (RNID, 2000), and which would be equally useful to all those working in healthcare. The guidelines are as follows:

- Remember to face patients when talking to them and check that they have understood.
- Try to reduce background noise, especially for hearing aid users.
- Avoid having bright light behind you, or equipment blocking the patient's view, as these make lip reading more difficult.
- Speak in a moderate rhythm, try not to change the subject abruptly, and rephrase if the patient has not understood.
- Keep a pen and paper handy in case you need to write anything down.
- Ask patients how they prefer to communicate, and mark their records so that surgery staff also know.
- Keep details of sign language interpreters handy (obtainable from the local health authority).
- Think about how patients in the waiting room know when it is their turn.
- Set guidelines for how to deal with hard of hearing and deaf patients so that all staff feel confident about communicating effectively.
- Be aware of technical aids such as induction loops for reception areas, and listening devices for the surgery.

Finally, remember, just being aware of the possibility that the patient you are speaking to may be deaf or hard of hearing will help to change the way you communicate with them.

References

Ballantyne, D. (1990) *Handbook of audiological techniques*, London: Butterworth-Heinemann.

Beecham, L. (2000) 'Medicopolitical digest', *British Medical Journal*, 320, 519.

Goffman, E. (1963). *Stigma – notes on the management of spoiled identity*, London: Pelican.

Lysons, K. (1996) *Understanding hearing loss*, London: Jessica Kingsley.

McCall, R. (1981) 'The effects of sudden profound hearing loss in adult life', *British Society of Audiology*, 10 April.

Royal National Institute for Deaf People (2000) *Communication guidelines*, London: RNID.

8 Marked on sight

Tony Wright

Introduction

The focus, brought about by the 'Psychology of the Mark' (see Jones *et al.*, 1984), on the interaction between people who are sighted and people who are blind and partially sighted – potential marker and marked respectively – comes as a distinctive point of departure from some previous contributions from the field of psychology. Understanding the complex realities and possibilities in this interaction requires appreciation of both sighted reactions to 'the blind' and the lived experience of serious sight loss, i.e. sight loss to a diagnosable degree: blind, partially sighted or legally blind.

Concealment and course of the mark

The complex intertwining of these elements of the psychology of the mark can defy clear demarcation. The innumerable possibilities for serious loss of sight occurring similarly defy complete categorisation. People born blind or blind from the earliest of ages, i.e. with no visual memory, can be said to be visibly blind all their lives. The possibility of an extreme form of concealment thrust upon a congenitally blind person is not unknown. People who are born with a congenital eye condition, which means the serious loss of sight later in life, i.e. those who have some visual memory, may or may not conceal their mark at different stages of their eye condition. The majority of people who are blind and partially sighted are so adventitiously, and predominantly through age-related eye conditions (Baker and Winyard, 1998). Despite this variety of the lived experience of serious sight loss, it is possible to apprehend the issues in relation to concealing, and the course of, the mark. To achieve this, an appreciation of the difference between the lived experience of serious sight loss and the possible (and prolific) reactions of sighted people is needed. Examples from my own counselling research (a narrative analysis) and the research and works of others, in relation to people who are blind and partially sighted, contribute to this chapter.

Table 8.1   **Helen's narrative: 'I didn't register anything'**

Lack of anticipation

1	I dismissed it
2	I think er…
3	I didn't register anything

Impact on daughter with explanation

4	And my daughter was with me at the time
5	and she nearly fell off the chair
6	because she was so shocked
7	we thought with the GP saying
8	it was the retina that had slipped [uhum]

Helen's attitude

9	I automatically
10	I was a bit apprehensive [uhum]
11	but I thought
12	'oh well whatever, it's got to be rectified'
13	so I went along with it [uhum]

Helen's reaction

14	When he said that I'd lost me sight
15	I think I er
16	I was numbed you know
17	inside
18	but I didn't say anything
19	didn't register anything
20	and I think…
21	well I came out stunned
22	'but I think… [stunned]

Decitudinal stance

23	You know it's like all the other things in my life
24	that I've dealt with it in a way that I've thought best
25	carry on you know
26	as though nothing has happened you know
27	but deal with it and
28	carry on doing the best I can
29	in the way I do it

Return to affect and resolution

30	So I felt stunned really and
31	I didn't feel any emotions or anything
32	it was just tuck them inside somewhere you know

A brief analysis

Helen's loss of sight has been a gradual one and is age-related. Helen's interview began with a lengthy chronicle of how her GP's referral led to over two years of medical treatment at the hands of seven consultants, potentially offering an improvement in her ability to see. Helen then slips into a narrative beginning with her dismissal of the detailed medical information imparted to her about her eyes. Helen is finally diagnosed as partially sighted.

Two years after seeing her GP, Helen has held onto his words about the possibility of her having a slipped retina (lines 7–8), which Helen knows can often be successfully treated. Despite waiting for treatment for age-related macula degeneration, Helen dismisses (line 1) the information given to her by the consultants. The emotionally charged atmosphere (lines 4–8) at the time she is told she has lost her sight is evidenced by the reported reaction of her daughter. Helen's attitude to potential restorative treatment (lines 9–13) which included 'a battery of tests' is then reported. However, her reaction (lines 14–22) is closer to trauma response, or even a response to being violated. Helen is numbed, or frozen, unable to register anything, doesn't speak and is stunned. Helen's shortened, slowed down and more staccato phrasing is also witness to the severity of her experience, recalled in this narrative. The shift from waiting for treatment and the hope of improved future eyesight is not only dashed, but a line has been crossed; Helen is now irrefutably visually impaired. She ignores (line 22) my repeating of the word stunned, despite the gap in conversation, and moves immediately on to how she decided to respond to being told she has lost her sight. As in the past, Helen falls back on her own way of dealing with things (lines 23–29), which are here spoken of somewhat ambiguously. What is made known is that Helen has dealt previously with traumatic events in her life. Paradoxically this is a mixture of carrying on as though nothing has happened, and yet dealing with it. Helen's resolution (lines 30–32) is to tuck her emotions away inside somewhere. Similar to her response to the medical information from the consultants, Helen dismisses the fact that losing her sight is a life changing and irreversible happening, unlike other traumas she has suffered, and is a change linked to the ageing process.

This narrative and brief analysis is sufficient to highlight the experiential issues pertinent to concealing, and the course of, the mark. Helen's narrative highlights a moment of crossing the threshold, from being a sighted person to becoming a person who is visually impaired. This threshold has two dimensions: (a) personal identity, of being a person who is visually impaired; and (b) others' awareness of being an individual who is visually impaired.

In Helen's example the threshold is crossed at the point of diagnosis and registration. The course of the mark, and issues of concealment or being visibly blind or partially sighted, converge, often with intensity, at such moments. Whether the threshold is crossed in such a traumatic and specific way, or whether it is a series of moments, possibly spread out over years before and after diagnosis and registration, there are some common experiential issues.

Helen's narrative clearly displays the lack of anticipation of serious and permanent loss of sight. Without the acknowledgement of being a person living with serious sight loss, concealment of the mark seems most likely. People living with a congenital eye condition which leads to a gradual loss of sight often across many years, such as retinitis pigmentosa, frequently conceal their mark as long as is possible, as in the case of Susan.

> ... you're always trying to appear that you're the same as other people that there's nothing different about you ... until obviously your vision becomes so bad that you can't pretend it's normal anymore. I don't know whether other people would be like that but the ones I know have always been the same as me, so it must be a normal reaction I think.

Kuusisto (1998) more fully reports his own experience of this link between personal identity; how others, especially the sighted, perceive him and the concealment and course of the mark. The following remark poignantly expresses this point: '... it is not hard to learn to use a cane – it is hard to think of oneself as a person who uses a cane. This to me is a question of identity' (Potok *et al.*, 1983). A significant part of crossing the threshold for the person who is blind or partially sighted, in addition to the personal identity issues, can be said to be one's identity in relation to others. Prior to blindness or partial sight being apparent through appearance, the use of a cane, a guide dog or low vision aids, select disclosure may occur. Becoming publicly visibly blind or partially sighted requires adaptation and adjustment. It seems many do not make this adjustment.

RNIB estimates (statistics available at the RNIB's website, www.rnib.org.uk), based on prevalence rates for 1996, record the following figures:

- UK total, visually impaired persons (registerable): 1,066,740
- UK total people registered blind and partially sighted: 354,153

Should these estimated figures be accurate, approximately two-thirds of all people in the UK who could register as blind or partially sighted choose not to do so. Concealing the mark and the degree to which any individual becomes visibly blind or partially sighted is a significant factor facing individuals and agencies concerned with appropriate service provision or care.

Once individuals living with serious sight loss make it over this first hurdle of crossing the threshold in terms of personal identity, other issues in the same area can be dealt with. This again is a highly individual path. Ainlay (1989) reports that, after an initial phase of concern about the meaning of becoming blind or partially sighted, those that become visibly blind or partially sighted turn to the more practical everyday concerns they now face. It is often this time of adjusting to the unseen environment which brings to the fore issues of concealment (Conyers, 1992).

This brief exposition of just some of the experiential issues related to the concealing and course of the mark is sufficient to show the importance of identity issues incurred through serious loss of sight. To illustrate the diversity of possible expression of the issues outlined, consider the statement 'I'm happy to be blind'. Some people who are or become blind or partially sighted do not conceal their mark at all. There is no end to the possible reactions to the intra-personal cognitive affective mix and the extra-personal *sitz-im-leben* incurred through serious sight loss. Issues of identity, reactions and attitudes to them are forged in a constellation of relationships, and this brings us to the response of the sighted to people who are blind and partially sighted.

Reactions of the sighted

The adventitiously blind and partially sighted, by definition, have visual memory and all but approximately 4 per cent of these have some functional vision. 'Blindness is often perceived by the sighted as an either/or condition: one sees or does not see' (Kuusisto, 1998).

Past psychological studies attempting to establish 'the psychology (or even the psychopathology) of the blind' have failed to do so. People who are blind or partially sighted share the same psychological make up as the rest of society. The attempt to understand the difference in life experience incurred through serious sight loss remains in its infancy. This tension of sameness and difference, in the life experience of people who are blind and partially sighted, is a core issue throughout, and there are manifold related identity issues for the individuals concerned.

> I didn't want to be different ... erm, because I construed at a very early age that you knew you were different because you were blind.
>
> (Research participant)

Managing to maintain a focus on the lived experience of serious sight loss can be said to be a failing of past psychological writings. 'Most of the traditional psychological theories or conceptualisations of blindness can be thought of as projections of the anxieties and hopes of sighted people' (Tobin, 1995: 74).

While understanding the cultural background of the reactions of sighted people towards people who are blind or partially sighted remains helpful, it is simply an understanding of sighted people's reactions. The experiential issue here for people, who are blind or partially sighted, is the attitude of sighted others. Without having to do, say or be anything, people who are blind or partially sighted have throughout history had people who are sighted attribute roles and meanings to them, individually and collectively; in other words, they are stigmatised. The person who is blind or partially sighted encounters something not of themselves through this process of erroneous attribution.

> In the difficult adaptation to the loss of sight, vision-impaired and blind persons frequently report that the most difficult part is coping with the attitudes of people in their environment (Monbeck, 1973). Thus the purpose of this article is to assist counsellors, teachers and other professionals who work with visually impaired persons to become more familiar with the cultural origins of the attitudes that their clients must come to terms with.
>
> (Wagner-Lampl and Oliver, 1994: 267)

Ward (1973) highlights a commonly experienced intense reaction to working with people who have visual problems on the part of sighted employees with little or no previous association. This intense reaction was recorded as lasting between one and two days, and occasionally longer. 'This reaction was characterized by the interns with the following terms: depression, frustration, trauma, fear, withdrawal, melancholy, sadness, fright, amazement, nervousness, helplessness, uneasiness, dizziness, sorrow, revulsion, pity, annoyance, guilt, shyness, self-consciousness, resentment, "lost", "fit-to-be-tied"' (Ward, 1973). What is of note here is the intensity and frequency of the response, not the particular form, which could be common or highly idiosyncratic. Feelings produced from immediate and sustained contact with people who are blind or partially sighted, fear of becoming blind oneself, and a more philosophical questioning about life and its meaning, are recorded as making sense of this intense reaction. This is particularly important in understanding the interaction between the newly blind or partially sighted person and those with whom they have most contact, including those closest personally.

This, coupled with symbolic meanings erroneously attributed to people who are blind or partially sighted, can easily combine in the internal life, the intra-personal cognitive affective mix, of the sighted person to produce a marking response to people who are blind or partially sighted. Dichotomous and contradictory symbolic meanings themselves reveal ambivalence towards people who are blind or partially sighted from some sighted people. On the one hand, sighted people can attribute terrifying fear of the dark, misery, helplessness and uselessness, the need for pity, a lack of adjustment, evilness, punishment for sins, and also the roles of fool and beggar. On the other hand, sighted people (and sometimes the same sighted people) can attribute to the blind or partially sighted powers beyond the norm, remarkable and better senses other than sight, deeper powers of insight, and moral superiority. Often these attributes are conceptualised as being compensatory gifts for the lack of sight (Tobin, 1995; Kent, 1989; Wagner-Lampl and Oliver, 1994).

Some examples

There is a seemingly endless supply of anecdotal examples of the potent mix of feelings and symbolic meanings expressed towards people who are blind or partially sighted by sighted people. The newly blind or partially sighted find themselves dealing with them across the full range of relationships and social contacts.

Consider, for example:

- the blind or partially sighted person asked to change tables at a restaurant because the people on the adjacent table do not like the sight of a blind or partially sighted person eating;
- the blind or partially sighted person refused service at a bar or café on the grounds that they are more likely to spill their drink and make a mess;
- the blind or partially sighted person waited on hand and foot by their family on the ground that they can do nothing for themselves;
- the blind person or partially sighted person accused of being not really blind;
- the blind or partially sighted person whose partner becomes withdrawn physically and sexually;
- the blind or partially sighted person accused of trying to tamper with or steal goods from a shop when in fact they are simply using low vision aids;
- the blind or partially sighted person treated as though they are stupid;
- the blind or partially sighted person talked about as though they are not there;
- the newly blind or partially sighted person ignored by sighted friends and/or neighbours;
- the blind or partially sighted person physically attacked as a 'soft' target;

- the partially sighted person whose bus pass is confiscated by the driver on the grounds that they are not blind and so must have stolen it;
- the sighted person who decides a blind or partially sighted person needs – and will have – their help, whether it is wanted or not;
- the sighted person who expects gratitude from the poor helpless blind or partially sighted person for their 'help'.

The list could easily be extended, both numerically and by the severity of responses possible. Concealing a visual impairment is an easier option than having to deal with any single such response, let alone a constellation of them. It is hardly surprising that many seriously visually impaired people simply do not take up the task of tackling such a degree of change in themselves and in others. This also explains the immense difficulty individuals can have in accessing appropriate services, as to do so would involve the acknowledgement to self and others that 'I am blind or partially sighted' (Wainapel, 1989). Such moments of acknowledgement are often accompanied by a backlog of emotions needing to be dealt with also, cf. Dodds (1993), especially in connection to learned helplessness.

There is a twofold issue here which seems ubiquitous and manifold in its expression: the ignorance of potential markers; and the identity issues of the potentially marked. People who are blind or partially sighted do not become so in a vacuum. Preceding 'blindness', considered as a mark, there are attitudes and behaviours on the part of the sighted which may be expressed on the level of personal response (gut reaction, and often fear) and the theoretical level (often incorporated into policy).

Among people who are adventitiously blind or partially sighted there is the added twist that, prior to their serious loss of sight, they too may have subscribed to the stuff of folklore, myth and legend, and may well be harbouring attitudes towards themselves based on these interjects. This may well account in part for the learned helplessness and concealment of the mark taken up by so many.

Healthcare

Rusalem, in his dated though seminal work *Coping with the Unseen Environment* (1972), typically does not include the general issue of healthcare for people who are blind and partially sighted. Throughout his work he records the attitudes and behaviours in a variety of settings of people who are sighted. The comprehensive picture is for a raising of awareness of the needs of people who are blind or partially sighted, an awareness he notes as lacking even within rehabilitation settings.

To my knowledge, this is an area requiring research to establish an accurate picture of the quality of healthcare provision. The lack of available research, coupled with the enormity of anecdotal material from people who are blind or partially sighted in respect of healthcare received (or not, as the case may be), leads easily to the formulation of a quite dismal picture of exclusion with many facets. That there is little available research itself seems suggestive of exclusion. Sighted healthcare workers are likely to be as prone to the 'sighted reactions' outlined above as any other portion of the population. Without raising healthcare providers' awareness of the needs of people who are blind or partially sighted, it seems reasonable to expect little change.

References

Ainlay, S.C. (1989) *Day brought back my night: ageing and new vision loss*, London: Routledge.

Baker, M. and Winyard, S. (1998) *Lost vision: older visually impaired people in the UK*, RNIB Campaign Report No. 6, London: RNIB.

Conyers, M. (1992) *Vision for the future: meeting the challenge of sight loss*, London: Jessica Kingsley.

Dodds, A. (1993) *Rehabilitating blind and visually impaired people: a psychological approach*, London: Chapman and Hall.

Jones, E.E., Farina, A., Hastorf, A.H. *et al.* (1984) *Social stigma, the psychology of marked relationships*, New York: W.H. Freeman.

Kent, D. (1989) 'Shackled imagination: literary illusions about blindness', *Journal of Visual Impairment and Blindness*, March, 83(3): 145–50.

Kuusisto, S. (1998) *Planet of the blind*, London: Faber and Faber.

Monbeck, M.E. (1973) *The meaning of blindness*, Bloomington: Indiana University Press.

Potok, A., Hancock, E., Krajczar, N.F. and Fearon, A.M. (1983) 'A question of identity', panel discussion, First General Session, *Proceedings from the 1983 Helen Keller Seminar*, New York: American Foundation for the Blind.

Rusalem, H. (1972) *Coping with the unseen environment*, New York: Teachers College Press.

Tobin, M.J. (1995) 'Blindness in later life: myths attitude and reality', *The British Journal of Visual Impairment*, July 13, 2: 69–75.

Wagner-Lampl, A. and Oliver, G.W. (1994) 'Folklore of blindness', *Journal of Visual Impairment and Blindness*, May 88(3): 267–76.

Wainapel, S.F. (1989) 'Attitudes of visually impaired persons towards cane use', *Journal of Visual Impairment and Blindness*, November 83(9): 446–8.

Ward, A.L. (1973) 'The response of individuals beginning work with blind persons', *The New Outlook*, January 67(1): 1–5.

9 Communication impairment and stigma

Emily McArdle

Introduction

The moment a person opens their mouth the listener is making judgements about them; about their status, social class, level of education and even personality. Close your eyes and think of a university professor; imagine them talking – what do you hear? It is likely that you imagine an older man talking in a Standard English (or Received Pronunciation) accent, probably with a high-pitched voice and a rapid rate of speech. Few of us will imagine someone with a strong Cockney accent, for example. We all have a set notion of how people speak and make assumptions about them based solely on their accent, voice, rate of speech, pitch/resonance and dialect.

Accent

Before considering the communication-impaired population it is useful to think about the prejudices faced by speakers with intact speech and language skills. As mentioned in the introduction, value judgements are made about people just from the way they talk. Plenty of research has been carried out into listener perceptions of accent and dialect (Honey, 1989). In one study listeners rated speech samples in terms of subjective attributes and, perhaps unsurprisingly, speakers with Received Pronunciation (RP) were rated with higher prestige than accented speakers (Giles and Powesland, 1975; see Table 9.1). Accented speakers on the other hand were more favourably evaluated in terms of social characteristics. Certain regional accents are consistently rated worse than others, with several studies showing that the four accents that are always rated unfavourably are London (Cockney), Liverpool (Scouse), Glasgow and Birmingham. It is also interesting to note that speakers of these most stigmatised accents themselves rate them negatively, consistently giving RP a higher rating (Honey, 1989). A study by Menzies (1999) concluded that her young Glaswegian subjects 'held underlying negative attitudes to their spoken vernacular'. In recent years we have seen companies locating their

Table 9.1 Personal characteristics of accented speakers

Accent	Attributed characteristics
Received pronunciation	More ambitious
	Intelligent
	Self-confident
	Determined
	Industrious
	Wealthy
Regional	Personal integrity
	Social attractiveness
	Less serious
	More talkative
	Good natured
	Humorous

Source: Based on Giles and Powesland, 1975.

customer services telephone centres in areas whose accent they feel the general public rates as helpful, friendly and less serious.

In legal settings defendants and witnesses with standard accents are seen as more credible than those with regionally accented speech, and doctors have been shown to assess the working-class individual less favourably than the middle-class person. Giles and Powesland (1975) suggest that 'it is possible that the doctor might place more reliance upon an account of symptoms related in a standard form of speech than upon similar descriptions given in a non-standard style'. Hein, cited by Wodack (1996), clearly showed that 'there are language barriers between doctors and patients attributable to differences in social class. Patients from a working-class background were treated with condescension'. This even resulted in differing treatment being proposed for the same symptom.

Student teachers were asked to form subjective impressions of eight (fictitious) children based on a photograph, a taped speech sample and a sample of work from each one. Subjects evaluated those children with 'good voices' significantly more favourably than those with 'poor voices'. They were judged to be better students, more intelligent, privileged, enthusiastic, self-confident and gentle. The way the children spoke was an important influencing factor in the teacher evaluations, even when combined with other cues (Seligman, Tucker and Lambert, 1972).

The pitch, volume and rate of our speech also give an impression. Loud voices can be associated with anger, high-pitched voices with grief and fast delivery with indifference. Our physical make-up, our state of health and our emotions affect voice quality. For example, people suffering with depression often have flat monotonous intonation and quiet volume.

Many actors have had success due to the deep and resonant qualities of their voices. Other famous people are attributed certain traits because of their voice and intonation. For example the snooker player Steve Davies was labelled as boring; was this because of his level intonation and slow speech rate? Some sportsmen have been figures of fun when the pitch of their voices has been incongruously high. In politics, too, the politician's accent can affect their popularity.

Speakers with normal speech, therefore, can face many prejudices because of the way that they speak. Consider life for the speech and language impaired population.

Speech and language impairment

There are an estimated 2.3 million people in Britain with some form of communication impairment (Royal College of Speech and Language Therapists, 1996). The varied types of disorder and their impact on a person's communication skills are shown in Table 9.2.

Table 9.2 Types of speech, language and communication impairment

Condition	Communication impairment
Acquired neurological disorders • Cerebro-vascular accident • Dementia • Neurosurgery • Progressive neurological disorders • Traumatic brain injury	• Dysphasia – difficulties understanding verbal/written expression • Dysarthria – weakness, slowing, incoordination or altered muscle tone causing speech and voice problems
Cerebral palsy	• Dysarthria • Language delay – comprehension and expressive language • Dysfluency – stuttering
Cleft lip and palate	• Resonance disorders – hypernasal speech • Articulation difficulties
Hearing impairment	• Language difficulties – comprehension and expressive language • Speech disorders • Resonance disorders
Ear, nose and throat • Head and neck surgery • Laryngectomy	• Voice • Articulation difficulties • Voice disorders
Learning disabilities (children and adults)	• Comprehension difficulties • Expressive language delay/disorder • Speech difficulties • Social communication difficulties

Table 9.2 Continued

Condition	Communication impairment
Mental health	• Social communication difficulties • Comprehension and expressive language difficulties • Dysfluency
Autism	• Social communication difficulties • Conversational skills • Social interaction skills • Comprehension of 'body language' • Eye contact and appropriate expression of emotion
Specific speech and language disorder (average cognitive ability)	• Comprehension difficulties • Expressive language difficulties • Grammar • Word recall • Speech disorder – unintelligibility
Speech and language delay	• Comprehension difficulties • Expressive language difficulties • Speech immaturities
Stutter (dysfluency)	• Blocking, prolongation or repetition of sounds, syllables or words

Concealability – the hidden disability

People with speech, language and social communication difficulties have a wide variety of impairments affecting many processes. For some people, communication impairment is part of another physical condition, and is therefore unconcealable. For example, somebody who has had a cleft lip and palate shows the physical scars, and a person who has cerebral palsy or a stroke may well have some difficulty walking. Somebody with a social communication difficulty may have impaired non-verbal behaviour that is instantly noticeable to others in the way they move, their facial expression and lack of eye contact.

Many people with communication impairment, however, have disabilities that do not have any physical signs. You cannot tell if someone has difficulty constructing a sentence or pronouncing sounds until they speak.

Some people have an articulation difficulty that is apparent as soon as they open their mouths to speak. This may be slurred speech caused by dysarthria following a stroke, or it may be something as minor as a lisp. People who have a stammer will often show this as soon as they begin to talk, particularly with someone new or in unfamiliar settings. However, there are some people who stammer so covertly that their life is an endless effort. They will avoid words they perceive to be difficult to say, therefore escaping an obvious block or repetition. This can be very successful until the time comes to introduce people by name, read aloud or perform similar inflexible tasks. A parent recently told me that her three-year-old daughter often gives her friend's name instead of her own, because she finds her own too difficult to speak fluently.

Children and adults who have voice disorders can also be identified quickly. The person who has had a laryngectomy will have a distinctive 'voice' quality, and the hoarseness caused by vocal abuse is also noticeable.

Expressive language disability is often less immediately obvious. Again, degrees of the problem make it more or less identifiable to the general population. Problems with language output can frequently be subtle, such as being unable to retrieve words quickly or to use complex sentence structure.

One of the most concealable communication impairments is comprehension disorder. It can be easy to fool people into thinking you have understood, particularly if you have good social skills. Some children and adults who have comprehension difficulties present with challenging behaviour, often disguising their inability to understand. It is easy to see why these types of problems coexist. Have you ever sat in a lecture or lesson where you could not follow what was going on or there was too much jargon? If so, did you listen attentively or switch off completely? Have you ever felt the confusion and panic when people talk to you in a foreign language they assume you understand? Many children withdraw from interacting with others because they feel constantly frightened when faced with a code that everyone else is 'in on' except themselves. No wonder, then, that these feelings of frustration can boil over into anti-social behaviour.

It is not clear how many disaffected people in the UK have communication problems. Certainly there is growing evidence of the prevalence of communication disorders among the prison population. Bryan and Forshaw (1998) cite the Polmont Young Offenders Survey (Johnson, 1994) in which 10–20 per cent of young offenders serving more than three months were found to have significant communication problems. This is a higher incidence than among the general population (approximately 4 per cent). Few speech and language therapists (32 in 1998) work with this population, and it is likely that many inmates will have language difficulties that are concealed.

Some research has been done into undetected language problems in children. Cross (1997, 1998) looked at the literature linking emotional and behavioural difficulties and language problems. She cites studies in which a high proportion of children with emotional and behavioural difficulties were found to have language problems that had previously been unde-tected (Cohen *et al.*, 1993; Giddan *et al.*, 1996).

For the most part people with communication impairment look just like the rest of the population, and it is only when they attempt to interact that their problems become apparent to the person with whom they are communicating. Even within the communication-impaired population there are degrees of concealability, with some people's problems being so well concealed that they have been overlooked altogether.

The very nature of communication impairment means that it is difficult for sufferers to make themselves heard as a disadvantaged group. Attempts to highlight the handicaps they face require the very skill that they lack. In this way their disability is concealed further from the general public.

How the communication impaired are stigmatised

As discussed at the beginning of this chapter, value judgements are made about a person from listening to the way they speak. Imagine, therefore, the impact of communication impairment.

The stigmatisation process begins early in life. From the time we are old enough to watch cartoons, we are fed the belief that speech difficulties are funny. Many cartoon studios have given their characters speech impedi-ments, for example Tweety Pie and Elmer J. Fudd have speech delays, and Sylvester and Daffy Duck have articulation disorders (all produced by Warner Brothers studios). What message is given when the articulate Bugs Bunny always manages to get the last laugh? Some comedy shows and films have encouraged the public to laugh at the stammerer and to find the struggle of that individual something that is amusing rather than disabling.

People with speech and language impairment face prejudice from all sections of the community. Even children stigmatise their speech- and language-impaired peers from an early age. Rice (1993) describes the rejec-tion of a young child with limited language by children he attempts to play with. It is not only other children who judge negatively. Rice gives evidence of language-impaired children being rated, incorrectly, by adults as having low intelligence simply because of their poor language skills.

During my professional career I have come across prejudiced assump-tions by those workers whom one would expect to be more enlightened. A worker employed to care for speech and language-impaired children commented that it was a shame that the father of a particular child was an alcoholic. Her basis for this assumption was his slurred speech and strange manner. The man in question was actually schizophrenic and on medica-tion that caused dysarthria. He had told me in the past how embarrassed he was about the way he spoke, probably for this very reason.

Within schools I have heard children described as 'naughty' because they can't understand, or 'lazy' because they have a speech delay or disorder. A teacher recently reported consistently disobedient behaviour of a pupil who had a severe language disorder. She told me that, no matter how many times he was told, he would not stop running both across the classroom and along the corridors of the school. The teacher described how she would shout 'Don't run!', a seemingly simple command. The child, however, was unable to understand negative instructions and, as he understood it, was being instructed to run! When the instruction was changed to 'Walk', this anxious-to-please four-year-old suddenly started to conform.

A final example illustrates the type of prejudice faced by speech-impaired individuals as they attempt daily activities. A client told me he had been thrown off a bus for being drunk when he asked for his fare. He, too, suffered from dysarthria, and that – together with general coordination problems following a stroke – had given the completely wrong impression. Any speech and language therapist would be able to recount stories such as these.

Until recently, much was supposed but little actually known about the impact of communication impairment on the lives of those experiencing it. In 1997 the Communications Forum commissioned a study entitled 'Living with Communication Impairment'. For this qualitative study a broad cross-section of people with different types and severity of communication impairment were interviewed by researchers from City University. They found striking commonalities in the accounts. Comments from the interviewees are grouped into themes, such as the consequences of communication impairment on work, school and finance; the impact on personal relationships; the environmental, structural and informational barriers faced; and vulnerability and stigma.

Many of the subjects felt their communication impairment had 'contributed significantly to difficulties experienced throughout their lives'. For those with long-term impairments, the feelings of failure and isolation often began at school. Participants described their problems finding suitable work and gave accounts that clearly show their feelings of anger and alienation. The impact on relationships is enormous. Many of the people interviewed felt detached and isolated. The subjects of this study gave accounts that displayed the prejudice, pity, ignorance and hostility they frequently faced, sometimes from supposedly more enlightened individuals.

> I have even had the experience when I've rung the hospital ... used my servox ... and I got through to the A & E by mistake. The nurse said 'What's your game? The dog got your voice?'
>
> (Jenny, 61, laryngectomy)

The concealability of language and speech impairment and the impact of this is discussed, and the study's authors conclude that 'ensuring that communication impairment ceases to be invisible will be a real step towards raising the social barriers' (Communications Forum, 1997).

The Communications Forum study therefore describes the feelings of isolation and social exclusion commonly faced by those with communication disorders.

Prejudice in legal settings

People with communication impairment can face prejudice within the legal system. The case of Mary Nevin highlights this. In 1997 Ms Nevin, who has multiple sclerosis, claimed that a care assistant had sexually assaulted her. Her evidence had been recorded on videotape because she has severe dysarthria and used an alphabet board to communicate. The judge threw the case out, ruling that the video was insufficient, as Ms Nevin could not be cross-examined on it in court (reported in *Royal College of Speech Language Therapy Bulletin*, November 1997). The speech-impaired population is therefore left vulnerable to exclusion from justice.

Barriers in healthcare

It is worrying that communication-impaired individuals have described attitudinal barriers in healthcare settings (Communications Forum, 1997). Most members of the general public find medical jargon extremely difficult to understand (Hein, cited in Wodack, 1996). Consider then the doctor–patient dialogue with respect to communication impairment. For a patient with a comprehension difficulty the language used in such settings can be impossible. Wodack (1996) describes non-communication-impaired patients as being 'afraid to ask questions'; add to this an expressive language or speech problem, coupled with loss of confidence and low self-esteem, and consider how hard it would be for such a patient to admit they can't understand.

For many people with communication impairment the environment of a healthcare setting can create barriers to the therapeutic process. Background noise can interfere with the intelligibility, formulation and comprehension of speech and language, as can the rate and timing of interactions. People with communication impairment need a significantly longer time to communicate their worries, needs and questions. This does not fit into a 'number crunching' conveyor belt approach to healthcare. There is little opportunity for people with speech and language impairment to communicate their dissatisfaction, since complaint procedures discriminate against those whose communication is poor.

When inclusion equals exclusion – the educational experience

Our early experiences of the world colour our attitudes, beliefs, self-confidence and relationships with others. For a young child, school is often their first independent encounter with the outside world and other people's attitudes. They can no longer rely on an adult to protect them from a judgemental society. Acknowledging that education has an impact on that person throughout their life can help us to understand why some patients can feel disadvantaged and excluded in many situations, including health-care environments.

In 1997 the government published its ideas for special educational needs provision in the UK in a document called 'Excellence for All Children'. It promoted inclusiveness so that, wherever possible, children would be educated in mainstream schools. For many children with a disability this has been good news. Previously condemned to segregation in a special school, they can now become fully integrated members of the community. For children with a specific speech and language disorder, however, this idea, if taken to the extreme, could spell disaster. Special educational provision for these children is usually special residential schools, language units attached to designated mainstream schools or extra support within the child's local school.

Parents feel very differently about these experiences. Some consider mainstream school to be 'a hostile environment' (Sambrook, 1999), whereas another mother explains that 'how much safer is she surrounded by friends who have chosen to be with her, than pupils thrown together only because they are on the same continuum of language difficulty' (Simpson, 1999).

In my experience, children with specific speech and language impairment do well in the semi-segregated language unit environment. The child is educated within a class of children with similar problems, thus eliminating the stigma of their communication impairment in situations where they must use language, but enjoys some of the benefits of mainstream school life. For example, one child with severely unintelligible speech moved from another area, where he had been receiving support within mainstream school, to a language unit. For several months after he first joined the class of twelve speech and language-impaired peers, he was passive in all group activities and would not answer questions. One year on, he has made some progress with his speech and his confidence has increased considerably. He is now a lively contributor to class discussions and a popular member of the school. One must question his previous experiences of life in the mainstream that so knocked his confidence and alienated him from the learning environment of school.

Thus the forced inclusion of children with speech and language disorder into a group of normally speaking peers can have far reaching consequences. Those children may receive the support they require to overcome their difficulties in a physical sense, but may not recover from the emotional effects of stigma.

As adults we like to socialise with people we feel are like us, people with whom we feel we have something in common. Many of the adult subjects of the Communications Forum study found meeting people who have similar difficulties to be a liberating experience. For some of them, this sort of stigma-free encounter changed their lives in ways that therapy had failed to do.

The curability of speech and language impairment

Provided there are no additional maintaining or causal factors, such as physical disability or learning difficulties, many childhood speech and language impairments can be remediated completely.

Children who have more severe problems can overcome their difficulties, but some go on to lead disaffected lives. Everingham and Matson (1996) describe the feelings of low self-esteem in speech and language-impaired adolescents. The Language Development Project (Clegg, Hollis and Rutter, 1999) has followed a group of boys with specific language disorder since 1960. Many of their subjects have residual, subtle language difficulties and an increased incidence of psychiatric problems, unemployment and lack of independence than are found in a control group.

Adults with communication disorders caused by accident or illness make improvements but rarely regain their previous communicative function. In some cases the best that can be hoped for is adaptation by the individual and those in their community. Those with voice problems and other transient conditions can make a complete recovery. However, others may suffer with communication impairments such as a stammer throughout their lives. An important part of the therapy process is the acceptance of this.

As the severity of a person's communication impairment diminishes given appropriate treatment, so the stigma they face can also diminish. However, subtle problems can be concealed and communication breakdown be wrongly attributed to other causes.

Overcoming the stigma

How can individuals with communication impairment overcome the stigma of these difficulties when prejudice about the way that people speak is entrenched in our society? People with speech and language impairment do not have the necessary communication skills to speak up for themselves and try and redress this inequality. Often their problems are concealed, which has made it all the more difficult to raise the awareness of the public. In the past, the Royal College of Speech and Language Therapists has organised public awareness weeks. Television documentaries have been made about conditions giving rise to communication impairment, which seem to make inroads into public education. Yet both children and adults with communication impairment continue to be stigmatised. There is clearly much progress to be made.

In a practical sense, it is the little things that people do that will ultimately make the difference for the speech and language impaired. In healthcare environments, improvements in the quality of interaction with communication-impaired patients can be made by giving them more time, checking that they have understood and focusing on what is being communicated rather than how it is said. This may be easier said than done in a pressurised working environment. It is not time consuming, though, for healthcare practitioners to appreciate the existence of communication impairment and to ensure that those individuals experiencing this disability are not further handicapped by prejudice. Access to healthcare is by its very nature a stressful experience for the patient, especially for those more vulnerable members of our community. It is our duty to minimise this stress.

Health workers must take the lead in reducing the stigma faced by communication-impaired members of the community – after all, they frequently cannot speak up for themselves.

References

Bryan, K. and Forshaw, N. (1998) 'Crime and communication', *Royal College of Speech and Language Therapists Bulletin*, 559: 7–8.

Clegg, J., Hollis, C. and Rutter, M. (1999) 'Life sentence: what happens to children with developmental language disorders in later life?', *Royal College of Speech and Language Therapists Bulletin*, 571: 16–18.

Cohen, N.J., Davine, M., Hordezky, M.A. *et al.* (1993) 'Unsuspected language impairments in psychiatrically disturbed children: prevalence and language and behavioural characteristics', *Journal of the American Academy of Child and Adolescent Psychiatry*, 32: 595–603.

Communications Forum (1997) *Living with communication impairment*, London: Communications Forum. Available online (accessed December 1999) http://www.communicationsforum.org.uk/information/lwci.shtml.

Cross, M. (1997) 'Challenging behaviour or challenged comprehension', *Royal College of Speech and Language Therapists Bulletin*, 545: 11–12.

—— (1998) 'Undetected communication problems in children with behavioural problems', *International Journal Language and Communication Disorders*, 33, supplement: 509–14.

Everingham, C. and Matson, G. (1996) 'Addressing the problem of low self-esteem in speech and language impaired adolescents', in *Caring to Communicate. Proceedings of the Golden Jubilee Conference, York, October 1995*, London: Royal College of Speech and Language Therapists.

Giddan, J.J., Milling, L. and Campbell, N.B. (1996) 'Unrecognised language and speech deficits in preadolescent psychiatric inpatients', *American Jnl of Orthopsychiatry*, 66: 1.

Giles, H. and Powesland, P.F. (1975) *Speech style and social evaluation*, London: Academic Press.

Honey, J. (1989) *Does accent matter?*, London: Faber and Faber.

Johnson, S. (1994) *A review of communication therapy with young male offenders*, Internal report, Scottish Prison Service.

Menzies, J. (1999) *An investigation of attitudes to Scots and Glasgow dialect among secondary school pupils*. Available online (accessed 3 December 1999): http://www2.arts.gla.ac.uk/COMET/starn/lang/menzies/menzie1.htm.

Rice, M.L. (1993) ' "Don't talk to him. He's weird" A social consequences account of language and social interactions', in A. Kaiser and D. Gray (eds), *Enhancing children's communication. Research foundation for intervention*, vol. 2, Baltimore: Paul H. Brooks.

Royal College of Speech and Language Therapists (1996) *Communicating quality 2*, London: Royal College of Speech and Language Therapists.

—— (1997) 'News', *Royal College of Speech and Language Therapists Bulletin*, 547: 6.

Sambrook, T. (1999) 'Inclusion: "the hardest lesson of all" ', *Royal College of Speech and Language Therapists Bulletin*, 567: 7–8.

Seligman, C.R., Tucker, G.R. and Lambert, W.E. (1972) 'The effects of speech style and other attributes on teachers' attitudes toward pupils', *Language in Society* 1: 131–42.

Simpson, D. (1999) 'Clare among her peers', *Royal College of Speech and Language Therapists Bulletin*, 567: 9–10.

Wodack, R. (1996) *Disorders of discourse*, London: Addison, Wesley, Longman.

10 The stigma of 'sexuality'
Concealability and course

David Evans

...and God said, 'be fruitful, multiply, fill the earth and subdue it'
(Genesis 1:28)

And thus it was that the stigma of sexuality was born.

Introduction

From time immemorial, homo sapiens has tried to make sense of life and existence. Paglia (1990) says that religion was created for just such a purpose. However, as far as sexuality is concerned, many religions incline towards a cultural enthronement of patriarchal, monogamous, procreative and familiacentric heterosexuality that proves hostile to difference (Usher and Baker, 1993; Foucault, 1984). Such differences incur the full wrath of the institutions that have set themselves up as pillars of society, and its moral guardians.

These 'pillars' include religion, out of which came law, politics, and concepts of marriage and organised family. Other 'pillars' include established institutions of state: education, armed forces and healthcare – particularly medicine and psychiatry. The popular and intentional promotion of these 'pillars' is interpreted through various forms of media, which tend to perpetuate the publicly predominant views of sexuality. There is little more than titillation, suspicious curiosity, or even overt hatred, of all that is 'other'.

The narrowness of sex

Sex and sexualities have been regulated and codified through the belief systems of these institutions. Sex is typically spoken of as though its 'natural' and 'normal' expression is exclusively concerned with procreative acts and the 'reproductive' organs. In this narrow view of humanity, sexuality is a mere compartment of life, of dubious importance outside of procreative intercourse. The current British approach to teenage and unwanted pregnancies is a prime example. This is two-fold: keep children and young people ignorant of the full implications of the 'facts of life' (Callery, 1998; Graham, 1998), or be overly preoccupied with providing pre- and post-coital contraception. The latter falls short of seeing sexual health and disease prevention as being any wider than *family* planning (Douglas *et al.*, 1997; Evans, 2000a).

Sexuality as 'orthos' (straight)

Sexuality is frequently presumed to mean heterosexuality, or 'orthosexuality', i.e. 'straight'. Other orientations are hidden, unless specifically referred to. Attitudes of many of the world's religions towards sex and (hetero-) sexuality can be positive and affirming. Sadly, there are also instances of the opposite too. This is especially so when sex is non-procreative, or when sexuality is other than heterosexual. It is the influence of such negativity that forms, and perpetuates, the stigma of sexuality.

Origins of sexual stigma

In the Judeo-Christian Bibles, so influential in the formation of Western civilisation, there are numerous examples of stigma attached to being a woman, to menstrual blood and to the 'desires' of sexual union. Pain, seen as integral to childbirth, is described as punishment for wrongdoing (Genesis 3:13). In addition, an instance of *coitus interruptus* (the so-called withdrawal method) by a man called Onan (Genesis 38:9) is embellished through the ages to include reference to all forms of non-procreative sex, including masturbation. The Victorian era saw Onanism falsely accredited with physical, as well as psychiatric, maladies (Howe, 1995).

In this worldview, women have generally been treated as having rights unequal to those of men. Partly from this inequality came condemnation of men who were thought to be feminine (effeminate) (Gorman, 1999) or take on a woman's role in sex (Leviticus 18: 22). This condemnation even occurred when the man had no choice in the matter, such as after having been raped by conquering soldiers in an act of utter brutality and humiliation (Donaldson, 1990). There are also biblical references to sex with animals, sacred and profane prostitution, pre-marital conception, extra-marital relations and infertility. As far as sex is concerned, there is nothing new under the sun.

Thus the stigmatisation of sex was created. Sadly, at the dawn of a new millennium, the origins of stigmatisation continue to be as deeply rooted in the very fabric of society as they have ever been.

Normal and natural

Sex and sexuality, devoid of stigma, tend to be seen in terms of being normal, natural, healthy, good, clean, wholesome and beautiful. Indeed, the celebration of such is regularly announced in the Births and Marriages columns of many newspapers. Yet it is the opposite that regularly inherits the marks and effects of stigma. As Jones *et al.* (1984) say, 'in an unthinking equation, it is apparent people believe that what is beautiful is good and what is ugly is bad'. Such ugliness can be internalised and intermingled with shame, so that the individual is never alone from the affects of stigmatisation, especially if the stigma commenced during early childhood years. It may then be carried throughout life, affecting people in different ways.

Goffman's seminal work *Stigma: notes on the management of spoiled identity* (1963, reprinted 1990) tends to refer to two major groups of people: the 'normals' and the 'stigmatised'. Jones *et al.* (1984) refer to 'markers' and the 'marked'. Although many authors on stigma do not address its relation to sex and sexualities, they do give examples of stigma's application to marked or stigmatised individuals.

Concealability and course

Jones *et al.* (1984) remark how stigmas may be concealed from public view, especially in early contact with 'marked' individuals. The process the stigma then follows is referred to as its 'course'.

The origins of a stigma may determine the response to it. If the source is outside of one's control, then appellations of 'innocent' or 'victim' are easily applied (Sontag, 1991). However, acquisition of certain stigmas may be treated as though the recipient has a choice. Choosing to accept the stigma is then perceived as a sign of (moral) weakness.

From badness to madness

Attitudes to sexual stigmas, pre- and post-Enlightenment, move from sinful or bad to mad (Davenport-Hines, 1990). For people who failed to repent of alleged immorality, or be adequately exorcised, religion was happy to use sadistic forms of torture, repression and execution (Dynes, 1990a). Examples of these practices happening in the year 2000, including execution for being gay, lesbian, bisexual or transgendered, are being investigated by Amnesty International (Bogues, 2000).

Psychiatry took over where religion's temporal power ended; just as where religion condemned, psychiatry pathologised. Psychiatry resorted to incarceration and techniques such as aversion 'therapy' more akin to a session with the Marquis de Sade than a healing treatment with a healing physician. Both psychiatry and psychoanalysis share an integral history, trying to 'cure' people of sexual diversity, or what they might call perversity (Lewes, 1989; Isay, 1993). Even as late as the twentieth century, the UK and Ireland used incarceration for people attributed with certain sexual stigmas. Such 'stigmas' include unmarried motherhood, consensual sexual 'crimes' and commercial sex work (Ferris, 1993; Thompson, 1994; Bloch, 1996). Stigma and sexuality continue to be intimate companions.

Altering the course

Stigma's course is not always linear, concealed at one point and revealed at another. Altering the course of a stigma may take place within individuals or society. Societal acceptance is evidence of a society comfortable with itself and unafraid of difference. Conversely, the more society enforces compliance of rigid identity, to that extent, diversity is stigmatised.

For stigmas of moral origin, the morals are usually from outside the person (Grey, 1993), and may be imposed upon the individual who chooses to conform or rebel. Moral condemnation can be internalised by individuals, leading to feelings of self-loathing and disgust (Goffman, 1990). Evidence shows that poor self-concept may predispose to risk-taking behaviours, which are detrimental to health, and may even lead to suicide (King, 1993; Kippax *et al.*, 1993; O'Hanlan *et al.*, 1997). Hatred of the stigma may also be turned outside of the self, such as punishments meted out to others possessing the same stigma. This may be seen in cases of 'puritanical' attitudes to sex, and homophobic bullying or 'queer bashing' in people rebelling against (homo-) erotic feelings within themselves (Meyer and Dean, 1998).

Stigma's course as disruptive

Disruptiveness is often related to the visibility of the mark and its affect on intra- and inter-personal relations. Take, for example, a physical blemish such as a birthmark, or a disabling characteristic. Pertinent questions include: how does the individual actually feel about the stigma? How does it enable or disable their relations with others? How much of a part does it play in affecting the expression of their sexual persona?

Advertising media campaigns routinely use 'beautiful', young, slim, white, financially viable, able-bodied and emotionally stable heterosexual models to sell products. The sheer invisibility of all other people, on grounds of not possessing these characteristics, can be an added burden for an individual in relating to others.

Conversely, before an encounter with a different (that is, a stigmatised) person, the more desensitisation that takes place the higher the chance that the perceived stigma will be diminished. For example, the total invisibility of public images of people with physical or learning disabilities having sex generally leads to the assumption that they are asexual (Adams, 2000). Exposure to images of sex involving people with disabilities frequently reveals attitudes of disgust or disapproval. However, this may be the first

step in raising awareness that people with disabilities are sexual. This reve-
lation can then be utilised to lessen the societal effects of negativity
towards the stigma (Graham, 1998).

The role of healthcare professionals in contributing to the stigmatising process

The primary contribution healthcare professionals (HCPs) make towards
stigma, and perpetuating its effects, stems from the fact that each HCP is a
member of a society, class, ethnic, culture and sometimes religious group,
which itself is frequently stigmatising. Just because a person dons a stetho-
scope and uses clinical jargon does not *de facto* render them
non-judgemental and accepting of sexual diversity.

Nursing (James *et al.*, 1994), medicine (Rose, 1994), psychotherapy
(Davies and Neal, 1997; Lewes, 1989) and psychiatry (McFarlane, 1998)
have all contributed to sexual stigmatisation. The education systems of the
caring professions have had a role to play, too (McHaffie, 1993; Evans,
1997; Crouch, 2000a). Here there is a general invisibility of issues of sex,
sexualities and sexual health, other than the mechanics of reproduction and
contraception, the pathologies of infertility and reproductive dysfunction,
or the treatment of sexual diversity as forensic perversion (ENB, 1999).

Not conforming to designated 'norms' frequently attracts characteristics
of stigma used as a punishing treatment of the individuals concerned.
Negative treatment imputes blame onto the individual (Jones *et al.*, 1984),
often seen as no more than they deserve because of the way they have
'chosen' to live. Blame may be overt, manifest in poor or unequal treatment
or in neglect and utter hostility. Such examples constitute a dereliction in
the duty to care, and in the right of respect of each individual client.

Blame may be evidenced in the way in which some are regarded as
innocent, deserving optimum treatment, while stigmatised individuals are
denied equal care (Sontag, 1991). The following contradictory remarks,
upon which attitudes to care may be based, are good examples: 'the causes
of certain conditions (e.g. syphilis) are associated with reprehensible
comportment and a squalid lifestyle' (Jones *et al.*, 1984). Compare with
Berkowitz and Callen (1983), who state that 'sex doesn't make you sick:
diseases do'.

The cultural enthronement of a particular expression of sex and sexuality essentially negates all that is contrary by rendering associated
healthcare needs invisible, and by perpetuating an unscientific hostility for
pathologising difference (Bloor, 1995).

The -isms and the phobias

The predominant ways HCPs contribute to the stigmatisation of sexuality
may be sub-divided under the following headings: sexism, heterosexism,

homophobia, biphobia and erotophobia. The use of the suffix -*phobia*, in many of these cases, is misleading, as they are more akin to the hatred of misogyny and racism than the phobic states defined by psychiatry (Evans, 1997). Limited examples will be given under each heading, although the list seems to be unending!

Sexism

Sexism is the imposition of power and rights of one sex (gender) over another. This is traditionally experienced with the imbalance of power relations and opportunities in life of male over female. Gynæphobia (fear of women) is quite different to sexist hostility towards women, misogyny, a term partly drawn from the Greek root verb 'to hate'. Many women have justifiable reason to complain of institutionalised inequalities. These traditionally refuse to see women with individual, unalienable rights, devoid of a dependant relationship on a man, or in relation to the continuation of the species.

In the world of healthcare, however, sexism can sometimes be inverted from that in society at large, with men's healthcare needs not always being as equally high profiled as women's. Male cancers, dangerous male-image ('macho') lifestyles, and a four-times higher suicide rate in men than women mean that men have health deficits which are inadequately addressed (Lloyd, 1996).

Also, as we have said, stigma around sexuality routinely attends people with physical and psychological disabilities (Grant and Roberts, 1998; Aylott, 1999). It is also particularly related to age, both young and old (Callery, 1998; Crouch, 2000b). Being discriminated against on grounds of more than one stigmatising attribute is a form of multi-oppression.

Heterosexism

Heterosexism is 'the unwarrantable social domination of heterosexuality over homosexuality and other minority sexual preferences' (Grey, 1993). This elevates unparalleled benefits in favour of patriarchal, reproductive, heterosexuality, while at the same time denying equality of rights and opportunities to all others.

Examples in healthcare begin with terminology and practices that presume all people are heterosexual. From this, provision of service is directed towards heterosexual (and reproductive) needs, with the denial of equal resources to sexually stigmatised people. A prime case is found in public, media and legal attitudes towards *in vitro* fertilisation and parental rights for lesbians (Alldred, 1998).

Homophobia

'Homophobia is a misnomer for hostility and hatred towards that which is perceived as a homosexual nature' (Evans, 1997). It is a misnomer in that the suffix -phobia belittles the reality of the abhorrence, and sometimes organised violence and annihilation, which same-sex sexual unions have had to suffer. Homophobia is institutionalised in healthcare when there is direct antagonism and discrimination against gay, lesbian and bisexual people. It is also institutionalised when their very existence, and clinical needs, are negated.

Homophobia is internalised by individuals to the extent that they turn the socialising processes of hostility towards themselves and others like them (Meyer and Dean, 1998).

With lesbians, homophobia takes a different slant (Kitzinger, 1989). Rather than the direct hostility meted out to gay, bisexual and other men-who-have-sex-with-men, it frequently takes the form of complete invisibility of clinical needs. Lesbians who never become pregnant are at higher risk of cancers related to nulliparity, yet the campaigns that address this are few and far between.

Lesbians and gay men are at higher risk of bullying, internalised oppression and reliance on substance excess like drugs and alcohol (Douglas *et al.*, 1997; Lock and Steiner, 1999). Gay men, and in particular the sub-population who are HIV positive, are at an even higher risk of suicide (O'Hanlan *et al.*, 1997).

Biphobia

This relatively new word points towards the fear – or, again, the hatred – of bisexual people (Dynes, 1990b; Davies, 1997). The marker is predominantly the heterosexual male (Kite and Whitley, 1998). Biphobia has different outcomes, dependant on whether it is directed towards males or females, and whether it originates from the heterosexual or gay and lesbian communities (McFarlane, 1998).

The stigma of sexuality and self-hatred

All of the above mentioned forms of stigmatisation, as well as ageism and disablism, can lead to mental illness such as internalised oppression and self-hatred, which in turn can include self-loathing and low self-esteem (Kowszun and Malley, 1997). People with low self-esteem are particularly at risk from unsafe sex and unsafe drug or alcohol use. Reasons include: (a) insufficient regard for themselves; (b) fear of rejection; and (c) craving for any form of love and affection from others.

The picture outlined in this chapter may appear somewhat bleaker than many people's experience would suggest. Yet evidence from authors referenced here shows ample sign of societal and personal stigma around the sexual aspects of life being detrimental to healthcare. With such a state of affairs, the question must be asked: what can be done to overcome stigma?

Overcoming stigma in the healthcare setting

A saying made popular by Britain's Prime Minister, Tony Blair, is 'Education! Education! Education!' Applying this motto to combat the stigma of sexuality in healthcare requires clinical practice based on Evaluative, Enlightening and Equality-enhancing education. Change in the clinical arena cannot take place without it being informed by learning, through research and evidence-based practice, which highlights the wholly discriminatory attitudes and behaviours surrounding the stigmas of sexuality, and ways to overcome them.

Evaluative education

'Reflection', 'critical analysis', 'evidence-based practice' and 'clinical governance': these are all popular healthcare terms. They aim to improve the services caregivers provide by constantly challenging received knowledge, and highlighting ways to improve or enhance it. Managers, clinical supervisors, counsellors, mentors, assessors and educational facilitators are equally part of this process.

Evaluation of current service provision will also show how accentuating stigmas, and perpetuating them, can have profoundly negative effects on the stigmatised, leading to detrimental mental health issues (McFarlane, 1998; Aylott, 1999). Evaluation, or audit, will show how early detection and desensitisation of stigmas to a wider audience, e.g. within a hospital setting, will ultimately be more cost-effective than dealing with the consequences. For example, health information campaigns using stereotypical images of 'beautiful' healthy models could also use alternative images. Inclusion, rather than exclusion, can have profound affects on those who are stigmatised, and on their psychological well-being.

Evaluation of learning, both in current clinical practice and for the future, highlights the need for more choice of services for individual clients suffering the affects of stigma. Such specialist or needs-focused services are required to be of a standard and quality comparable to 'mainstream' services, and to be offered as an alternative to them, allowing consumer choice. Specialist services should in no way be seen as letting mainstream services carry on with their traditional forms of stigmatisation; specialist services can act as a benchmark for quality control, and a resource of excellence.

Enlightening education

Education that is enlightening is integral to challenging and overcoming the negative effects of sexualities' stigmas. Education does not simply mean putting on an awareness course, or an anti-discrimination session. It includes personal analytical reflection on practice to improve care delivery (Crouch, 2000b). It means auditing the needs of stigmatised people: staff and service users, identifiable groups and individuals.

Areas where stigma is perpetuated, and in need of urgent challenge are shown in Table 10.1 opposite.

Sexual health resources must be equally accessible to all – the good, the bad and the aesthetically challenged – as well as to non-reproductive people. People in some of these groups are routinely missed in preventative screening programmes that are often aimed at the young, able-bodied, intelligent and more familiacentric women with children (Weston, 1994; Evans, 2000b).

Enlightening education, such as reflection on practice, will also help in the desensitisation of stigmas, challenge inappropriate attitudes and behaviours and replace them with effectively therapeutic positive images. Such campaigns target groups based on clinical need, not because they are society's majority.

Finally, there is a need for more 'talk therapies', which try to help individuals overcome the harmful effects of being stigmatised. These include forms of redress for people who have been neglected and abused by the healthcare system.

Equalising education

Combating stigma through this model requires the process and outcomes of the education to inform policies of equality. This equality is for opportunities, rights and privileges, including the celebration of difference. It is also for a quality of service relationship and provision. In this scheme of equality there is no room for discrimination. A prime example of discrimination is the way people with disabilities have their rights to partnership, sex and procreation regularly taken away from them by a paternalistic system which presumes to operate in the client's best interests.

Education and practice that pay regard to difference and the harmful effects of stigma will also aim to remove all vestiges of discrimination. This will include a re-evaluation of the ways in which healthcare has traditionally favoured the majority in society, and actively discouraged or discriminated against those who are stigmatised. Relevant issues include guaranteeing personal safety, free from discrimination by staff and other service users; lobbying for legislation to protect against discrimination on grounds of sexual difference, e.g. (dis-)ability or orientation; and measures to tackle bullying on the same level as racism.

Table 10.1 Stigma in healthcare: identifying and challenging

Identifying and correcting stigma in healthcare	
Lack of safer sex education, skills and resources for sexually active young people (especially those with differing needs and under the unequal ages of consent).	Address clinical need, not preconceived assumptions about who should or should not be sexually active.
Lack of sex and sexuality awareness for stigmatised people, especially those with physical or learning disabilities.	Encourage multi-professional awareness and protocols for facilitating wholeness of being, including sexual self.
Failure to take the sexual health implications of stigma seriously when addressing other healthcare needs, e.g. body (image) surgery or debilitating illness.	Incorporate equally relevant information, services, counselling etc., to address sexual health worries, concerns and adaption to changed sexual persona.
Reluctance of many lesbians to use GP services, due to heterosexist environment.	Awareness training for all staff, addressing needs of people from sexual minorities.
Reluctance of many gay men to use GP services, due to sexual orientation being used to discriminate against them for insurance and mortgages.	Challenge government and insurance industry that require doctors to break confidence and discriminate on grounds of gender and orientation.
Inequalities in the Mental Health Act, such as legal rights for next-of-kin (marriage, or six months co-habiting for heterosexual partners, five years for same-sex couples).	Challenge government for instigating inequality and discrimination; encourage service providers to incorporate policies of equality without discrimination.

Stigmatising and excluding	*Non-stigmatising and inclusive*
Documentation using sexist and heterosexist language, e.g. presuming a partner is of the opposite sex and the relationship is marriage.	Using terms like 'partner', and allowing the client to define the gender and relationship.
Presuming that unmarried people 'naturally' want to get married (i.e. that being single isn't a chosen option).	Define clinical provision in line with need, e.g. cervical screening for women who have not been pregnant: including disabled, lesbian and celibate women.
Stereotyping problems with sexual imagery, e.g. that commercial sex workers are 'carriers of disease', and that gay men with bowel problems have caused it through anal sex.	Demythologise the causes of sexual/sexual health problems: see the whole person, not just sex acts.
Attributing mental health problems to sexual stigma, or orientation, and therefore not addressing the real problems.	Treat stigma and mental health issues openly and seriously.

Making the model work

Certain criteria are essential for this model to work. They include addressing the sex issues of life positively, appropriately and commensurately; therapeutically challenging the stigmas with clinical expertise and knowledge, and proficiently applying practical skills to deal with others. Without these criteria, the 'markers' will go on marking (stigmatising), and those suffering the negative affects of stigmas will have been denied an opportunity for healing, growth and development from the very professions committed to holistic care and therapy.

Conclusion

This chapter has explored the aspects of concealability and course of stigma, described by Jones *et al.* (1984) in specific relation to sexuality. The exploration highlighted instances where this stigma is particularly relevant to the world of healthcare and healthcare professionals. Examination of these issues was brief, and by no means exhaustive. The reader is encouraged to explore matters further, in relation to their own clinical life and practice.

Finally, the chapter proposed a model that can be adapted and used to fit many situations where stigma negatively affects the therapeutic encounter. It is hoped that this brief chapter is a springboard for further work in overcoming the stigmas of sexualities.

References

Note bene All biblical references are taken from *The Jerusalem Bible* (1984) Standard Edition, London: Darton, Longman and Todd.

Adams, J. (2000) 'Sex and politics', in H. Wilson and S. McAndrew, *Sexual health – foundations for practice*, London: Baillière Tindall.
Alldred, P. (1998) 'Making a mockery of family life? Lesbian mothers in the British media', in G. Dunne (ed.), *Living difference: lesbian perspectives on work and family life*, New York: Harrington Park Press.
Aylott, G. (1999) 'Is the sexuality of people with a learning disability being denied?', *British Journal of Nursing*, 8, 7: 438–42.
Berkowitz, R. and Callen, C. (1983) *How to have sex in an epidemic: one approach*, New York: News From The Front Publications.
Bloch, I. (1996) *Sexual life in England past and present*, Hertfordshire: Oracle Publishing.
Bloor, M. (1995) *The sociology of HIV transmission*, London: Sage.
Bogues, M. (2000) 'Saudi Arabia reportedly executes six men for sodomy', http://www.ilga.org./~/nine_saudi_arabian_national_are.htm (28 July 2000).
Callery, P. (1998) 'Sex and children in the past and the present', in T. Harrison (ed.), *Children and sexuality – perspectives in healthcare*, London: Baillière Tindall.

Crouch, S. (2000a) 'Sexual health 1: sexuality and nurses' role in sexual health', *British Journal of Nursing*, 8, 9: 601–6.

—— (2000b) 'Sexual health 2: an overt approach to sexual health education', *British Journal of Nursing*, 8, 10: 669–75.

Davenport-Hines, R. (1990) *Sex, death and punishment – attitudes to sex and sexuality in Britain since the Renaissance*, London: Fontana.

Davies, D. (1997) 'Working with people coming out', in D. Davies and C. Neal (eds), *Pink therapy: a guide for counsellors and therapists working with lesbian, gay and bisexual clients*, Buckingham and Philadelphia: Open University Press.

Davies, D. and Neal, C. (eds) (1997) *Pink therapy: a guide for counsellors and therapists working with lesbian, gay and bisexual clients*, Buckingham and Philadelphia: Open University Press.

Donaldson, S. (1990) 'Rape of males', in W.R. Dynes, *Encyclopedia of Homosexuality*, Chicago and London: St James Press.

Douglas, N., Warwick, I., Kemp, S. and Whitty, G. (1997) *Playing it safe: responses of secondary school teachers to lesbian, gay and bisexual pupils, bullying, HIV and AIDS education, and Section 28*, University of London: Institute of Education.

Dynes, W.R. (1990a) 'Buggery', in: W.R. Dynes (ed.), *Encyclopedia of homosexuality*, vols 1 and 2, Chicago and London: St James Press.

—— (1990b) 'Bisexuality', in W.R. Dynes (ed.), *Encyclopedia of homosexuality*, vols 1 and 2, Chicago and London: St James Press.

ENB (1999) *Post-registration studies programmes – list of institutions with approval to conduct the programmes*, circular, London: English National Board for Nursing, Midwifery and Health Visiting.

Evans, D.T. (1997) *The psychic shadows of HIV and AIDS: and the role of social representations in post registration nurse education*, University of Wales: MPhil Thesis (unpublished).

—— (2000a) 'Speaking of sex: the need to dispel myths and overcome fears', *British Journal of Nursing*, 10, 9: 650–5.

—— (2000b) 'Sexual health the process: primary care', in H. Wilson and S. McAndrew, *Sexual health: foundations for practice*, London: Baillière Tindall.

Ferris, P. (1993) *Sex and the British – a twentieth century history*, London: Michael Joseph.

Foucault, M. (1984) *The history of sexuality*, vol. 1, London: Penguin.

Goffman, E. (1990) *Stigma: notes on the management of spoiled identity*, London: Penguin Books.

Gorman, M.R. (1999) 'Male homosexual desire', in R.A. Nye (ed.), *Sexuality*, Oxford: Oxford University Press.

Graham, G. (1998) 'Promoting young people's sexual health', in T. Harrison (ed.), *Children and sexuality – perspectives in health care*, London: Baillière Tindall.

Grant, J.M. and Roberts, J. (1998) 'Psychological development: sex and sexuality in adolescence', in T. Harrison (ed.), *Children and sexuality – perspectives in healthcare*, London: Baillière Tindall.

Grey, A. (1993) *Speaking of sex: the limits of language*, London: Cassell.

Howe, J. (1995) 'A natural remedy: giving patients permission to masturbate', *Nursing Standard*, 9, 29: 46–7.

Isay, R. (1993) *Being homosexual: gay men and their development*, London: Penguin.

James, T., Harding, I. and Corbett, K. (1994) 'Biased care? Lesbians and gay men', *Nursing Times*, 90, 51: 29–31.

Jones, E.E., Farina, A., Hastorf, A.H. *et al.* (1984) *Social stigma: the psychology of marked relationships*, New York: W.H. Freeman.

King, E. (1993) *Safety in numbers – safer sex for gay men*, London: Cassell.

Kippax, S., Connell, R.W., Dowsett, G.W. and Crawford, J. (1993) 'Sustaining safer sex: gay communities respond to AIDS', *Social Aspects of AIDS Series*, London: The Falmer Press.

Kite, M.E. and Whitley, B.E. Jr (1998) 'Do heterosexual women and men differ in their attitudes toward homosexuality?', in G.M. Herek (ed.), *Stigma and sexual orientation – understanding prejudice against lesbians, gay men and bisexuals*, London: Sage.

Kitzinger, C. (1989) *The social construction of lesbianism*, London: Sage.

Kowszun, G. and Malley, M. (1997) 'Alcohol and substance misuse', in D. Davies and C. Neal (eds), *Pink therapy: a guide for counsellors and therapists working with lesbian, gay and bisexual clients*, Buckingham and Philadelphia: Open University Press.

Lewes, K. (1989) *The psychoanalytic theory of male homosexuality*, London and New York: Quartet.

Lloyd, T. (1996) *RCN men's health review*, London: Royal College of Nursing.

Lock, J. and Steiner, H. (1999) 'Relationships between sexual orientation and coping styles of gay, lesbian, and bisexual adolescents from a community high school', *Journal of the Gay and Lesbian Medical Association*, 3, 3: 77–82.

McFarlane, L. (1998) *Diagnosis: homophobic – the experiences of lesbians, gay men and bisexuals in mental health services*, London: P.A.C.E.

McHaffie, H.E. (1993) *The care of patients with HIV and AIDS: a survey of nurse education in the UK*, Edinburgh: Institute of Medical Ethics, Department of Medicine, University of Edinburgh.

Meyer, I.H. and Dean, L. (1998) 'Internalized homophobia, intimacy and sexual behaviour among gay and bisexual men', in G.M. Herek (ed.), *Stigma and sexual orientation – understanding prejudice against lesbians, gay men and bisexuals*, London: Sage.

O'Hanlan, K.O., Cabaj, R.P., Schatz, B. *et al.* (1997) 'A review of the medical consequences of homophobia with suggestions for resolution', *Journal of the Gay and Lesbian Medical Association*, 1, 1: 25–40.

Paglia, C. (1990) *Sexual personae: art and decadence from Nefertiti to Emily Dickinson*, London and New Haven: Yale University Press.

Rose, L. (1994) 'Homophobia among doctors', *British Medical Journal*, 308, 26: 586–7.

Sontag, S. (1991) *Illness as metaphor: AIDS and its metaphors*, London: Penguin.

Thompson, B. (1994) *Sadomasochism – painful perversion or pleasurable play?*, London: Cassell.

Usher, J.M. and Baker, C.D. (eds) (1993) *Psychological perspectives on sexual problems – new directions in theory and practice*, London: Routledge.

Weston, A. (1994) *Sapphic sickness: a study of the healthcare experiences of women patients who disclose their sexual identity as lesbian*, Brunel University: MSc Dissertation (unpublished).

11 HIV and AIDS

Caroline Carlisle

Introduction

> They [neighbours] came last night and smashed all the front windows.
> I don't know how they found out about it [HIV status] and now my
> daughter is suffering too. I'm too terrified to go out, I really don't
> know how much longer I can carry on...
>
> (Val, March 1986)

> I feel as if I'm at the edge of a cliff ... I want to be able to hang on but
> I don't think I'm strong enough to go on fighting. If they [brother and
> family] walk out on me again ... well, what's the point. I just can't
> promise you I won't harm myself again...
>
> (Jane, October 1999)

Over a decade spans the statements of the two HIV-positive women above
which I have taken from my patient case notes. I am often asked if attitudes have changed towards people affected by HIV and AIDS over the
years due to increased knowledge and awareness, and I am sure in many
respects there have been improvements in our understanding and consequently in the ways in which HIV-positive people are viewed. But the field
of my clinical practice means that I see only those individuals who are not
coping, who are emotionally damaged by HIV and who often suffer the
effects of stigma. It is unfortunate that my caseload has not lessened over
the years and that the problems of prejudice and stigmatising attitudes
remain. Although society now has greater information and understanding
of the transmission and effects of HIV, the problem of prejudice still exists,
and Goffman warns that 'familiarity need not reduce contempt' (Goffman,
1963: 70). Indeed, recent research still identifies the ways in which society
can reject the need for services for those with AIDS and that the NIMBY
(Not In My Backyard) syndrome still exists (Takahashi, 1997).

This chapter provides the reader with an insight into the ways in
which people affected by HIV and AIDS are affected by stigma and social

exclusion, and suggests ways that health professionals could deliver sensitive and supportive healthcare.

HIV and AIDS

The year 1981 has been identified retrospectively as the time when the first reports of a new set of symptoms, one that was eventually to be called Acquired Immunodeficiency Syndrome (AIDS), appeared in North America (Powell, 1996). Incidents of a rare form of pneumonia, *pneumocystis carinii* pneumonia (PCP), and an equally rare form of cancer, Kaposi's sarcoma (KS), were documented in young homosexual men. These men were also immunodeficient. By 1983, the virus now known to lead to AIDS was isolated. This virus was given various names, but the internationally accepted term today is the human immunodeficiency virus (HIV).

The majority of people who are exposed to HIV and become infected can be asymptomatic for a number of years due to the long incubation period of the virus.

During this asymptomatic period, antibodies to HIV are developed, sometimes up to six months after infection (Powell, 1996), but these antibodies do not prevent progression of the disease process. The infected individual is also potentially infectious to others, both prior to the development of antibodies and when antibody-positive. Although asymptomatic, a test to detect these antibodies can be carried out.

In HIV infection the body's normal reaction to infection is inhibited and the subsequent effect on the body can be wide ranging. Most of the physical symptoms which can eventually develop are the indirect result of damage to the immune system by HIV. Some of these physical symptoms are obvious to the person infected but not necessarily to other people. Initial symptoms can include persistent generalised lymphadenopathy, fevers and night sweats. Opportunistic infections can present in such forms as herpes zoster and oral candidiasis. The range of potential infective organisms is wide and can affect many body systems, causing gastro-intestinal, central nervous, renal and dermatologic manifestations. The incidence of later opportunistic infections can vary according to geography, PCP being common in the industrialised world but less so in Africa, where tuberculosis is the most common opportunistic problem (Lucas *et al.*, 1993). In addition, HIV can have direct effects upon the body; for example, the effect on brain cells can lead to HIV encephalopathy. Brain function can then be impaired to various degrees, ranging from lack of concentration to personality changes and disorder of motor function. KS remains an important complication of HIV infection (Beiser, 1997) and presents as dark, purplish or brown lesions which can be located on the face, arms, legs or in the mouth. KS lesions can also involve visceral organs such as the lungs, liver and gastro-intestinal tract, and can lead to signs and symptoms dependent on the site of the lesion, such as obstructions, enteropathies, and pulmonary involvement such as cough and dyspnoea (Ungvarski and Staats, 1995). Later signs and symptoms such as KS can be very obvious to other people, and even if the person infected should wish to hide their diagnosis, this may well be impossible.

The past few years have seen a growing optimism with regard to the prognosis of people living with HIV, and a growing number remain not only free of AIDS but are also asymptomatic (Rutherford, 1994). Much of the optimism rests on the increasing confidence in the use of combination antiretroviral drug therapy. Triple combination therapy as a first-line treatment for all people with HIV is now practised in many centres, and there is a belief that this approach should be the standard of care for HIV drug therapy in infected people (De Cock, 1997). The fact remains, however, that as yet there is no cure for AIDS and prospects for a cure remain uncertain (Cohn, 1997). This uncertainty remains a strong influence on the way in which HIV and AIDS impact psychologically on those people who are infected and affected. The lack of a cure also affects the way in which the virus is viewed by society. The fear which can be engendered by diseases for which there is no cure or which lead inexorably to death can create emotional and behavioural reactions which are not always rational in origin (Sontag, 1991). Discrimination is one such reaction which faces people affected by HIV, and stigmatising societal responses are the product of complex beliefs, many of which are rooted in views around sexuality and sexually shared infections.

The stigma of HIV and AIDS

HIV can affect all individuals regardless of gender, sexual orientation, age or race, and does not solely affect the homosexual population among whom the virus was originally identified (Fan *et al.*, 1994). The fact that the early history of HIV and AIDS was closely associated with already discriminated-against groups within society, homosexual men and drug users, led to a societal response which was based on judgemental attitudes and further discrimination (Pollak, 1992). This societal response has been tenacious even in the face of intense educational campaigns and growing awareness of the nature and spread of the virus. The tendency to view HIV and AIDS as something which happens to other people, and particularly to people who are 'different' either in their behaviour or their sexual orientation, can lead to a stigmatising response by society.

Death, although no longer the taboo it was in the past, still retains fear for many people in industrial societies (Marris, 1996). AIDS confronts the non-infected with the reality of death, and so they are reminded about their own mortality; this challenge engenders a distancing–stigmatising response. Stereotyping also highlights prevailing societal prejudices, and greatest prejudice is shown towards persons suffering from an infectious illness that primarily affects marginal persons (Dukes and Denny, 1995).

The means of contracting HIV, the spread of the disease and the media portrayal of it as affecting marginal groups leads to an infected person facing stigma in more than one way. The double stigma experienced by infected gay men – being HIV positive and being gay – is also experienced by others who are part of a marginal group, for example drug users and sex workers. Of course, simply being HIV-positive can lead others to assume one has other associated stigmatising traits: the assumption that an HIV-positive man must also be gay.

Sociologists have also highlighted societal responses which have led to the search for scapegoats and thus distinctions to be drawn between the 'innocent' and the 'guilty' (Paicheler, 1992), the latter being those people infected by virtue of their own sexual or drug related behaviour rather than 'innocently' by such means as infected blood products or blood transfusion. 'Innocent victims' can also experience stigma, however, due to biophysical changes in the HIV disease trajectory (Alonzo and Reynolds, 1995). Hence the fact of being unable to hide the effects of late-stage HIV disease, e.g. KS lesions, can in itself produce a stigmatising response from others.

It follows that issues of 'concealability' and trajectory or 'course' are important considerations in relation to the potential for social exclusion of people affected by HIV and AIDS.

Concealability and course of HIV and AIDS

Viral infections are not visible; only the manifestations of the effect of the virus on the body can be seen by others. There is now evidence that an individual may remain free of AIDS twenty-five years after the initial infection (Rutherford, 1994). This lengthy asymptomatic period is one where the virus can be transmitted to others through such means as sexual activity and shared 'works' in drug use. This concealed nature of HIV infection is of basic importance when considering society's reaction to those infected. Nowhere is this more evident than in the requirement to reveal HIV status, or to be tested for presence of the virus, in certain circumstances such as life insurance or travel. The fact that a negative result of an HIV test does not guarantee that an individual is free of disease has not changed the insistence that certain people are required to be tested or to reveal that they have been tested.

People infected by HIV conceal for two main reasons: to hide their positive status; and to keep secret the means by which they became infected. In his explanation of stigma, Goffman (1963) calls this need to appear normal as 'passing'. The need to 'pass' as normal is taken on board at an early stage by the positive person, and part of pre- and post-HIV test counselling involves an exploration of who the individual may wish to tell about the test and the possible consequences of revealing that one has tested positive or negative. From the point of diagnosis, therefore, a positive person is aware of the difficulties and potential for judgement and rejection because of HIV status. Although there are a variety of diseases which are stigmatising, it is important to distinguish the case of someone stigmatised for a purely physical trait such as facial disfigurement from that when the stigma actually brings with it judgements which are related to a stereotype. It is suggested that people 'tend to impute a wide range of imperfections on the basis of the original one' (Goffman, 1963: 16). So the HIV positive person may be stigmatised not solely for being positive, but also for suppositions regarding their sexual lifestyle, sexual orientation, and other stigmatising characteristics such as drug use. The most obvious example is the already-mentioned one of assuming that someone who is HIV-positive is gay. This can of course work in reverse; disclosing the fact that one is gay may bring with it judgements from others on the strong possibility that one is also HIV-positive and indeed sexually promiscuous.

It has been noted that the tactic of concealing a positive status is not an entirely adequate strategy for avoiding the pain of illness-related stigmas (Alonzo and Reynolds, 1995). Fear of discovery can be high and, even although HIV status is concealed, the very act of this concealment can lead to restricted social interaction and be a barrier to the development of intimate relationships.

Although HIV-positive people can gain much support and care if they choose to reveal their status, the fear of judgement and rejection by others means that the issue of concealment is an important one. The stigma associated with HIV and AIDS can have the effect of polarising individuals within families into those who will accept the positive person and those who will reject them (Powell-Cope and Brown, 1992). It is also important to note that partners or family members who care for a positive person may themselves experience the same effects of the stigma. This 'courtesy stigma' (Goffman, 1963) can result in further isolation of the family affected by HIV and AIDS, thus limiting their support networks when both emotional and physical help is needed. This situation is further compounded when a positive person begins to redefine themselves in ways which arise from society's image of them, and so view themselves from the other's perspective and apply a negative evaluation to their situation (Alonzo and Reynolds, 1995).

Current partners, who may be the main source of physical and emotional support to the HIV-positive person, can be adversely affected in a number of other ways. When someone shares the diagnosis of HIV or AIDS, a partner may begin to question the person's sexual fidelity, develop worries regarding their own HIV status, and become fearful of a future which may require them to care for someone who is ill and who may die. This can place a great strain on the relationship. Partners will also have to consider whether they need to 'keep a secret' and to whom they may look for support without experiencing 'courtesy stigma'.

It can be seen, therefore, that there are a number of forms of judgement in place. These can be viewed as enacted stigma, e.g. being deliberately

ignored by family members, and felt stigma, e.g. the feelings of abandonment and isolation related to the enacted stigma. This sense of being
judged can also involve aspects of self-judgement, in that a person can
view him or herself as being deserving of some form of judgement or rejection by others. The moral overtones in this situation, where the
self-fulfilling prophecy of labelling someone as deviant can mean that the
person begins to view him or herself in a different and judgemental light
(Becker, 1963), are important when considering the psychological and
emotional health of a positive person. It should also be noted that the
loneliness and lack of social support is an additional factor which can
result in instances of parasuicide and successful suicide (Starace, 1995;
Catalan and Pugh, 1995).

Concealing HIV status can have a significant effect on whether or not an
HIV-positive person seeks appropriate healthcare. Stigma and social exclusion can limit access to health and social services, and this is equally true of
seronegative partners who often feel they are 'invisible' to the services to
which their seropositive partners have access (Van der Straten *et al.*, 1998).

Concealability is compromised, however, as the course of HIV
progresses to a symptomatic stage. The plethora of signs and symptoms
related to opportunistic infections and KS can challenge the positive
person's ability to conceal the true nature of the syndrome.

'Course' relates to the potential of the features of an attribute to change
over time and thus affect the extent of stigmatisation (Jones *et al.*, 1984).
The appearance of such signs as extreme weight loss, debility, HIV
encephalopathy or KS means that an HIV-positive person or their partner
may have to face telling others of the diagnosis or become involved in
more elaborate efforts towards concealment. Even the management of the
course of HIV by combination therapy can threaten concealability due to
the need to take large amounts of tablets and the presence of unwanted
side-effects.

In order to maintain concealability, individuals affected by HIV and
AIDS use a number of strategies. Lying about the diagnosis to others,
particularly outside of the immediate care-giving relationship, is notable.
So alternative diagnoses, such as forms of cancer or disorders of the
nervous system, can provide a plausible explanation for neighbours,
acquaintances, and even other family members.

Decisions by the person with HIV or AIDS regarding drug therapy and
treatment can also lead to judgements from other people. Society expects
individuals to avail themselves of all treatments, and therefore 'concurrence with social demands brings approval and better acceptance' (Jones
et al. 1984: 40). There are many instances, however, when people affected
by HIV and AIDS do not necessarily take up traditional or accepted forms
of treatment, most particularly that of combination therapy. Some HIV-
positive individuals prefer to use complementary therapies, and this tactic
is often not well understood by healthcare professionals.

Finally, it should be noted that those who live with HIV and AIDS do not purely comprise people infected with the virus. For every person *infected* with HIV there exists a network of people who, by virtue of their family or emotional ties, are also *affected* by the virus. It is recognised that any disease or illness affecting one member of a family can exert an effect on other members of that family and cause changes in support systems, role expectations and interpersonal relationships (Arnold and Boggs, 1995). It can be argued that an HIV-positive person at least has the choice of being able to reveal their status and the means by which they contracted the virus to the person closest to them and who is providing care to them. Many of these carers, however, have been unable to reveal their situation to someone with whom they could talk to openly and honestly due to the need to maintain the confidentiality of their partner or family member. Many carers are in great need of emotional support. Even in the gay community, when others know of the situation, the person closest to the HIV-positive individual may well feel marginalised at the time of death. Any denial by the family of origin (the biological family) of the significant place which the partner had in the life of the positive person can be a source of great emotional pain for the carer.

A summary of the issues related to stigma and social exclusion is highlighted in Table 11.1. Some suggestions related to the provision of healthcare are also provided.

Table 11.1 Managing the stigma of HIV in healthcare settings

Effect of stigma or social exclusion	*Considerations for provision of care*
The potential for stereotyping an HIV-positive person or person with AIDS, e.g. an HIV-positive man being labelled as gay.	Avoid making assumptions beyond the fact of HIV-positive status.
Partners and informal carers such as family members may experience or be concerned about 'courtesy stigma'.	Acknowledge potential need for emotional support among partners who may also feel socially excluded.
Social exclusion may lead to restricted support networks for the HIV-positive person and their family.	Be aware that usual family and support networks may be lacking. Care planning may require more extensive parameters involving home care, social support, etc.
Potential for low self-esteem and self-judgement within the HIV-positive person.	Implement a non-judgemental approach and positive valuing process in interactions with the HIV-positive person.
The HIV-positive person and their partner/family may lie about the diagnosis to others.	Confidentiality is important, with careful and sensitive information giving to others. The positive person should be in control of 'who knows', and this can be guided on a need-to-know basis.

It is important for healthcare workers to remember that people affected by HIV and AIDS can have healthcare needs which have nothing to do with the fact that they may be HIV-positive. HIV or AIDS need not always be the priority, and those infected have many other facets to their health and life which do not revolve around HIV. If healthcare needs are planned using a patient- or client-centred approach with a shared and negotiated agenda, this will avoid feelings of being stereotyped and labelled for the HIV-positive person.

Conclusion

Stigma and social exclusion related to HIV and AIDS have numerous effects, most notably in relation to the effect of concealment on the potential for lack of emotional support throughout the whole of the disease trajectory. Even where the HIV-positive person has been open about the diagnosis, social exclusion exists in many forms. As at the commencement of this chapter, the last word should be with those primarily affected. Jane (pseudonym) has been bereaved through HIV-related illness, and her social exclusion continues on beyond her husband's death.

> They should have been there [when he was alive]. I mean I felt they should have been there when I needed them and now it's too late … I just could not forgive them. And I've resented it so much when he was dead. They came back and said 'Well, it's OK now because he's not here.' I am socially acceptable again and I've no time for that!

References

Alonzo, A.A. and Reynolds, N.R. (1995) 'Stigma, HIV and AIDS: an exploration and elaboration of a stigma trajectory', *Social Science and Medicine*, 41, 3: 303–15.

Arnold, E. and Boggs, K. (1995) *Interpersonal relationships: professional communication skills for nurses*, second edn, London: W.B. Saunders.

Becker, H.S. (1963) *The outsiders: studies in sociology of deviance*, New York: The Free Press.

Beiser, C. (1997) 'HIV infection – II', *British Medical Journal*, 314: 579–83.

Catalan, J. and Pugh, K. (1995) 'Suicidal behaviour and HIV infection – is there a link?', *AIDS Care*, 7, Supplement 2: S117–S121.

Cohn, J.A. (1997) 'Recent advances: HIV infection – I', *British Medical Journal*, 314: 487–91.

De Cock, K. (1997) 'Guidelines for managing HIV infection', *British Medical Journal*, 315: 1–2.

Dukes, R.L. and Denny, H.C. (1995) 'Prejudice toward persons living with a fatal illness', *Psychological Reports*, 76: 1107–14.

Fan, H., Conner, R.F. and Villarreal, L.P. (1994) *The biology of AIDS*, third edn, London: Jones and Bartlett.

Goffman, E. (1963) *Stigma: notes on the management of spoiled identity*, London: Penguin.

Jones, E.E., Farina, A., Hastorf, A.H. *et al.* (1984) *Social stigma: the psychology of marked relationships*, New York: W.H. Freeman and Company.

Lucas, S.S., Hounnou, A., Peacock, C. *et al.* (1993) 'The mortality and pathology of HIV infection in a West African city', *AIDS*, 7: 1569–79.

Marris, V. (1996) *Lives worth living: women's experience of chronic illness*, London: Harper Collins.

Paicheler, G. (1992) 'Society facing AIDS', in M. Pollak, G. Paicheler and J. Pierret (eds), *AIDS: a problem for sociological research*, London: Sage.

Pollak, M. (1992) 'Attitudes, beliefs and opinions', in M. Pollak, G. Paicheler and J. Pierret (eds), *AIDS: a problem for sociological research*, London: Sage.

Powell J. (1996) *AIDS and HIV-related diseases: an educational guide for professionals and the public*, London: Plenum Press.

Powell-Cope, G.M. and Brown, M.A. (1992) 'Going public as an AIDS family caregiver', *Social Science and Medicine*, 34, 5: 571–80.

Rutherford, G.W. (1994) 'Long term survival in HIV-1 infection', *British Medical Journal*, 309: 283–4.

Sontag, S. (1991) *AIDS and its metaphors*, London: Penguin.

Starace, F. (1995) 'Epidemiology of suicide among persons with AIDS', *AIDS Care*, 7, Supplement 2: S123–S128.

Takahashi, L.M. (1997) 'The socio-spatial stigmatization of homelessness and HIV/AIDS: toward an explanation of the NIMBY syndrome', *Social Science and Medicine*, 45, 6: 903–14.

Ungvarski, P.J. and Staats, J.A. (1995) 'Clinical manifestations of AIDS in adults', in J.H. Flaskerud and P.J. Ungvarski (eds), *HIV/AIDS: a guide to nursing care*, third edn, London, W.B. Saunders.

Van der Straten, A., Vernon, K.A., Knight, K.R. *et al.* (1998) 'Managing HIV among serodiscordant heterosexual couples: serostatus, stigma and sex', *AIDS Care*, 10, 5: 533–48.

12 The stigma of epilepsy
Implications for clinical management

Gus A. Baker and Ann Jacoby

Introduction

Epilepsy is one of the most common neurological disorders, with an age-adjusted incidence of between 20 and 70 per 100,000 and a prevalence of 4–10 per 1,000 (Chadwick, 1994). It has been estimated that around 50 million people worldwide have epilepsy. In more than three-quarters of people with epilepsy, seizures begin before the age of 18 years (Porter, 1993). Though in the majority of cases there is no identifiable cause for epilepsy, it can be the result of virtually any major category of serious disease or disorder of humans, including congenital malformations, infections, tumours, vascular diseases, degenerative diseases or injury. The overall prognosis for remission as demonstrated by epidemiological studies (Annegers, Hauser and Elvebeck, 1979) is very good, and it is likely that the early course of epilepsy is a good predictor of eventual outcome.

Recent advances in the clinical management of epilepsy including the evaluation of drug kinetics, interactions, efficacy and toxicity, and the preference for monotherapy rather than polytherapy, have resulted in seizure remission in at least 60–80 per cent of patients. A proportion of patients, however, will continue to have seizures, which are refractory to optimal anti-convulsant therapy. Having continuous seizures is likely to mean that patients will have to attend hospital regularly, take large doses of antiepileptic medication and suffer the secondary psychosocial handicaps associated with chronic epilepsy.

Epilepsy as a stigmatising disorder

Despite being rendered seizure-free with optimal anti-convulsant therapy, a significant proportion of patients will face uncertainty about their condition and its prognosis. This is of particular importance in respect of whether or not they continue to see themselves as a person with epilepsy, and the implications that has for their day-to-day lives. The label of 'epilepsy' is still considered by many, both with and without the condition, as stigmatising, and carries with it both statutory and informal restrictions.

In the UK, for example, people with epilepsy are barred from holding a driving licence unless they meet specific criteria regarding the control of their seizures. There are also a number of occupations that prevent admission for those with epilepsy, including the armed forces, police, fire brigade, heavy goods vehicle driving and flying (Craig and Oxley, 1988). Legitimate discrimination, however, only forms a small proportion of the barriers faced by people with epilepsy. Prospective employers in many occupations may hold negative beliefs and attitudes about epilepsy that will influence their policy towards recruitment of people with such a condition.

Why is epilepsy considered such a stigmatising disorder? According to a number of authors, stigma and discrimination have been the defining social responses to epilepsy throughout history (Hermann and Whitman, 1986). There are a number of examples in the literature suggesting that epilepsy has long been considered a disease to be feared and shunned and that its treatment was a reflection of this (Tempkin, 1971). In ancient times, epilepsy was considered to be a result of demonic possession and madness and still is, in the developing countries. A number of important scientific discoveries in the late 1800s led to its establishment as a disorder of the brain, but despite this advance its more sinister images persisted.

In US statute, epilepsy has been associated with terms such as *idiotic, feebleminded and imbecile* (Commission for the Control of Epilepsy and its Consequences, 1978: 647). This prejudice resulted in a number of laws in the 1930s and onwards, in respect of people with epilepsy, governing prohibition against marriage, eugenic sterilisation, adoption of children with epilepsy and compulsory institutionalisation for those with uncontrolled seizures. According to Dell, these laws only continued to reinforce the notion that people with epilepsy were 'undesirable, dangerous and somehow mentally deficient and capable of passing along that deficiency to their offspring' (Dell, 1986: 189).

Given the reaction to epilepsy throughout history, it is not surprising that people with epilepsy may adopt negative views about themselves and their condition. West (1986), however, has argued that the meaning of epilepsy is defined not only by those with the condition but by the ideas of those without the condition. Schneider and Conrad (1983) have suggested that there are a number of participants involved in the process of giving a meaning to epilepsy and these include the person with epilepsy, their family members, friends, work associates and the health professionals treating them. Scambler and Hopkins (1986) have argued that, through the experience of seizures, people with epilepsy develop a special view of the world underpinned by the stigma associated with it. Though they may lead relatively normal lives, they retreat into their own special view of the world in the presence of witnessed seizures. Scambler and Hopkins's work was important because it made the distinction between the concept of enacted stigma – an episode of discrimination – and perceived or felt stigma – an oppressive fear of enacted stigma. Scambler (1989) reported that people with epilepsy were much more likely to experience felt than enacted stigma, a finding reinforced in a subsequent large-scale quantitative study of people with well-controlled epilepsy (Jacoby, 1994). Jacoby reported that only 2 per cent of subjects could recall any actual occurrence of discrimination in the workplace, but a third of them believed that having epilepsy made it more difficult for them than for those without the condition to find employment. In a more recent European study of over 5,000 people with epilepsy, Baker *et al.* (2000a) documented that 51 per cent of the sample reported being stigmatised, 18 per cent of whom reported feeling severely stigmatised. A number of factors were found to be predictive of scores on a self-completed stigma scale, including age of onset, marital status, worry, feelings about life as a whole, general health and duration of epilepsy. Interestingly, the relative importance of these variables differed across countries (Baker *et al.*, 2000b).

Concealability of epilepsy

Epilepsy represents what Goffman (1990) termed 'an undesired differentness'. A number of studies have highlighted that individuals' beliefs about the social meaning of epilepsy not only affect their attitudes towards their diagnosis but also their subsequent behaviour (Schneider and Conrad, 1983; Scambler, 1989). Scambler (1989) reports that, because of the potential stigma of epilepsy, many people in his study attempted to negotiate a less intimidating diagnosis, rejecting the label 'epilepsy' for fear of the intolerance and discrimination resulting from lay ignorance. Once a diagnosis had been accepted, the most common strategy of dealing with it was concealment. In Schneider and Conrad's (1983) study, epilepsy was managed by a range of behaviours which included elaborate methods for controlling and concealing information, strategies for preventing seizure occurrence, restricting activities and avoiding situations with high risk of exposure, and informing others in advance about the possibility of a seizure and lying. Dell (1986) considered the effect of concealment and suggested the following:

- The concealment of epilepsy often results in severe emotional damage.
- Stress is often a result of concealing stress.
- In the course of maintaining secrecy for many years, the secrecy itself can be a negative influence.
- A person with concealed epilepsy is still *discreditable* because at any time his secret might be revealed.
- Concealment often leads to avoidance of social interaction.
- Information management becomes the central interpersonal problem in concealment, and this can lead to less desire for intimacy.
- Parental coaching for concealment results in disability, dependence and feelings of incompetence.

According to Dell the effect of concealment is, in the long term, a much less healthy option than openness. Further, maximum disclosure may be an important positive strategy for coping with epilepsy. It is important also to note that Dell recognises that the negative effects of epilepsy are dependent on the affected person 'buying into' the devaluation.

Course of epilepsy

Between 60 and 80 per cent of people diagnosed and treated for epilepsy will attain long-term remission (Annegers, Hauser and Elvebeck, 1979). For the majority of these, remission will occur immediately or shortly after commencing treatment. Once a person has been considered seizure-free for some time, it is then reasonable for them to consider withdrawing from antiepileptic drug treatment. For the remaining 20–40 per cent the outlook is less positive, with some people developing epilepsy resistant to antiepileptic drug treatment. A small proportion of those with intractable epilepsy may go on to be considered as candidates for the epilepsy surgery programme. The outcome of surgery has been relatively successful, with between 60 and 70 per cent of patients rendered seizure-free. For those patients achieving seizure freedom through surgery the prognosis in terms of their psychosocial functioning is usually very good (Kellet *et al.*, 1997).

Within the framework of a large cross-sectional study of an unselected community sample we were able to examine the clinical course of epilepsy and its relationship to psychosocial functioning, including patient-perceived stigma. Our results clearly demonstrated that individuals with frequent seizures had significantly poorer scores on an epilepsy stigma scale than those with infrequent or no seizures (Jacoby *et al.*, 1996). These results were in accordance with previous findings for people with well-controlled epilepsy (seizure-free for at least two years) who reported very low levels of stigma (Jacoby, 1994). A recent Europe-wide study of people with epilepsy (Baker *et al.*, 2000b) also reported differing levels of stigma dependant on whether people with epilepsy had active seizures or were seizure-free (see Table 12.1).

Previous studies have highlighted that the occurrence of seizures acts as a continuous reinforcer of the label 'epilepsy'. Achieving seizure control, either through antiepileptic drug treatment or surgery, is therefore a key factor in minimising the stigma and the negative psychosocial conse-quences associated with it.

The contribution of health workers to the stigmatising process

In the case of epilepsy, doctors, whose role it is to act as interpreters of the disease, confer the diagnosis. In doing so, they determine whether a person

Table 12.1 Reported stigma in epilepsy by seizure type and frequency

	Score on stigma scale			
	0	*1*	*2*	*3*
Seizure type:	*(n2418*)*	*(n1027)*	*(n616)*	*(n920)*
Tonic-clonic only (%)	56	21	9	14
Tonic-clonic plus others (%)	39	22	16	23
Others only (%)	54	19	10	17
Seizure frequency:	*(n2508)*	*(n1054)*	*(n629)*	*(n939)*
None in last year (%)	63	19	8	10
Less than one per month (%)	52	22	11	15
One or more per month (%)	33	21	17	29
All respondents (%)	49	21	12	18

Note: *Figures in brackets are numbers on which percentages were calculated

with symptoms becomes labelled as a person with epilepsy. Physicians are generally well aware of the pejorative image of epilepsy and so, West (1979) has noted, may make use of clinical uncertainty to avoid or stall from labelling an individual as 'epileptic'. Unfortunately, it appears that doctors can themselves be prejudiced against people with epilepsy (Schneider and Conrad, 1983), and as a consequence pass on their own misconceptions to the patient, the patient's family and the general public. Many physicians will also manage the person with epilepsy using the medical model where the emphasis is on treating the seizures while ignoring the social issues. This phenomenon has been reported in a number of studies where physicians appeared uninterested, insecure, hurried and unable to discuss the wider issues relating to the non-medical management of the condition (Taylor, 1982; West, 1986). In reviewing the services for people with epilepsy in the UK, Chadwick (1990) has argued that one of the reasons for the relatively poor services is that there 'is a certain stigma that still attaches to epilepsy and that this penetrates to professionals as much as it is prevalent in the community as a whole'.

Overcoming the stigma of epilepsy

There are a number of ways in which minimising the impact of epilepsy and reducing its stigma can be achieved. These include: better education and training for healthcare professionals; a multidisciplinary team approach to care; better information and education for people with epilepsy and their families; and more vociferous campaigns to educate society about the condition. In this section the authors will briefly discuss each approach.

Educating and training health professionals

It has been argued that physicians lack the motivation, training or time to elicit patients' own perspective on epilepsy and as a consequence tend to concentrate on the clinical management of the condition. In essence this means that little attention is paid to the patient's experience of their epilepsy or how they can develop strategies for coping with their condition and its psychosocial sequelae. It would appear from the relevant research that what patients want is to be listened to by their doctors about issues that cause them the most concern, and these usually relate to the impact that epilepsy is having on their day-to-day lives. Clinicians have a significant role in influencing the process of accommodation by being aware of the timing of their communications about diagnosis of epilepsy, since diagnosis marks the beginning of a protracted and sometimes lifelong process of adjustment. A number of authors have highlighted the role of the clinician in aiding the adjustment process through rational drug therapy, combined with treatment for possible psychological or psychiatric sequelae of epilepsy, or medication or psychosocial factors (Hermann and Whitman, 1991; Scambler, 1993). It is only reasonable to accept that not all of the demands and expectations of people with epilepsy are going to be met by even the most caring physician. However, there is no doubt that patients are much more likely to be satisfied with their services when they view their physician as someone who is empathic, interested and willing to try and understand the problems they face.

One important innovation in the management of epilepsy has been the development of the role of the epilepsy specialist nurse. This has been primarily to liaise between general practitioners in the community and the hospital-based epilepsy services. They have also taken the lead in responding to requests from patients and their families for better information about both medical and non-medical issues relating to the management of their condition. The epilepsy specialist nurse can act as coordinator of care, liasing between a number of health, social and educational services. Some of them will possess counselling skills and consequently will be able to provide counselling and behavioural treatment where necessary.

Better information and education for people with epilepsy and their families

It is important for people with epilepsy and their families both that they should have a good understanding of their condition, and that any unhelpful beliefs they might hold about their condition are demystified. The importance of recognising the connection between misconceptions about epilepsy and psychosocial functioning has been well documented (Mittan, 1986). Hills and Baker (1992) demonstrated how possession of accurate information about epilepsy was significantly related to level of well-being: people with epilepsy who were more informed about the management and treatment of their condition perceived themselves as being more in control, and consequently had significantly better psychological profiles than those who were less informed. This finding was supported in a recent Europe-wide study of people with epilepsy and their carers (Baker *et al.*, 2000b).

In some circumstances, people with epilepsy may feel so overpowered by the impact of their condition that they require professional help. A small number of epilepsy centres will have a psychologist who is able to provide counselling or cognitive–behavioural treatment. Cognitive–behavioural therapy involves shaping the way people think, feel and behave. In using this approach in people with epilepsy, the rationale would be to help them minimise the impact of their condition on their daily lives. Interventions aimed at the cognitive level emphasise the importance of providing new information about the illness or its management. Cognitive–behavioural techniques are also implemented to modify the underlying core beliefs people have about their condition, which may cause psychological impairments. Tan and Bruni's (1986) use of group-based cognitive–behavioural therapy, though it did not significantly reduce seizure frequency, did result in an increase in ratings of well-being in patients with epilepsy. Families should also be considered as important targets for demystifying beliefs about the epilepsy, its cause and its management. It is important to ensure that the person with epilepsy and their family are encouraged to discover for themselves much of the necessary information they require to make sense of their condition and its management, since this process of empowerment will be beneficial in the process of adjustment (Mittan, 1986).

A number of authors have advocated that people with epilepsy should disclose their condition. Dell (1986) has reviewed the benefits of disclosure and recorded the following observations:

- Being open about epilepsy to relatives, teachers and schoolmates can ultimately dispel fallacies.
- If the average person with epilepsy 'comes out', it helps the average person without epilepsy to understand better.
- Disclosure can be therapeutic for the teller.
- Disclosure broadens public acceptance and lowers stereotypes.
- The sense of stigmatisation is broken down with disclosure.
- Maximum disclosure seems to yield the most tolerant response.

Educating society about epilepsy

Increasing public awareness forms a significant role for the epilepsy support organisations. One such organisation, The British Epilepsy Association, helps people with epilepsy and their families by:

- providing an information and advice service;
- organising talks, seminars and conferences and providing source material in the form of pamphlets, videos and newsletters;
- Supporting a national network of local self-help groups;
- Campaigning on behalf of people with epilepsy and acting as an advocate for individuals facing problems with employment, benefits, legal and insurance matters;
- Combating negative attitudes and prejudice by improving understanding of epilepsy;
- Funding social research.

While organisations such as this should be praised for their efforts in raising awareness among the public, a significant amount of ignorance about epilepsy among the lay public still exists. Recently, a number of campaigns initiated both nationally and internationally have been launched and it is hoped that these will help further the cause of people with epilepsy. However, as already mentioned, one of the most significant means of influencing the attitudes of the lay public is for individuals with epilepsy to act as their own advocates.

Conclusions

The stigma of epilepsy is a complex phenomenon with multiple origins. A number of authors have cited the importance of parental reaction to the diagnosis, e.g. shame and concealment (Austin, 1996; Schneider and Conrad, 1983), while others have highlighted the importance of the reaction of others (Hills and Baker, 1992). The severity of the condition and the personality of the individual may also affect how he or she responds to direct or indirect experiences of discrimination (Baker *et al.*, 2000a). The attitudes and beliefs of healthcare professionals and the beliefs and understanding of the lay public will also contribute to both enacted and perceived stigma. From all these sources, people with epilepsy face both formal and informal barriers that will ultimately limit the choices they come to make about their lives. Reducing the stigma of epilepsy requires a collaborative effort involving the person with epilepsy, their family, health professionals, epilepsy support organisations and legislative bodies, to change the way epilepsy is viewed by themselves and by society. At the heart of this, is a requirement that the person with the condition must be helped to think, act and behave in a way such that the impact minimises their condition and maximises their quality of life.

References

Annegers, J.F., Hauser, W.A. and Elvebeck, L.R. (1979) 'Remission of seizures and relapse in patients with epilepsy', *Epilepsia*, 20: 729–37.

Austin, J.K. (1996) 'A model of family adaptation to new-onset childhood epilepsy', *Journal of Neuroscience Nurses*, 28: 82–92.

Baker, G.A., Brooks, J.L., Buck, D. and Jacoby, A. (2000a) 'The stigma of epilepsy: a European perspective', *Epilepsia*, 41: 98–104.

Baker, G.A., Jacoby, A., De Boer, H. *et al.* (2000b) 'Patients' understanding and adjustment to epilepsy: interim findings from a European Study', *Epilepsia*, 40: 26–9.

Chadwick, D.W. (ed.) (1990) *Quality of life and quality of care in epilepsy*, Royal Society of Medicine Round Table Series 23.

—— (1994) 'Epilepsy', *Journal of Neurology, Neurosurgery and Psychiatry*, 57: 264–77.

Commission for the Control of Epilepsy and its Consequences (1978) *Plan for nationwide activity on epilepsy*, (DHEW Publication No. NIH 78–276), Washington, DC: U.S. Government Printing Office.

Craig, A. and Oxley, J. (1988) 'Social aspects of epilepsy', in J. Laidlaw, A. Richens and J. Oxley (eds), *A textbook of epilepsy*, third edn, Edinburgh: Churchill Livingstone.

Dell, J. (1986) 'Social dimensions of epilepsy: stigma and response', in S. Whitman and B.P. Hermann (eds), *Psychopathology in epilepsy: social dimensions*, Oxford: Oxford University Press.

Goffman, E. (1990) *Stigma: notes on the management of spoiled identity*, London: Penguin.

Hermann, B.P. and Whitman, S. (1986) 'Psychopathology in epilepsy: a multi-etiological model', in S. Whitman and B.P. Hermann (eds), *Psychopathology in epilepsy: social dimensions*, Oxford: Oxford University Press.

—— (1991) 'Neurobiological, psychosocial and pharmacological factors underlying interictal psychopathology in epilepsy', in D. Smith, D. Treiman and M. Trimble (eds), *Advances in Neurology. Vol. 55: Neurobehavioural problems in epilepsy*, New York: Oxford University Press.

Hills, M.D. and Baker, P.G. (1992) 'Relationships among epilepsy, social stigmas, self-esteem and social support', *Journal of Epilepsy*, 5: 231–8.

Jacoby, A. (1994) 'Felt versus enacted stigma: a concept revisited', *Social Science and Medicine*, 38: 269–74.

Jacoby, A., Baker, G.A., Steen, N. *et al.* (1996) 'The clinical course of epilepsy and its psychosocial correlates: findings from a UK community study', *Epilepsia*, 37 (2): 148–61.

Kellet, D., Smith, D.F., Baker, G.A. and Chadwick, D.W. (1997) 'Quality of life after epilepsy surgery', *Journal of Neurology, Neurosurgery and Psychiatry*, 63 (1): 52–8.

Mittan, R.J. (1986) 'Fear of seizures', in S. Whitman and B.P. Hermann (eds), *Psychopathology in epilepsy: social dimensions*, Oxford: Oxford University Press.

Porter, R.J. (1993) 'Classification of epileptic seizures and epileptic syndromes', in J. Laidlaw, A. Richens and D.W. Chadwick (eds), *A textbook of epilepsy*, fourth edn, Edinburgh: Churchill Livingstone.

Scambler, G. (1989): *Epilepsy*, London: Tavistock.

—— (1993) 'Coping with epilepsy', in J. Laidlaw, A. Richens and D.W. Chadwick (eds), *A textbook of epilepsy*, fourth edn, Edinburgh: Churchill Livingstone.

Scambler, G. and Hopkins, A. (1986) 'Being epileptic: coming to terms with stigma', *Social Health and Illness*, 8: 26–43.

Schneider, J.W. and Conrad, P. (1983) *Having epilepsy: the experience and control of illness*, Philadelphia: Temple University Press.

Tan, S.Y. and Bruni, J. (1986) 'Cognitive–behavioural therapy with adult patients with epilepsy: a controlled outcome study', *Epilepsia*, 27 (3): 225–33.

Taylor, D.C. (1982) 'The components of sickness: diseases, illnesses and predicaments', in J. Apley and C. Ounsted (eds), *One child*, London: Heinemann Medical.

Tempkin, O. (1971) *The falling sickness*, Baltimore: John Hopkins Press.

West, P. (1979) 'Investigation into the social construction and consequences of the label "epilepsy" ', PhD Thesis, University of Bristol.

—— (1986) 'The social meaning of epilepsy. Stigma as a potential explanation for psychopathology in children', in S. Whitman and B.P. Hermann (eds), *Psychopathology in epilepsy: social dimensions*, Oxford: Oxford University Press.

13 Burns and social stigma

Sue Kaney

Introduction

Burn injuries are often sudden, tragic and emotive. Such injuries result in pain and in many cases require surgery. In cases of severe burns injuries, involving large areas of the body, physical disfigurement, scarring and disability may result. Advanced surgical techniques and nursing care ensure that patients with large burns now have a better chance of survival. However, the future is uncertain and the patient may have many issues to confront in their long-term psychological adjustment. Psychological issues facing the burns patient involve reaction to acute pain, threat to survival, hospitalisation, medical and surgical procedures, post-traumatic stress disorder (PTSD), depression, anxiety and stigmatisation.

Caring for the burns patient now involves a range of procedures including use of skin substitutes, early excision and grafts and the use of topical antibacterial agents to prevent infection (Patterson et al., 1993). Patients suffering smoke inhalation and burns caused by the inhalation of flames and hot gases now receive cardiovascular and respiratory support, which has also increased survival rates (Heimbach, 1983; Grube et al., 1988).

Psychological survival

For the burns patient, recovery times may vary. The size, depth and site of the burn and the treatment required will determine the length of stay in hospital. The length of stay can vary upwards from 24 hours. Treatments can range from simple dressing and monitoring of heart rate in a patient with a minor electrical burn to full-blown intensive care unit treatment, ventilation and major surgery. Psychological adjustment begins from the moment the patient realises they have survived a frightening, painful and potentially life-threatening situation.

A number of challenges face the burns patient once they have survived. The first major challenge for the patient with a large burn involving the face is coming to terms with a changed identity or different face. For some patients this is a most distressing time. Helping patients to deal with this distress will be addressed later in this chapter. The second challenge for the patient to overcome is the reaction of others to their changed identity. Patients often notice that visitors to their bedside recoil in shock at their changed facial appearance. The third step on the road to survival and rebuilding a future is facing the world outside the environs of the hospital ward. This step involves dealing with the stigma that is often attached to looking different from the rest of society.

The theory of stigma will not be addressed here. However, two concepts are important for the burns patient. They are concealability and course.

Concealability

Concealability is the degree to which the scar or mark is visible to other people with whom the burns patient has to interact. It is a dimension upon which it is possible to place any given mark or condition from which an individual may suffer; thus it is possible to place burns patients on the dimension of concealability.

Burn injury patients fall into categories, as displayed in Figure 13.1.

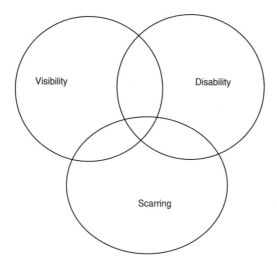

Figure 13.1 Categorisation of burn injuries

For some patients, their burn injury causes scarring but this is not visible and it causes no disability. For other patients their burn causes disability but minimal scarring. At the intersection of the three circles are those patients for whom their burn injury causes severe scarring, is highly visible and therefore not concealable, and they suffer a physical disability as a result of the injury.

Case study: John

John, a 40-year-old electrician married with two children, sustained an electric shock when a circuit breaker failed. He was working on a machine at the time and touched wiring that was live. He received an electric shock to his right hand. His hand was not burned. However, the shock exited from his right shoulder leaving an exit burn some two inches in length. This was a minor burn. John was admitted to the burns unit overnight to monitor his heart rate. The burn was treated conservatively and he was discharged home the following day.

John has not worked since the accident. He complains of severe pain in his right hand and arm. He has not used his right hand since the accident. His arm and right shoulder are stiff and painful. His appearance is similar to that of a patient who has suffered a left hemispheric stroke, and paralysis is obvious in the right side. John carries his right arm across the front of his body with the palm of his right hand facing upwards. John also suffers with PTSD.

This case illustrates the point that, for some burns patients, the burn scarring is not noticeable or visible. However, the effect of the burn is to disable, and this aspect is highly visible and not possible to conceal.

While such cases have important psychological and social consequences for the patient, perhaps of more concern are the patients for whom facial scarring cannot be concealed.

The burns patient with facial scarring has to come to terms with the change in his or her own identity. We know what our own face looks like, and most of us check our identity every day by looking in the mirror. For the patient with a facial burn, looking in the mirror is a big shock. Some patients never come to terms with the change in identity they see when they view their face. The physical change in features can be profound. Patients can respond to this change in a variety of ways. Some patients can adjust and view their changed identity as part of their personality. For others the change is unacceptable, and their personality changes along with their facial features. An example of this type of personality change is given in the case below.

Case study: Billy

Billy was a 16-year-old who was severely burned while inhaling petrol fumes. He suffered an inhalation burn and scarring to his chest, face and head. Billy lost all his hair and his ears. After many months of surgery Billy was given prosthetic ears and seen by the hospital wigmaker. Billy opted for a long blond wig which covered his ears but was not in keeping with his original hair colour. He refused advice on how to wear the hair piece. He went out of his way to shock people with his burn scars.

This case illustrates how some patients never come to terms with their scarring and change of identity when it cannot be concealed. The reverse process happens for these patients who are also often psychologically distressed. They advertise their difference in a way that is shocking and, to some people, frightening. This inability to adjust was tested by Goldberg *et al.* (1974). In this study, children with facial scars from burns were compared with children with congenital heart disease on measures of adjustment. While the children with heart disease had a much worse physical prognosis than the children with facial scars, they were better adjusted than the children with facial scarring. The children with heart disease could see themselves having jobs, relationships and a future, whereas the facially scarred children did not view themselves as having jobs, careers or relationships.

Some patients, however, respond very positively and use their changed identity to help others and promote a change in social attitudes to people with changed identities. In his book *Changing Faces* (1997), James Partridge describes his own recovery from a burn injury which 'changed his face'. Partridge argues that there are two types of disfigurement that take place following a burn injury. First, there is the personal disfigurement. This relates to the change in the mental picture that the patient has of themselves. This change is often accompanied by a change in behaviour, and by thoughts and feelings about the way the person feels about themselves. It can include feeling a sense of low self-esteem, as the face is 'now so blemished and battered'.

Second, Partridge describes social disfigurement. This is the way the disfigurement is viewed by others and can alter the way in which people interact or behave towards the disfigured person. The way in which the disfigured person copes with the reactions of others will be considered later in the chapter.

Course

Patients with a burn injury face a difficult and uncertain course with the scarring or disfigurement they may have. Many factors can influence the course of disfigurement or scarring. To some extent, course will be determined by the nature of the injury. It may also be influenced by the factors which caused the scarring, for example if the burn was self-inflicted the individual may feel degraded, remorseful or feel that they deserve the pain and scarring. These are complex issues which are not separate from the course of the mark but can influence the outcome for the patient.

Listed below is a classification of burn injuries which will serve to illustrate the problems associated with the course of healing and concealability of the injury. Burns are classified according to depth of injury, in other words the level of tissue destruction.

- Superficial burns involve damage to the outer layer of skin and usually result from short contact with a source of heat, for example an iron. These burns result in reddening of the skin and blistering. They will normally heal within a week to ten days.
- Partial-thickness burns are deeper, damage the nerve endings and are extremely painful. A scald from hot water is an example of a partial thickness burn. Healing can take two to three weeks. Deeper partial-thickness (deep dermal) burns usually require skin grafting and take longer to heal.
- Full-thickness burns completely destroy all the layer of the skin, including hair follicles and nerve endings, and may even destroy underlying structures such as bone, tendon and muscle. These injuries are usually caused by longer contact with a very high temperature such as flame, electrical burns or chemicals. These burns cause major concern for the plastic surgeon and nursing staff, because they do not heal. Infection is always a great risk and such injuries need to be cleaned and covered with skin at the earliest opportunity.

Altering the course of a scar

Treatment is usually lengthy for the patient with full-thickness burns. The course of treatment can be broken roughly into three stages. First, cover as much of the injury as possible with skin. Second, deal with any major facial or bodily abnormalities. Third, try to cosmetically improve facial features and thus reduce the disfigurement. Partridge (1997) calls this the 'operation–dressing–operation cycle'. Following each operation, skin grafts need time to heal. Patients can often be immobile for sometime to promote healing and give grafts the best possible chance of taking. During this time dressings also have to be changed and this can be a painful procedure. Most burns units now employ advanced forms of analgesia and in some cases anaesthesia to aid this process and ease patients through the cycle.

Plastic surgery is the most common form of invasive procedure to improve the appearance of scarring following a burn injury. Plastic surgery and, increasingly, microsurgery can reconstruct the face, making it presentable. This is a difficult concept for many patients to grasp. For some patients they believe that continued surgery is the answer. On this view the question becomes how much surgery is necessary to restore the face? Some patients will have surgery every time the surgeon suggests that an improvement can be made, or they will request that surgery be carried out to improve their features. Others will not wish to continue on the operation–dressing–operation cycle. However, plastic surgery cannot restore the face to its pre-injury state. There will always be some residual scarring that will remain with the patient. The main aim of plastic surgery is to give the patient a face that neither repels, nor invokes pity. A face – albeit marked – that they can continue to live with. Given that a perfectly restored face is not a possibility, patients who decide on further surgery have to consider a number of issues. First, can further surgery improve their appearance? Second, is surgery necessary if perfection cannot be obtained? Finally, what will they have to forego to undergo surgery?

The role of the team in burn injuries

The course of a burn injury scar will also be influenced by a number of people from the burns unit team, such as plastic surgeons, nurses, physiotherapists, occupational therapists, psychologists and prosthetics technicians.

Staff on a burns unit and dressing clinic are used to seeing the disfigurement that can result from a burn injury. Staff respond to patients in a positive manner and very rarely show outward signs of repulsion at the injuries they see. While this is an appropriate professional response from the staff of the unit, the same response cannot be expected from family, friends or outsiders. The environment of the burns unit is 'safe' in this respect. For patients, the worst time can be just prior to discharge, when fears about going home, resuming life and meeting the responses of outsiders are prevalent.

Staff on the unit can help with these fears. Many patients, once their grafts are stable, are sent home for the weekend. This helps the patient adjust to their home environment. Staff can ease this process by explaining to patients about being back in the home environment. Activities of daily living are to be encouraged, including meeting with friends and family. Patients should also be encouraged to go out when they are home. There is always a danger that patients who are facially disfigured and scarred simply replace the hospital environment with the home environment and never venture out. At home, some hospital routines will have to be maintained, such as dressing changes and physiotherapy exercises, and these have to be built into daily routines.

On returning to hospital, patients usually feel very tired and relieved that the first stage towards going home has been achieved. Once back on the ward, the burns patient may have to undergo further surgery in consultation with their plastic surgeon and so begin the cycle of surgery and recovery once more. Throughout this process the patient, trying to come to terms with their scarring, may fluctuate in mood between optimism and anxiety. The role of team members is vital in noting such changes in behaviour and counselling the patient. In some cases psychological disturbance may be too intense. Staff may not feel they have the time nor skills necessary to deal with such problems. Severe psychological problems need to be referred to the clinical psychologist or psychiatrist attached to the unit.

Overcoming the stigma of disfigurement

Once a patient is discharged from the unit the challenges begin. The first problem to overcome is facing society with a changed appearance. Everyone the person meets is going to notice their face. People will stare rather than glance and pass by. Name calling and verbal abuse are not uncommon. The person with a changed appearance may also be very sensitive to the behaviours of those around them. In turn, the person's behaviour and view of themselves may influence how others react to them.

Case study: Jill

Jill was a 16-year-old who survived a house fire which left her with a badly disfigured hand. Despite extensive surgery her fingers were badly misshapen, and she described them as 'gross sausages'. She eventually underwent further surgery to have two fingers removed. When she went home, local children taunted her about her hand. Her response was to use her disfigured hand to frighten the local children. She also used to enjoy watching the shock on people's faces when she waved her hand around at the local disco. In the small community where she lived she eventually got a reputation for being a frightening person. Few people related to her and her family found it difficult to remain in the area.

The public image that the person displays can influence the responses of other people in society. Moreover, the 'normal' facial expressions that most of us take for granted can often become distorted in the person with a facial disfigurement. For example, a smile may not be recognisable as such, and a frown may not convey the message that its wearer wants it to convey. Similarly, a disfigured or distorted facial appearance can alter society's perception of the individual's character. Disfigurement and distortion are often associated with stupidity, poor/low mental ability, evil, cruelty, nastiness, greed and selfishness. Literature has for many years propagated these social stereotypes with such books as 'Dracula' and 'Frankenstein', while movies such as 'Nightmare on Elm Street' epitomise the vileness and horror of someone who is both burned *and* evil beyond belief.

The individual with altered facial appearance has to contend with these images that are unwittingly strengthened by the media through advertising. Only beautiful, clever, thin, attractive, unmarked and blemish-free individuals appear in television commercials and magazine advertising. Failure to meet such high standards by those with facial disfigurement stigmatises them as being social failures, below average intelligence and of dubious character.

Challenging these myths and standing up for their rights can be a full-time occupation for the facially disfigured individual. The media can sometimes help by highlighting cases of discrimination in the workplace, at school and in social settings. The main task of defeating social stigma rests with all of us. By learning from the facially disfigured, interacting with them and dispelling myths, they will once again be able to resume their place in society.

References

Goldberg, R.T. (1974) 'Adjustment of children with invisible handicaps: congenital heart disease and facial burns', *Journal of Counselling Psychology*, 21: 428.

Grube, J.J., Marvin, J.A. and Heimbach, D.M. (1988) 'Therapeutic hyperbaric oxygen: help or hindrance in burn patients with carbon monoxide poisoning?', *Journal of Burn Care and Rehabilitation*, 4: 249–52.

Heimbach, D.M. (1983) 'Smoke inhalation: current concepts', in T.L. Watchel, N. Kahn and H.A. Franks (eds), *Current topics in burn care*, Rockville, MD: Aspen.

Partridge, J. (1997) *Changing faces: the challenge of facial disfigurement*, third edn, London: Changing Faces Publications.

Patterson, D., Everett, J., Bombadier, C. *et al.* (1993) 'Psychological effects of severe burns injuries', *Psychological Bulletin*, 113: 363–78.

Part II

Applications to practice

Section II: Deviance

14 Exclusive language?

Rachel E. Perkins and Julie M. Repper

> Language sets everyone the same traps: it is an immense network of easily accessible wrong turnings.
>
> (Ludwig Wittgenstein, quoted in Cartwright, 1998)

Introduction

Debates about language often seem irrelevant to busy clinicians: mere semantics, an affectation of political correctness. However, the implications of language cannot be so readily dismissed. More than simply convenient tags or labels, the words we use define the quality and value of that which is named and deny the existence of that which is not (Daly, 1978). Much of the language that is traditionally used in the mental health arena perpetuates exclusion.

> Historically, language has been the principal tool that has served to separate people with labels of differentness by defining the needs of these people with a label as fundamentally different from those of other citizens. In this way, language keeps oppression intact. Therefore an important way to change these negative, stigmatized beliefs and behaviours is to change the language.
>
> (Carling, 1994: 2)

The language we use defines the ways in which we think about mental health problems and the people who experience them. It thus has implications for the way in which they are treated, both within and outside services. Words are not 'right' or 'wrong', in and of themselves, but they all carry implications which must be debated.

The language of passivity: patienthood and exclusion

Numerous different terms have been used to describe people who experience mental health problems. Within services it has long been the habit to define people in terms of their diagnosis: a schizophrenic, a manic depressive. Reducing a person to nothing more than their difficulties is one of the most damaging and dehumanising forms of language. It denies the existence of any facet of the person, any relevant roles or characteristics, other than their diagnosis (Chamberlin, 1984; Brandon, 1991).

Even if we wish to describe someone as 'having schizophrenia', this does not make them 'a schizophrenic'. Small though this difference may seem, its implications are far-reaching. Defining a person as merely a collection of problems and dysfunctions engenders hopelessness in both the person labelled and the one who does the labelling. Such a form omits to label any positive assets and possibilities for the person, abilities, interests and opportunities, so these go unheeded and cannot therefore be fostered and developed. The person labelled, for example, 'schizophrenic', is under pressure to adopt a self-conception consistent with the way in which they have been labelled (Scheff, 1975).

Someone so labelled has two options. On the one hand, if the person accepts the definition of themselves as 'just a schizophrenic', then they are likely to see themselves as no more than the problems which this label implies. Mental health services are replete with people who have 'given up' because they have come to understand their situation as hopeless and ceased to believe in the possibility of leading a valued life. On the other hand, if the person rejects being defined simply as a collection of problems, they are likely also to reject the services which so labelled them and denied the other facets of their individuality. There is much popular concern about people who reject the help which they are offered, and much consideration of ways to ensure compliance (Perkins, 1999). Yet is not such rejection of services a rational act if the price of acceptance means abandoning the possibility of having a satisfying and fulfilling life?

At a collective level, the term most commonly used to describe those who experience mental health problems remains that of 'mental patient'. This term, borrowed from the arena of physical ill health, implies that those with mental health difficulties have an 'illness' and remain 'patients' until such time as they are 'cured'.

There are many who reject the notion that mental health problems are 'illnesses' with the clear organic pathology that the term implies (see, for example, Szasz, 1973). Such authors cite the elusive nature of the supposed underlying physical pathology associated with 'mental illnesses' (Mosher, 1999). They argue that assumptions of organicity generate exclusion by differentiating the 'mad' from the 'sane'. The thoughts and feelings of the 'mad' can therefore be discounted as manifestations of their supposed pathology and their behaviour is assumed to be beyond their control. Thus social control and coercion are legitimised in the form of removal of freedom and choice, compulsory detention and treatment.

On the other hand, there are those who argue that illness constructions serve to demystify madness. If mental illness is seen as just as understandable and treatable as physical illness, then the fear that 'madness' engenders in the general population, and the social exclusion which results from it, can be reduced (National Alliance for the Mentally Ill, 1996). However, the ways in which society constructs illnesses of the body and illnesses of the brain may be quite different. For example, Nieradzik and Cochrane (1985), in a study of public attitudes, found that deviant behaviour is more likely to be tolerated if the perpetrators are not assigned the label of 'mental illness'. When told that a behaviour resulted from mental illness, people were more likely to say that they did not want to live in the vicinity. When they were told that exactly the same behaviour resulted from difficult life experiences they were less likely to reject them in this way.

It is noteworthy that the now-popular term 'mental health problems' is still firmly grounded within an illness perspective. What is a 'health problem' if it is not an illness? Whether or not mental health problems are seen as 'illness', there are other difficulties with the 'patient' identity.

The role of patient is not a positively valued one. Patients are valued only for the other roles which they may also occupy: mother, worker, footballer. A patient identity may be functional in relieving a person of the responsibilities of other roles (going to work, looking after children) for brief periods of sickness. However, if a person has longer-lasting problems, then the role of patient tends to become permanent and take the place of all other roles. When the patient role becomes pervasive in this way, the inherent passivity, lack of personal agency, self-determination and value implied by the role become destructive. They are seen as dependant upon the ministrations of professionals and their prescriptions to restore health. As the term implies, they must wait patiently for the cures to take effect. Because they are ill, patients are deemed incapable of engaging in ordinary activities and are therefore excluded.

The exclusion associated with labelling problems as 'illnesses' and people as 'patients' permeates psychiatry. Having defined the patient as different from 'ordinary citizens' – absolved from ordinary roles and responsibilities – mental health professionals are supposed to provide services which meet their 'needs' (Department of Health, 1995). However, the language of needs in psychiatry is quite different from that in the general population. Needs identified in the general population have varied from basic physiological requirements for food, shelter, warmth and safety, through social needs for love and belonging, to social status and self-actualisation (Maslow, 1970). The needs of 'mental patients' to which services must respond have been defined quite differently. One text defined them as self-neglect, social withdrawal, slowness and overactivity (Sainsbury Centre for Mental Health, 1997). Other psychiatric needs assessments talk of needs for specific service inputs: medication, training, day care, hostels etc. (Phelan *et al.*, 1995). Difference is reinforced and exclusion ensured.

> A new breed of human (or should I say sub-human) is born: one who,
> quite unlike any other member of the species, has a 'need' for day-
> centres, group homes and the like. Needs and ways of meeting those
> ways become confused and segregation is all but guaranteed (after all,
> it is only the mad who need such places).
>
> (Perkins, 1999: 7)

If patients are ill then they 'need' therapy. Therefore all help tends to be construed as some form of therapy: work therapy, gardening therapy, social therapy. The language of therapy serves to devalue even the limited range of activities in which patients are permitted to engage, and to differentiate these from ordinary pursuits.

For example, the work done by most citizens is for the benefit of others, whether it be paid employment or non-paid labour such as child-rearing. The worker contributes to society by producing goods or delivering services that are valuable to others. Of course, the worker benefits via deriving a wage, social status, identity and a sense of personal worth from their labours, but the *raison d'être* of employment (and the reason why it confers these benefits on those who engage in it) is producing something that has social value. Work therefore connects the individual to the society in which he or she lives.

The exclusion from the labour market, at least in part resulting from constructions of the community of 'mental patients' as 'ill' and unfit for work, is reflected in extraordinarily high rates of unemployment. The 1995 Labour Force Survey showed that only 13 per cent of that community were employed. However, occupation is considered to have therapeutic value, therefore 'mental patients' may be provided with 'therapeutic work'. This semantic sleight of hand – 'work' to 'work therapy' – completely changes the meaning and purpose of, and therefore the value attached to, the activities performed. 'Work therapy' is done primarily for the benefit of the individual worker – to improve their mental health. The product becomes relatively irrelevant, with the major consideration being the therapeutic value of the process. In fact, the product may actually have value and a place in the economy; for example, the packing and assembly tasks carried out in much 'therapeutic work' are contracted from local businesses. Yet the person who performs these tasks is devalued and excluded from the general labour market when it is labelled 'work therapy', a value clearly symbolised by the appallingly low level of earnings which they receive for this therapy.

It is not only the case that mental patients are deemed passive recipients of the therapeutic ministrations of expert professionals; the language used to describe their experiences was invented by these experts, and their allied researchers: people who typically have never experienced the phenomena they seek to describe. The language in which madness is described is exclusively one of problems and dysfunctions (Chadwick, 1997), delusions, hallucinations, ideas of reference, passivity phenomena. A brief glance at accounts provided by those who have experienced mental health problems reveals the limitations, and the dehumanising effect, of such professional descriptors. O'Hagan (1996) provides a stark illustration of the contrast between the rich language of experience and poverty of professional discourse. She contrasts entries she made in her diary during an admission to a psychiatric hospital with medical notes made by her psychiatrist. For example, her medical notes recorded: 'Flat, lacking in motivation. Sleep and appetite good. Discussed aetiology. Cont. LiCarb. 250mg qid. Levels next time.'

The account O'Hagan wrote in her diary on the same day was quite different:

> Today I wanted to die. Everything was hurting. My body screaming. I saw the doctor. I said nothing. Now I feel terrible. Nothing seems good and nothing good seems possible.
> I am stuck in a twilight mood
> where I go down
> like the setting sun
> into a lonely black hole
> where there is room for only one.
>
> (O'Hagan, 1996: 46)

The professional language of psychiatry not only reinforces social exclusion, it also excludes people from the right to define their own experiences.

The language of agency: recovery and inclusion

Those who have themselves experienced mental health problems are beginning to challenge the professional language of mental illness. They have begun to reclaim a language and associated understanding of madness based on the expertise of experience.

> Alas, even the briefest perusal of the current literature on schizophrenia will immediately reveal to the uninitiated that this collection of problems is viewed by practitioners almost exclusively in terms of dysfunction and disorder. A positive or charitable phrase or sentence rarely meets the eye.
>
> (Chadwick, 1997: xii)

Chadwick (1997), a psychologist with a diagnosis of schizophrenia, criticises such deficit-focused definitions and descriptions of schizophrenia. He outlines the ways in which these both:

- generate biased accounts by failing to entertain the possibility, and recognise research, which suggests that the 'psychosis-prone mind' may access states of mental clarity and profundity, empathy and creativity, inaccessible to 'standard-minded' people; and

- ignore the psychotic tendencies of numerous influential people – statesmen, scientists, scholars, composers, writers and artists.

Similarly, Jamison, a clinical psychologist and prestigious Professor of Psychiatry with a diagnosis of manic-depression, has extensively researched the creativity and contribution of people with such a diagnosis (Jamison, 1989, 1993, 1995).

Both Chadwick (1997) and Jamison (1996) emphasise the deleterious implications of the language of problem and dysfunction for the ways in which people with such diagnoses are treated.

> Deficit-obsessed research can only produce theories and attitudes which are disrespectful of clients and are also likely to induce behaviour in clinicians such that service users are not properly listened to, not believed, not fairly assessed, are likely treated as inadequate and are also not expected to be able to become independent and competent individuals in managing life's tasks ...
>
> (Chadwick, 1997: xii–xiii)

Pursuing a similar theme, Deegan (1988) has criticised the professional language of treatments and cures. 'Patients', she argues, are not passive recipients of treatment who 'get cured' or 'rehabilitated' in the same way as a television set may 'get repaired' or a car 'gets tuned up'. A cure-based perspective denies all hope to those whose problems cannot be eliminated in the language of the 'chronic patient'.

People with mental health difficulties, whether these can be reduced by 'treatment' or not, are active agents in an ongoing process of their own recovery. Adopting a perspective grounded in the language of 'disability' rather than that of 'illness', Deegan draws explicit parallels with physical disability and argues that those who are disabled by ongoing physical or psychiatric problems face the challenge of rebuilding valued, satisfying and contributing lives despite the continued presence of their difficulties.

'Recovery' is an alien concept in a traditional psychiatry imbued with a language of the passivity of treatments and cures and the hopelessness of chronicity when these fail to remove the disabilities and dysfunctions on which its science is based (Coleman, 1999).

> Recovery does not refer to an end product or result. It does not mean that one is 'cured'. In fact recovery is marked by an ever-deepening acceptance of our limitations. But now, rather than being an occasion for despair, we find our personal limitations are the ground from which spring our own unique possibilities. This is the paradox of recovery, i.e. that in accepting what we cannot do or be, we begin to

discover who we can be and what we can do. Thus recovery is a process. It is a way of life. It is an attitude and a way of approaching the day's challenges.

(Deegan, 1992: 3)

As with constructions of disability in the domain of physical impairment, there are no assumptions that the person who, for example, has a severed spine must be 'cured' to live a valuable and fulfilling life. Recovery involves considering issues of growth and access to opportunities – the adaptations and accommodations that are necessary to make a reality of inclusion (Perkins and Repper, 1996, 1998a).

We are pressing back against the tide of hopelessness. We are learning that those of us with psychiatric disabilities can become experts in our own self-care. Can regain control over our lives, and can be responsible for our own individual journey of recovery; we are learning that the environment around people must change if we are to be expected to grow.

(Deegan, 1992: 5)

The language of recovery implies active agency, choice and control on the part of the individual in rebuilding their life, with the restoration of hope and dignity that this implies.

In trying to move away from the language of 'patienthood', those who experience mental health difficulties have experimented with different labels. In place of 'patients' we have seen users, survivors, consumers and recipients. Although there are many similarities between these labels there are also important differences (Perkins and Repper, 1998b).

The terms 'users', 'consumers' and 'clients' indicate that the person chose to use or consume services, or to consult as a client. This is misleading. Most people do not have a meaningful choice over what they receive. There is nowhere else to go if you do not like what is on offer in your local service, and the mental health legislation ensures that some of those who do not voluntarily accept what is offered can be compelled to do so. In recognition of the absence of choice, some prefer the term 'recipient' to describe those in contact with mental health services.

'User' is a term more often adopted by those whose aim is to improve the quality of that which they use – mainstream services. This term, like 'recipient', is problematic in its failure to name those who, despite their mental health problems, have not used, or actively avoid, mental health services. The term 'survivor' is a construction used by those who see the mainstream mental health system as irremediable and seek to create radically different alternatives; by those who see themselves as having 'survived' the traumatic experiences of mainstream psychiatry. However, the language of survival fails to acknowledge those who have not survived:

those who have died and those whose lives have been irreversibly damaged by, for example, decades of incarceration in 'old, long-stay back wards'. There are also questions around whether survival is enough. A recovery perspective, for example, goes beyond mere survival, to development and growth.

In order for language to be inclusive, it is important that those with mental health problems retain the right to define themselves; however, explicit consideration of the politics of the chosen language is also vital. What are the implications of the words used (choice and compulsion, surviving and thriving, etc.)? Who is excluded by not being named (those who avoid services, those who fail to survive, etc.)?

Throughout this chapter, we have used the term 'mental health problems' – this too must be problematised. Apart from the 'illness' implications of the term 'mental health', the word 'problems' excludes, by failing to name, the possibility of benefits and assets, and the positive associations of madness.

> It would seem almost impossible to give positive value to mad people when you will not give positive value to their madness.
>
> (Campbell, 1998: 246)

Language and the challenge to exclusion

In promoting positive value, two distinct languages can be discerned (Perkins, 1999). On the one hand, there have been attempts to bridge the void between the 'mad' and the 'sane' in a language of 'distress'. On the other hand there has been a celebration of difference via the language of 'mad pride'.

The language of distress implies a 'continuum'. Everyone gets distressed, but people may be more or less distressed, for longer or shorter periods, with greater or lesser impacts on their lives, and for more or less obvious reasons. In the face of discrimination and exclusion, the desire to minimise difference that is inherent in a language of distress is understandable. However there are problems.

Numerous research studies have shown that, in our society, very clear dividing lines are drawn between understandable distress and apparently incomprehensible madness (Repper and Brooker, 1996; Repper *et al.*, 1997). 'Sane' citizens do not recognise a continuum of misery, but clearly distinguish ordinary misery and despair that is seen as an understandable response to adversity, from the extraordinary thoughts, feelings and behaviour that have been labelled madness. The continuum language of distress also fails to name the very real social disadvantages, loss of rights and personhood, rejection and ridicule of those who cross society's madness divide.

To be mad is to be defined as 'other', not a cosy extension of the everyday experience of distress. A construction of madness as distress denies the reality of difference, and therefore obviates the need for all communities to accommodate that difference. It denies the fact that madness is not always distressing. It denies the expertise of those who have experienced madness. After all, if everyone has experienced distress then everyone has that wisdom.

(Perkins, 1999: 6)

Instead of minimising difference, the language of 'mad pride' celebrates that difference and demands inclusion and citizenship for those defined as different.

The problem is not that difference exists, but the value attached to that difference – when black, gay, mad means 'less than' with all the denial of rights that this entails.

(Perkins 1999: 6)

In criticising a language which minimises difference, parallels can be drawn with the combating of black and lesbian/gay oppression. A language which denies difference – 'acting white', 'passing as straight', 'they're just the same as everyone else except for who they choose to sleep with, the colour of their skin, the extent of their distress ...' – may do little to diminish exclusion.

The question is whether social inclusion can be better fostered, and citizenship promoted, by minimising difference with the language of distress or celebrating difference via the language of mad pride.

Within the user–survivor movement, people have embarked on a process of 'consciousness raising' directed towards understanding experience, and developing a language that describes not merely oppression but identity. Whether in 'madness' or 'distress', there must be a recognition of the power of language to combat exclusion:

To advance the opportunities for people to come together to find their common voice and help potential allies change their basic negative assumptions.

(Carling, 1994: 2)

References

Brandon, D. (1991) 'User power', in P. Barker and S. Baldwin (eds), *Ethical issues in mental health*, London: Chapman and Hall.

Campbell, P. (1998) 'Listening to clients', in P.J. Barker and B. Davidson (eds), *Ethical Strife*, London: Arnold.

Carling, P. (1994) 'Language: a tool for change', *Tempo*, 3, 1: 2.

Cartwright, J. (1998) *Leading the cheers*, London: Hodder and Stoughton.

Chadwick, P.K. (1997) *Schizophrenia: the positive perspective*, London: Routledge.

Chamberlin, J. (1984) 'Speaking for ourselves: an overview of the ex-psychiatric inmates movement', *Psychosocial Rehabilitation Journal*, 515: 3–11.

Coleman, R. (1999) *Recovery an alien concept?*, Gloucester: Handsell.

Daly, M. (1978) *Gynaecology: the meta ethics of radical feminism*, London: The Women's Press.

Deegan, P. (1988) 'Recovery: the lived experience of rehabilitation', *Psychosocial Rehabilitation Journal*, 11: 11–19.

—— (1992) *Recovery, rehabilitation and the conspiracy of hope*, Burlington, VT: Centre for Community Change through Housing and Support.

Department of Health (1995) *Building bridges: a guide to arrangements for inter-agency working for the care and protection of severely mentally ill people*, London: HMSO.

Jamison, K.R. (1989) 'Mood disorders and patterns of creativity in British writers and artists', *Psychiatry*, 32: 125–34.

—— (1993) *Touched with fire: manic depressive illness and the artistic temperament*, New York: The Free Press.

—— (1995) 'Manic depressive illness and creativity', *Scientific American*, February: 46–51.

—— (1996) *An unquiet mind: a memoir of moods and madness*, London: Picador.

Maslow, A. (1970) *The assessment of need*, London: Viking.

Mosher, L. (1999) *Recovery – an alien concept*, paper presented at conference of the same name, 18 November 1996, Chamberlin Hotel, Birmingham.

National Alliance for the Mentally Ill (1996) *Open your mind*, Washington DC: NAMI.

Nieradzik, K. and Cochrane, R. (1985) 'Public attitudes towards mental illness – the effect of behaviour, roles and psychiatric labels', *International Journal of Social Psychiatry*, 31, 1: 23–33.

O'Hagan, M. (1996) 'Two accounts of mental distress', in J. Read and J. Reynolds (eds), *Speaking our minds*, Milton Keynes: Open University.

Perkins, R.E. (1999) 'Madness, distress and the language of inclusion', *Open Mind*, 98: 6.

Perkins, R.E. and Repper, J.M. (1996) *Working alongside people with long term mental health problems*, London: Chapman and Hall. Reprinted 1999 by Stanley Thornes, Cheltenham.

—— (1998a) *Dilemmas in community mental health practice – choice or control* Oxford: Radcliffe Medical Press.

—— (1998b) 'Different but normal: language, labels and professional mental health practice', *Mental Health Care*, 2, 3: 90–3.

Phelan, M., Slade, M. and Thornicroft, G. (1995) 'The Camberwell assessment of need', *British Journal of Psychiatry*, 167: 589–95.

Repper, J.M. and Brooker, C. (1996) 'Attitudes towards community facilities for people with serious mental health problems', *Health and Social Care in the Community*, 4, 5: 290–9.

Repper, J.M., Sayce, L.E., Strong, S. *et al.* (1997) *Tall stories from the back yard. A national survey of local NIMBY opposition to community mental health facilities*, London: Mind Publications.

Sainsbury Centre for Mental Health (1997) *Pulling together: the future roles and training of mental health staff*, London: Sainsbury Centre for Mental Health.
Scheff, T.J. (1975) *Labelling madness*, Englewood Cliffs, NJ: Prentice Hall.
Szasz, T.S. (1973) *The manufacture of madness*, London: Paladin.

15 Race, stigma and stereotyping

The construction of difference in forensic care

Mark Stowell-Smith and
Mick McKeown

Introduction

Into the new millennium, the large institutions of public service are faced
with urgent demands to address more effectively and sensitively the
needs of minority ethnic groups within contemporary multicultural
society. Among other contextual factors, this is set against a backdrop of
the MacPherson Report into the handling by the Metropolitan Police of
the Stephen Lawrence investigation (Home Office, 1999) and recent
media sensationalism surrounding the issue of asylum seekers. The
MacPherson recommendation that all public services must tackle the
thorny issue of institutionalised racism rests uncomfortably against the
racialised government rhetoric and attendant public furore over incoming
refugees. Both of these issues collide in the practice of healthcare professionals attempting to provide services to diverse ethnic groups, including
émigré victims of political and economic oppression, and working in a
system which has typically striven to solve recruitment crises by
poaching the workforce of developing nations.

The institutions of psychiatry have had a particularly chequered
history in dealing with minority groups, no more so than in contemplation of the notion of race. Identified problems are mirrored in
mainstream psychiatric services, but are most prominent within the
forensic sector, where we have chosen to concentrate our attention.
Concerns have been voiced over differential rates of detention, diagnosis
and treatment, and the contribution of racism to unwholesome occupational cultures and episodes of abuse. Our concentration upon the
forensic sector is in one sense 'Goffmanesque', in that scrutiny of the
'extreme' can serve to illuminate features of the mainstream or even
more general social interaction. Similarly, the position of black men of
Afro-Caribbean ethnicity in forensic services has been focused on because
this group in many ways exemplifies most vividly the application of
racist stereotypes. Though the analytic framework we favour is heavily
influenced by social constructionist theorising, there are various connections with Goffman's original work on stigma (Goffman, 1963), not least

in his imaginative challenge to forms of social science attached to simplistic notions of 'facts' and 'truth'. Constructionist perspectives differ from the interactionist theories which typify previous accounts of stigma and identity by privileging language and text as a foundation for social power relations.

In this chapter we suggest that the explanations usually proffered are insufficient to wholly account for the anomalous treatment of black men in psychiatry, and present an analysis which emphasises the social construction of difference. This point will be argued with reference to two pieces of interpretative research of our own which have examined subjective understandings of the position of black men in relation to mental health and psychiatric services, and the medico–legal construct of psychopathy, respectively. Our discussion of these studies explores the employment of particular constructions of race which imply a sense of black otherness set in juxtaposition to an idealised white self. These racialised social constructions resonate with the features of similar public representations of black people which have served various political ends from colonial times through to the discriminatory practices of the twentieth and early twenty-first centuries. The reliance upon the arbitrary signifier of skin colour to demarcate social difference and status is central to the function of these devices for categorising and grading people, and ultimately discrediting them (Goffman, 1963).

For Goffman, the very visibility of skin colour suggests that those groups who have their race attributed this way are more readily stigmatised, and, in effect, de-humanised. Thus rendered less than human, the discredited person is laid open to any manner of discriminatory practices. The people responsible for the application of the stigma are then able to rationalise this inherently irrational state of affairs by constructing a 'stigma theory' which supplies an ideological explanation for their actions (Burns, 1992). It is the forms that such discourse takes, and its effects in the psychiatric system, specifically forensic care, to which we now turn.

Race and forensic psychiatry

The issue of race in relation to psychiatric practice usually arises in the context of discussions around perceived inconsistencies in psychiatric epidemiology. Most notable is the over-representation of ethnic minority groups within certain diagnostic categories, especially in the case of schizophrenia (Cochrane, 1977; Carpenter and Brockington, 1980; Littlewood and Lipsedge, 1982; Ineichen *et al.*, 1984; McGovern and Cope, 1987; Harrison *et al.*, 1988). Associated concerns have been expressed about a tendency within services to concentrate black men in particular at the hard end of psychiatry. They are more likely than their white counterparts to be coercively introduced (Rogers and Faulkner,

1987; Francis, 1989; Home Office, 1992), detained under sections of the
Mental Health Act (Littlewood and Lipsedge, 1982; Barnes *et al.*, 1990),
within secure environments (Bolton, 1984; Norris, 1984; Jones and Berry,
1986; Moodley and Thorneycroft, 1988; Noble and Rodger, 1989;
McKeown and Stowell-Smith, 1996), subject to physical treatments
(Littlewood and Cross, 1980; Chen *et al.*, 1991) and use of restraint or
seclusion (Flaherty and Meagher, 1980; Lawson *et al.*, 1984; Mason,
1995). In the extreme, allegations of explicit personal and implicit institutionalised racism have been raised, and implicated in service failings,
incidents of abuse, and deaths in custody (HMSO, 1992; Prins, 1993).

These issues do not solely arise as problems for psychiatry; they are
paralleled within the criminal justice system. Again, in contrast to similarly situated whites, black men are more likely to be stopped and
searched (Browne, 1990), committed to trial at the Crown Court (Shalice
and Gordon, 1990), receive a custodial sentence (Home Office, 1989;
Hudson, 1989), or receive a psychiatric disposal (Browne, 1990). Thus
black people are criminalised and psychiatrised to a greater degree than
white people, and are consequently disproportionately represented in
hospital and prison populations. For instance, Afro-Caribbeans constitute
10.7 per cent of the male prison population despite accounting for only
1.2 per cent of the total population of Great Britain, with the respective
corresponding figures for ethnic minority groups, as a whole, being 15.5
per cent and between 4 and 5 per cent (NACRO, 1991). Boast and
Chesterman (1995) have argued that the criminal justice system and
psychiatric services operate together in concentrating black people within
secure hospitals.

Accounting for the discrepancies

Commentaries upon the issue of race in psychiatry typically account for
the differential treatment of black people in one of two ways. On the one
hand, the over-representation of black people in psychiatric institutions is
attributed to an actual higher incidence of severe mental illness among
black people (Rwegellera, 1977; Dean *et al.*, 1981; Cochrane and Bal,
1989). Such explanations either rely upon a perceived biologically determined vulnerability or an emphasis upon the role of environmental stress
factors specific to the experience of being black in Britain (Odergaard,
1932; Bagley, 1971; Littlewood and Lipsedge, 1982; Harrison *et al.*, 1988;
Glover, 1989; Frederick, 1991). The alternative standpoint focuses on the
part played by ethnocentricity in exaggerating the incidence of black
mental disorder (Littlewood and Lipsedge, 1982; Mercer, 1986; Fernando,
1991), calling into question the objectivity of the entire diagnostic process
(Littlewood, 1990; Fernando, 1991).

A third path to understanding the treatment of black people within
forensic psychiatry is contemplation of the role of language in the

construction of social groups and relations. Such a perspective privileges language and text as more than just a system for describing objective reality. Rather, discourse is seen as having a constitutive role in bringing things into being. In this sense, the notion of race itself offers an illuminating example of the way in which versions of reality and selfhood are constructed in language. This constructionist view is employed here in discussing research of our own which has focused upon black men in relation to particular points of contact with psychiatry (Stowell-Smith and McKeown, 1999a, 1999b).

Locating mental health in black and white men

The first study utilised Q methodology (Stephenson, 1935; Stainton Rogers, 1995) to elicit discursive accounts expressed by a range of interdisciplinary psychiatric practitioners who were asked to consider the position of black men with respect to mental health and service provision. The participants were requested to complete two Q sorts, relating to understandings of mental health and policy or to treatment prescriptions respectively. They were split into two groups, with one group required to sort the respective statements as if they were applicable to a white man, and the others to do so as if for a black man.

Thirteen interpretable factors were found in this study, and are described in detail elsewhere (Stowell-Smith and McKeown, 1999a); here we offer some general observations arising from our interpretation of these accounts. With respect to understandings of mental health, the white factors were largely anti-biological, and tended to emphasise notions of individuality and internally experienced psychopathology. In contrast, the black accounts de-emphasised the importance of individual psychological phenomena, with one supporting a biological understanding of causation of mental disorder, linking this with race. In downplaying the internal worlds of prospective psychiatric service users, the black factors stress the role of external, extra-psychic determinants of psychological distress and psychiatric morbidity. Similarly, the white policy accounts focused their attention upon the impact of treatment interventions upon individuals and intra-psychic experiences, towards the attainment of a state of mental well-being framed in terms of personal autonomy. The most desirable treatments are seen as talking therapies, delivered in non-institutional community settings. In one account, dangerousness is seen as a consequence of a disturbed mind, with psychiatry welcomed as having a curative and protective role with such individuals. Conversely, the black policy factors have a strong critical and anti-interventionist edge to them.

An overall comparison between the factors elicited from the two conditions of instruction reveals a distinction between the ways in which the mental health of black men and white men were constructed by the

participants. Broadly speaking, the mental health of black men was identified in relation to external reality, in contrast to that of white men
which was characterised in relation to internal reality. These relationships
were exemplified in the black accounts' engagement with a critical focus
upon macro issues, such as society, culture and the role of institutions,
compared to the prominence of intra-psychic phenomena within the white
accounts.

Race, the self, and psychopathy

The second piece of research employed discourse analysis to examine the
seemingly paradoxical under-representation of black men in the legal classification of psychopathy (Stowell-Smith and McKeown, 1999b).
Discourse analytic methods have been utilised by researchers sympathetic
to post-structuralist ideas in the reflexive and interpretative analysis of
texts, paying attention to the structuring effects of language (Burman,
1991). This approach was employed in the analysis of admission reports of
people admitted to a special hospital under the medico–legal category of
psychopathy. The relevant documentation was scrutinised for eighteen
white and eighteen black subjects, matched with respect to diagnostic,
admission and discharge characteristics. The textual analysis allowed the
description of two distinct sets of discursive structures at work in these
admission reports, one mostly associated with the white reports, the other
mostly associated with the black reports.

The narration of white psychopathy was a discourse which emphasised
the internal world of the subject. Characteristically, there would be a
storying of the patient's life events and history in tandem with a commentary upon his internal experience of these events, positing a causative
relationship between one and the other. Hence, in these accounts, the
dangerous behaviour of the white subjects is determined by their internal
experiences. There would be a tendency in these reports to focus upon the
role of previous psychological trauma in the commission of offending, to
the extent that in some reports the offence was represented as a form of
strangled communication. Certain descriptions showed evidence of the
reality of the offence paling into insignificance besides the detailed discussion of the patient's internal world such that it could seem to almost
disappear.

In contrast, the discursive accounts of black psychopathy narrate
dangerousness differently. This discourse shifts the focus onto outer experience, with the offence presented as the culminating act of an escalating
pattern of behaviour, with minimal attention paid to the person's psychological state. Here the internal world of the subject is de-emphasised with
diagnostic inferences made almost exclusively on the basis of the
behaviour. In a reversal of the accounting for white psychopathy, wherein
the offending behaviour was obscured, in this discourse the subjects them-

selves could almost disappear as a dynamic centre of awareness, over-whelmed by the narration of behaviour.

Black men as 'other'

The results of this research can be discussed with reference to previous work which has theorised the construction of race and the powerful role played by such discourse in historical and contemporary social relations. From such perspectives, Western psychiatry stands accused of forging an unholy alliance between scientific materialism and imperialist racism (Fernando, 1991). Dalal (1993) has suggested the dominance of a partic-ular stereotypical view of non-Europeans, which has its origins in the sixteenth-century European project to colonise the rest of the world. The moral justification for colonialism required a way of differentiating the coloniser from the colonised, resulting in a conceptual demarcation between us and them; self and other:

> Colour was used as the primary visible signifier to distinguish 'us' from 'them'. In order to do this properly it was necessary for the hallucinatory whitening of all the peoples of Europe including the Roman, the Greek, the Celt, and of course Jesus Christ, so that they could be distinguished from 'the coloured'.
>
> (Dalal, 1993: 278)

Thus, for Dalal, race is socially and politically constructed in a partic-ular time and place. The race construct is then available to serve a purpose in the maintenance of iniquitous power relations, primarily by under-scoring a sense of difference and separateness:

> the production of 'representations' of the Other, images and beliefs which categorise people in terms of real or attributed differences when compared to the Self. There is therefore, a dialectic between Self and Other in which the attributed characteristics of Other refract contrasting characteristics of Self, and vice versa.
>
> (Miles, 1989: 10)

Such depictions of minority groups as alien and separate have often been conjoined with a wider set of representations of black men as a threat. For Miles (1989: 14), these representations can be traced to Greco-Roman views of the African as a 'barbarian ... [who] was seen to lack the capacities of intelligible speech and reason, capacities that were considered to be the quintessence of Roman culture'.

One of the ways in which notions of differentness have been expanded has been the contrasting of versions of otherness with an idealised version of the self (Henriques *et al.*, 1984). Geertz (1979) describes this white, Western, male self as a:

> bounded, unique, more or less integrated motivational and cognitive universe, a dynamic centre of awareness, emotion, judgement and action, organised into a distinctive whole and set contrastively against other such wholes and against a social and natural background.
>
> (Geertz, 1979: 229)

In stark contrast to this psychologised white selfhood, Fanon (1986) has remarked upon depictions of black men which stress aspects of physicality, constructing them as hypersexual beings of low intelligence. Similarly, Rutherford (1988) has remarked upon the extent to which black masculinity is viewed essentially as physicality, divorced from emotions and cognitive faculties. Psychoanalytic theorists have suggested that such racial distinctions provide a vehicle for the projection of unwanted aspects of the ideal white self into the denigrated black subject (Timimi, 1996).

However, if the race construct is stripped of its representational power, its status as a biological entity of use in demarcating social groups becomes absolutely devalued. Similarly, ethnocentric beliefs in the superiority of one's own culture are difficult to sustain by appealing to biological science. The genetic evidence for a biological taxonomy of race is extremely weak, with greater genetic diversity within the accepted classificatory racial groups than can be found between them. Such findings have led Jones (1981) to conclude that 'the idea of racial type – and, some would argue, of 'race' itself – is no longer a very useful one in human biology'.

Although the very idea of race is contested, non-white minority groups cannot avoid being allocated to various racial categories, wherein they become subject to discrimination. The perceived racial differences are thus socially defined, reflecting the differential experiences of people in particular political and material situations. Clearly, any apparent differences are explicable in terms of the pertaining social relations, precluding their attribution to essential (racial) qualities (FitzGerald, 1993).

Otherness and forensic psychiatry

Despite the debunking of the race construct, concerns over race and racism remain live issues for the institutions of forensic psychiatry. A possible conclusion is that, even though race is empty of conceptual validity, its appeal and utility for the organisation and delivery of forensic practice is more enduring. The characteristic integration of black men as both 'other' and 'threat' reveals the way in which forensic psychiatry might itself be informed and circumscribed by culturally available discourse. An argument can be developed making the case for the influence of wider social representations of black otherness within the micro-practices and social relations of forensic psychiatric institutions. A dialectic or reciprocal exchange of knowledge, understandings and representations can be posited at the intersection of professional and lay domains (Parker *et al.*, 1995). The leakage of medicalised language and practices into popular usage and culture has been commented on and described in terms of a psychological complex (Rose, 1990; De Swann, 1990). Similarly, lay discourse and practices seep into the psychiatric arena, as evidenced by the research discussed here.

Potent and extreme examples of the infiltration of forensic psychiatric practices by racialised lay representations are furnished in some of the more recent critical commentaries upon secure institutions. In the case of the 1992 Ashworth Hospital Inquiry, perhaps more worrying is the standpoint of managers post-inquiry that the 'cultural' problems of the institution have been resolved by recourse to values-based staff training, such that the Inquiry Report was seen, four years on, as an historical and, by implication, redundant document in certain quarters (McKeown and Stowell-Smith, 1996). The reports into the deaths in custody of numerous young black men in Broadmoor prison suggest the pervasive impact of the stereotypical view that black patients inherently pose a greater risk of violence or aggression than their white counterparts. The prominence of such views was such that the official account of the circumstances surrounding the death of Orville Blackwood and his unfortunate peers was subtitled 'Big, Black and Dangerous' (Prins, 1993).

In the current NHS climate of evidenced-based practice, the idea that irrational and discriminatory constructs might inform the care and management of forensic patients casts into doubt the assumed scientific objectivity and neutrality of forensic psychiatry and its various practitioner groupings. Of course, forensic psychiatry is not alone in this, there being numerous examples of objectively unsupportable racist stereotypes within the wider scientific community and in other carceral domains (for instance, the transatlantic controversy between psychologists propounding and disputing a genetic, and racially demarcated, determination of intelligence, reported in the *Guardian* newspaper in 1996). More recently, there were calls for the resignation of the Director of Prisons for his assertion, supposedly based on research findings, that the deaths in custody of black prisoners were due to their inherent vulnerability to strangulation while being restrained (*Guardian*, 1998).

Conclusions

A social constructionist perspective on the institutional handling of race within forensic psychiatry allows us to focus attention on the construction of difference. A powerful example of this is the demarcation on racial lines of different versions of selfhood; a split between an idealised post-enlightenment view of the white self, set apart from a pejorative view of black subjectivity as 'otherness'. If the starting point for psychiatry generally, and hence specifically for forensic psychiatric practices, is the psychopathology of white, Western selves, then the anomalous treatment of black patients is at least partially understandable in these terms. Thus, black men become more likely to be treated for disorders such as schizophrenia seen to have a biological (physical) basis, and given biochemical (physical) treatments. Concurrent with this, the emphasis on black physicality as threat leads to a concentration of black men at the hard end of psychiatric services, subject to increasing rates of physical (bodily) interventions such as restraint and seclusion, and carceral disposal. The seemingly paradoxical under-representation of black men in the archetypal forensic category of psychopath is rendered less incomprehensible by contemplating the extent to which black 'others' fail to fit the paradigm of self and mind (abnormal or otherwise), necessary to be so described. Such constructions of difference deserve more attention in the planning and delivery of forensic care, the training of practitioners, and analyses of discrepancies in treatment.

Overt racism and discrimination within psychiatric services is easy to spot and can be combated by strong management and progressive trade unions, both of which have been lacking in the tainted history of some forensic institutions. The forms of indirect, institutional racism highlighted in the MacPherson Report can be less easy for organisations and professionals to acknowledge and identify, insidious in their actions and effects, and hence difficult to remedy. One set of responses has focused upon raising awareness and sensitivity towards authentic cultural differences between various ethnic groups and how these may be expressed in terms of genuine health need, or misinterpreted by relatively insensitive personnel or services. A range of training and policy initiatives has been urged, largely at the level of shifting the values of individuals and organisations or targeting some of the most obvious anomalies in treatment. Alternately, separate services for black people have been advocated, at least as a short-term solution (Fernando *et al.*, 1998). Most informed commentators agree that any solutions which focus solely upon the level of service provision will be inadequate to the task in hand. Racism in wider society and its relationship to structural and legal processes needs to be tackled systematically. In doing so, the power of language in sustaining iniquitous social relations should not be neglected.

A point for sober reflection in this respect is provided by one of the pivotal moments in the evidence given to the MacPherson Inquiry. In the immediate aftermath of the murderous assault on Stephen Lawrence, two passers-by provided comfort by the roadside and whispered to Stephen that he was loved as his life ebbed away. Despite this heartbreaking kindness, the couple later admitted that their first reaction was to hesitate to get involved, because the presence of two black men (Stephen was accompanied by his distressed friend Duwayne) caused them to 'sense danger'.

This minor vignette within a set of altogether more tragic and vicious events, an exemplary honest appraisal in hindsight of a fleeting moment in time, suggests the persuasiveness of a stereotype of black men as 'other' and threat, and the magnitude of the challenge to turn this around.

References

Bagley, C. (1971) 'Mental illness in immigrant minorities in London', *Journal of Biosocial Science*, 3: 449–59.

Barnes, M., Bowl, R. and Fisher, M. (1990) *Sectioned: social services and the 1983 Mental Health Act*, London: Tavistock.

Boast, N. and Chesterman, P. (1995) 'Black people and secure psychiatric facilities: patterns of processing and the role of stereotypes', *British Journal of Criminology*, 35: 218–35.

Bolton, G. (1984) 'Management of compulsorily admitted patients in a high security unit', *International Journal of Social Psychiatry*, 30: 77–84.

Browne, D. (1990) *Black people, mental health and the courts*, London: NACRO.

Burman, E. (1991) 'What discourse is not', *Philosophical Psychology*, 4: 325–41.

Burns, T. (1992) *Erving Goffman*, Routledge, London.

Carpenter, I. and Brockington, I. (1980) 'A study of mental illness in Asians, West Indians and Africans living in Manchester', *British Journal of Psychiatry*, 137: 201–5.

Chen, E., Harrison, G. and Standen, P. (1991) 'Management of first episode psychotic illness in Afro-Caribbean patients', *British Journal of Psychiatry*, 158: 517–22.

Cochrane, R. (1977) 'Mental illness in immigrants in England and Wales: an analysis of mental hospital admissions, 1971', *Social Psychiatry*, 12: 25–35.

Cochrane, R. and Bal, S. (1989) 'Mental hospital admission rates of immigrants to England: a comparison of 1971 and 1981', *Social Psychiatry and Psychiatric Epidemiology*, 24: 2–11.

Dalal, F.N. (1993) 'Race and racism: an attempt to organise difference', *Group Analysis*, 26: 277–90.

Dean, G., Walsh, D., Downing, H. and Shelley, E. (1981) 'First admissions of native-born immigrants to psychiatric hospitals in south east England, 1976', *British Journal of Psychiatry*, 139: 506–12.

De Swann, A. (1990) *The management of normality*, London: Routledge.

Dolan, B., Polley, K., Allen, R. and Norton, K. (1991) 'Addressing racism in psychiatry: is the therapeutic community model applicable?', *The International Journal of Social Psychiatry*, 37: 71–9.

Fanon, F. (1986) *Black skin, white masks*, London: Pluto.

Fernando, S. (1991) *Mental health, race and culture*, Basingstoke: Macmillan in association with MIND Publications.

Fernando, S., Ndegwa, D. and Wilson, M. (1998) *Forensic psychiatry, race and culture*, London: Routledge.

FitzGerald, M. (1993) 'Racism: establishing the phenomenon', in D. Cook and B. Hudson (eds), *Racism and criminology*, London: Sage.

Flaherty, J. and Meagher, R. (1980) 'Measuring racial bias in inpatient treatment', *American Journal of Psychiatry*, 137: 679–82.

Francis, E. (1989) 'Black people, dangerousness and psychiatric compulsion', in A. Brackx and C. Grimshaw (eds), *Mental health care in crisis*, London: Pluto.

Frederick, J. (1991) *Positive thinking for mental health*, London: The Black Mental Health Group.

Geertz, C. (1979) 'From the natives' point of view: on the nature of anthropological understanding', in P. Rabinow and W. Sullivan (eds), *Interpretive social science*, Berkeley: University of California Press.

Glover, G. (1989) 'Why is there a high rate of schizophrenia in British Caribbeans?', *British Journal of Hospital Medicine*, 42: 48–51.

Goffman, E. (1963) *Stigma: notes on the management of spoiled identity*, Harmondsworth: Penguin.

Guardian (1996) 'The gene genies', *Guardian 2*, 1 May: 2–3.

—— (1998) 'Anger at gaffe over black's jail death', news item, 27 March: 5.

Harrison, G., Owens, D., Holton, A. *et al.* (1988) 'A prospective study of severe mental disorder in Afro-Caribbean patients', *Psychological Medicine*, 18: 643–57.

Henriques, J., Holloway, W., Urwin, C. *et al.* (1984) *Changing the subject: psychology, social regulation and subjectivity*, London: Methuen.

HMSO (1992) *Report of the committee of inquiry into complaints about Ashworth Hospital*, London: HMSO.

Home Office (1989) *Statistical bulletin: the ethnic group of those proceeded against or sentenced by the courts in the Metropolitan Police District in 1984*, London: HMSO.

—— (1992) *Discussion paper. Services for people of black and ethnic minority groups: issues of race and culture*, Department of Health/Home Office, London: HMSO.

—— (1999) *The inquiry into the matters arising from the death of Stephen Lawrence*, London: HMSO.

Hudson, B. (1989) 'Discrimination and disparity: the influence of race on sentencing', *New Community*, 16, 1: 112–38.

Ineichen, B., Harrison, G. and Morgan, H. (1984) 'Psychiatric admissions in Bristol: 1. Geographical and ethnic factors', *British Journal of Psychiatry*, 145: 600–4.

Jones, G. and Berry, M. (1986) 'Regional secure units: the emerging picture', in G. Edwards (ed.), *Current issues in clinical psychology*, vol. 4, London: Plenum.

Jones, J. (1981) 'How different are human races?', *Nature*, 293: 188–90.

Lawson, W., Jerome, A and Werner, P. (1984) 'Race, violence and psychopathology', *The Journal of Clinical Psychiatry*, 45: 294–7.

Lewis, G., Croft-Jeffreys, C. and David, A. (1990) 'Are British psychiatrists racist?', *British Journal of Psychiatry*, 157: 410–15.

Littlewood, R. (1990) 'From categories to contexts: a decade of the new cross-cultural psychiatry', *British Journal of Psychiatry*, 156: 308–27.

Littlewood, R. and Cross, S. (1980) 'Ethnic minorities and psychiatric services', *Sociology of Health and Illness*, 2: 194–201.

Littlewood, R. and Lipsedge, M. (1982) *Aliens and alienists: ethnic minorities and psychiatry*, Harmondsworth: Penguin.

McGovern, D. and Cope, R. (1987) 'The compulsory detention of males of different ethnic groups', *British Journal of Psychiatry*, 150: 505–12.

McKeown, M. and Stowell-Smith, M. (1996) 'Ashworth's record on race', letter to the editor, *Nursing Times*, 92: 38, 26.

Mason, T. (1995) *Seclusion in the special hospitals: a descriptive and analytic study*, London: Special Hospitals Service Authority.

Mercer, K. (1986) 'Racism and transcultural psychiatry', in P. Miller and N. Rose (eds), *The power of psychiatry*, Cambridge: Polity Press.

Miles, R. (1989) *Racism*, London: Routledge.

Moodley, P. and Thorneycroft, G. (1988) 'Ethnic group and compulsory detention', *Medicine, Science and the Law*, 28: 324–8.

NACRO (1991) *Briefing: race and criminal justice*, London: NACRO.

Noble, P. and Rodger, S. (1989) 'Violence by psychiatric in-patients', *British Journal of Psychiatry*, 155: 384–90.

Norris, M. (1984) *Integration of special hospital patients into the community*, Aldershot: Gower.

Odergaard, O. (1932) 'Emigration and insanity', *Acta Psychiatrica Neurologica Scandanavica*, Suppl. 4.

Parker, I., Georgaca, E., Harper, D. *et al.* (1995) *Deconstructing psychopathology*, London: Sage.

Prins, H. (1993) *Report of the committee of inquiry into the death in Broadmoor Hospital of Orville Blackwood and a review of the death of two other Afro-Caribbean patients: big, black and dangerous?*, London: Special Hospitals Service Authority.

Rogers, A. and Faulkner, A. (1987) 'A place of safety', *MIND's Research into Police Referrals to the Psychiatric Services*, London: MIND.

Rose, N. (1990) *Governing the soul: the shaping of the private self*, London: Routledge.

Rutherford, J. (1988) 'Who's that man?', in R. Chapman, and J. Rutherford (eds), *Male order: unwrapping masculinities*, London: Lawrence and Wishart.

Rwegellera, G. (1977) 'Psychiatric morbidity among West Africans and West Indians living in London', *Psychological Medicine*, 7: 317–29.

Shalice, A. and Gordon, P. (1990) *Black people, white justice? Race and the criminal justice system*, London: Runnymede Trust.

Stainton Rogers, R. (1995) 'Q-Methodology', in J.A. Smith, R Harre and L. Van Langehoven (eds), *Rethinking methods in psychology*, Buckingham: Open University Press.

Stephenson, W. (1935) 'Correlating persons instead of tests', *Character and Personality*, 4: 17–24.

Stowell-Smith, M. and McKeown, M. (1999a) 'Locating mental health in black and white men: a Q-methodological study', *Journal of Health Psychology*, 4: 209–22.

—— (1999b) 'Race, psychopathy and the self: a discourse analytic study', *British Journal of Medical Psychology*, 72: 459–70.

Timimi, S. (1996) 'Race and colour in internal and external reality', *British Journal of Psychotherapy*, 13: 183–92.

16 The mentally disordered offender

Looking-glass monsters: reflections of the paedophile in popular culture

Dave Mercer and Tuxephoni Simmonds

Introduction

The inclusion of the mentally disordered offender in a healthcare text dealing with human difference, 'otherness' and exclusion is both persuasive and problematic. Collectively, those individuals who transgress legal *and* moral codes face a double stigma, typically characterised as a *sickness* of mind and spirit. Their treatment or management is often enacted within institutions of maximum security that are geographically, socially and symbolically remote from the society against which they have offended. It is not unusual for their crimes to attract widespread reportage and condemnation, as the 'monsters' of tabloid headlines. Here is the first contradiction of their 'moral career', as shameful pariah and public persona – of secrecy and scrutiny. In an age of psychiatric revisionism, democracy and de-institutionalisation, forensic provision signifies a vestige of the era of the asylum, whose inhabitants occupy a sinister world. It is a world where care must compete with containment, custody and control; where the patient is a prisoner; where the client is coerced; and where rehabilitation and reform are inseparably linked to wider debates about screening and surveillance of the social body. Faced by the spectre of the 'dangerous individual', then, stigma is inevitable and functional. Or, is it?

This chapter will suggest that benchmarking good practice in forensic provision requires a deeper level of analysis which engages critically with professional knowledge, media representations and public attitudes. At the very least we must begin to understand the dynamic process that constructs the mentally disordered offender as a complex interplay between 'mad-men' (and women), 'mad-doctors' and the mass media. We need to explore the fear and loathing which accompanies a psychiatric diagnosis of the criminal, the public panic and professional despair surrounding treatment, transfer and recidivism. One starting point might be to challenge the representation of the disordered offender as an homogenous population; and to note that many of those who encounter criminal justice and mental health services, without extreme or serious offences, are themselves victims of violence and abuse. And this is indeed so.

In contrast, though, we have chosen to take the path less travelled in outlining an alternative perspective, focusing on the paedophile to illustrate the argument. For, with little doubt, this group of offenders challenges faith in behavioural science, confuses personal feelings and professional agendas, and ultimately leads us to question the ethics of medical intervention. Bluntly stated, the forensic care-plan is one strategy aimed at protection of the self and the soul. If some offenders threaten physical safety, others offer a glimpse into the darkest recesses of desire; bad men may terrify us, but they also give flesh to our dreams. Where the medico–legal discourses are conjoined in the arena of 'dangerous sexualities', categories of sexual deviance – as departures from material norms – symbolise 'regimes of truth'. At a practice level, the policing of *passion* is a powerful illustration of treatment as a political tool, where stigma is an unpleasant side-effect.

Theorising sexuality, from pathology to postmodernity

Early critics of the therapeutic state (Kittrie, 1971) drew attention to the way that an expansion of psychiatric intervention had replaced traditional mechanisms of punishment. Behaviours viewed as 'deviant', such as interpersonal violence, sexual assault and child abuse, became the focus of treatment and the territory of experts. In each case, though, the medicalisation process mirrored an established pattern of basing diagnosis upon the infraction of moral or ethical codes; removing both the actor, and the act, from any larger social or sexual context. Neutralised by the language of 'mental hygiene', the political dimension of pathology was obscured (Goffman, 1961), and the deviant embraced more firmly within the social body. If this stigmatisation of the 'non-person' began with the involuntary confinement of the 'mentally ill' (Foucault, 1967), it was reinforced through the collaboration of law and psychiatry. Indeed, the partnership between these two powerful institutions derives from a similarity, rather than a difference, in their 'cryptonormative' functions (Leifer, 1969). Nowhere is this view of interconnectedness seen to be more justified than in relation to the shocking and bizarre crimes of the sexual offender, as a distinct *class* of deviant: 'At this point, forensic psychiatry meets up with the most important discourses on perverse sexuality, namely sexology and psychoanalysis' (Cameron and Frazer, 1987).

By focusing on the pioneering work of Krafft Ebing and Freud, Cameron and Frazer (1987) offer a feminist critique of dominant explanations of sexual murder. Differentiating between 'descriptive' (biologic) and 'interpretative' (psychic) accounts, they illustrate the gendered and cultural assumptions which constructed both nineteenth-century forensic science and criminology. From these insights we can begin to explore the discursive practices that manufacture, and manage, distinctive 'sub-species' of being within a Foucauldian (1981) analysis of sexual power/knowledge.

In his critique of the 'repressive hypothesis', Foucault (1981) reconceptualised the sexual subject by noting how the 'secret' of sex had become enshrined in a proliferation of instructional discourses, supported by the elaborate practices of *'scientia sexualis'*. This 'psychiatrisation of perverse pleasure' sees the sexual body as a site of regulation, control and surveillance where power, rather than residing in the juridical application of legislative sanction, operates through the internalisation of knowledge and ideas as 'truth': 'Through them we find our innermost sexual souls cleansed through the verbalisation of desires and practices in medical, psychiatric, criminal, educational, sociological, philosophical and historical examinations' (Evans, 1993: 19). In the realm of offending behaviour, diagnostic typologies are merged with criminal identities in the construction of such non-citizens as the 'sex' prisoner (Foucault, 1977).

The explosion of discourses about sex and sexuality have become a characteristic of contemporary popular culture, to the extent that there is now talk about the sexualisation of advanced capitalist societies. Technological advances of the late twentieth century, which have mediated this mass marketing of sexual interests and commodities, are consistent with the descriptor of postmodernity: 'Not just in pornography as narrowly defined, but also in mainstream Hollywood cinema and prime-time television drama, newspapers and magazines, pop music and video, advertising and fashion photography, images of sexuality and their meaning abound' (McNair, 1996: 2). Here, traditional distinctions and categories are eroded, singular accounts and explanations are challenged, and a diversity of discourses and scripts compete in any attempts to understand social or sexual realities. The materialist contradiction, between public consumption of sexual production and the personal choice of an alternative lifestyle, has witnessed an escalation of political resistance aimed at recognition and citizenship. Crystallised by the struggle to de-medicalise and validate homosexuality through the 'gay rights' movement (Bayer, 1981), an increasing number of minority groups have confronted the norm of procreative heterosexuality in advocating a 'different kind of loving' (Brame *et al.*, 1997).

As a consequence of these trends, the hidden worlds of the sexual 'outsider' have lost their obscurity through social discourse: 'Of these, a small number become a special focus of attention and these frequently provoke an intense response; their appearances are not merely sanctioned severely, but their dangers advertised and their potential suspected, and actual practitioners are aggressively pursued' (Simon, 1996: 125). Against a backdrop of real risk and moral panic around child abuse and child pornography, the paedophile has emerged as an icon of evil in populist reports of sexual crime (Spargo, 1999).

Paraphilia, perverse pleasure and the policing of passion

Regardless of trenchant critique, dominant ideologies about sexuality have proved remarkably resistant in the domain of forensic practice. The distinction between 'fixated' and 'regressed' paedophiles, first introduced by Krafft Ebing, retains clinical currency. Indeed, sociological studies are singled out as blameworthy for making the therapists' job more difficult (Prendergast, 1991); it is suggested that an awareness of socio-cultural sexual difference represents collusion with perpetrators, rather than a challenge to unravel complex sexual metaphors. If the importance of addressing sexuality is now recognised in the delivery of forensic nursing care (Evans and Clarke, 2000), paedophilia remains as one item on a checklist of 'paraphilic behaviours'. The problem facing healthcare workers and clinicians in this area is not difficult to comprehend. In rejecting the 'codified system which arranges sexual acts on a continuum from "perverse" to "normal" and talk instead of "diversity", progressive thinkers leave only the divide between consensual and non-consensual sex-acts' (O'Connell-Davidson and Layden, 1998). Where sexual attraction is focused upon the pre-pubescent child, who cannot legally give consent and lacks those semiotics of the body which signify the erotic, an empathic response is not untypically compromised (Simon, 1996).

A major achievement of wider feminist challenges to the medicalisation of sexual crime (Dobash and Dobash, 1992) has been enacted at a policy level in terms of provision, across the criminal justice system, for victims and survivors of male violence. It has also been noted, though, that as sexual violence has been allocated a central position in theorising patriarchal power the 'gaze' has remained firmly fixed on the experiences of women. The neglect of critical inquiry into the social world of perpetrators, it is argued, leaves unquestioned the dominant psychiatric explanations of disease and pathology. Confronting the androcentric bias which characterises most of the empirical work in this area, Scully calls for an exploration of the 'reality' of the 'real experts' by critically invading and examining the social constructions of men who rape (Scully, 1990). A similar approach to interviewing convicted rapists in the USA (Kellett, 1995) revealed a series of discourses that perpetuated gender hatred and offending, while acting as defensive strategies in the justification of those behaviours. If individual accounts of sexual offending are rooted within a larger discursive domain, and the identity of the 'sex offender' is played out in the institutional structures of law and psychiatry, there is a need to access the narrative voices of prisoners and detained patients.

The kind of research outlined above signals an advance on bio-essentialism generally, and affords a new way to approach the sexuality of the paedophile by focusing attention on the 'sexual scripts' that invest actions and actors with erotic content (Simon, 1996). If this perspective promises a larger project around the social construction and management of desire, it has not been without its critics. Indeed, in an acrimonious retort to recent legislation relating to the possession of child pornography in Canada, Doidge (1999) singles out the 'insidious' writings of Foucault as providing a 'haven for perversion' in the 'muddy waters' of postmodernity. This kind of narrow reading, failing to see history as a way of 'diagnosing' the present (Kendall and Wickham, 1999), does however direct attention to the discourses which construct 'contingencies' of the 'erotic' (child) and 'innocent' (childhood); focusing on campaigns to 'de-stigmatise' and 'decriminalise' adult–child sexual relations, and the need to protect young people from sexual abuse.

It has been noted that the 'voice' of the paedophile has been silenced by shame, stigma and the fear of imprisonment. Or, that the few 'stories' which do enter the public domain are communicated in the language of media outrage or medical ownership (Plummer, 1995). In opposition to this hostile or clinical reporting of 'sexual abuse' is a narrative strand that advocates 'child love' and 'sexual citizenship for children', expressed largely through the political pamphlets of groups such as PAL (Paedophile Action for Liberation) and PIE (Paedophile Information Exchange) (PIE, 1978; O'Carroll, 1980; CAPM, 1982). Social taboo, legal sanctions and tabloid sensationalism guarantee a powerful resistance to these articulations of 'damned desire': 'All the fashionable literature on marginality/outsiders/silenced voices allows no space for these marginal voices to be heard. They were an embarrassment to even the most liberal of voices. They should be silenced' (Plummer, 1995: 119).

This brief review of forbidden sexualities is central to the stuff of forensic practice, yet it has a resonance for healthcare agents in a much wider sense – shifting attention from the role of social control to social surveillance. An image of the paedophile, through the 'psychiatrisation of perverse pleasure', is reflected in the 'pedagogisation of childhood' (Foucault, 1981). Thus, 'Children become defined as pre- or a-sexual, innocent beings with, however, a sexual potential that must be protected by a wide range of guardians, doctors, teachers, nurses and, of course, parents' (Evans, 1993: 17). The next section of this chapter moves on to explore these ideas in the context of current concerns for healthcare workers, concluding with a specific focus on the institutional management of the sexual offender; a journey from the public world of media representations to the private world of the prison and special hospital.

The dreamchild, the pageant queen and pornography

Contemporary literature attests to the enduring themes of predatory abuser and seductive child (Nabokov, 1955; Prager, 1999). It is a well rehearsed 'fiction', in which the reader is offered a romantic version of illicit love (Ray, 1998) or the horrific description of sadistic child rape (Bukowski, 1983). In an increasingly sexualised 'pomo' (postmodern) marketplace, incest has become the stuff of chic, and allegedly empowering, fantasy: 'The word "father" has become virtually synonymous with "sex offender" ' (Califia, 1994). Perhaps the tragic death of tiny beauty pageant queen JonBenet Ramsey (Wecht and Bosworth, 1998), as a metaphor for innocence defiled and destroyed, is brought into focus when viewed through the 'historical lens' of nineteenth-century textual and visual discourses. A legacy of art and prose has manufactured the erotic 'dreamchild', with paedophilia located at the cultural centre of desire and denial: 'Demonizing this figure at the same time we call loudly for his presence, asserting his marginality as we proclaim his importance, dissociating as we make his alliance, we anoint as we execute the pedophile' (Kincaid, 1994: 5).

A feminist critique has condemned this commodification of children's sexuality, linking desire with fantasy production, for promoting exploitation and abuse: 'The implication is that children are available sexually and that youth is the most desirable form of sexuality' (Elliot, 1992: 219). It is an insidious and de-sensitising process that erodes the barriers of acceptability and, unwittingly perhaps, reinforces the claims of the paedophile as pornographer. If these connections become much more transparent in relation to the 'childification' of adult women in the commercial sex industry, it has been suggested that child pornography has received too little critical attention from anti-pornography campaigners. Thus it seems that 'a percentage of the general public finds these forms of sexual violence plausible enough for "fiction", but unbelievable and unacceptable in reality, regardless of the testimony of child and adult survivors' (Kelly, 1992: 114).

Despite a growing body of experimental and experiential evidence to support a correlation between pornography and harm, from social science research (Russell, 1993: Dines *et al.*, 1998) to therapeutic work (Lee, 1988; Wyre, 1992), the actual use of pornography by incarcerated sexual offenders remains contested (Langevin *et al.*, 1988). In relation to child pornography, as a permanent record of actual abuse, the focus of analysis and action needs to shift from the 'effect' to the 'production' of sexually explicit materials and the independent oppression of children as 'non-persons' (Kelly, 1992). Referring to both 'situational' and 'preferential molesters', Tate (1990) claims that 'there can be no real understanding of paedophilia without a corresponding grasp of child pornography, and certainly no examination of child pornography can ever take place outside the confines of paedophilia'. Without denying the very real risks of sexual and emotional abuse, this uncompromising equation between illegal materials and offending behaviours stifles even cursory discussion of 'sexual liberty', and illustrates the manipulation of law and morality in the manufacture of public prejudice and moral panic: 'Rejection and disgust is simple, understanding difficult, entering into another's feelings impossible' (Brongersma, 1988). More productively, we might question the research tradition that seeks the paedophile only in the prison and asylum; challenges a broad range of cultural representations that act as sexual scripts in the construction and mediation of sexual desire; and explores ways of empowering young people to express their sexuality outside the role of 'passive victim'.

Health and social care agents charged with the responsibility of 'child protection' might well recognise the constructs of 'innocent' and 'passive victim', and the implications of a pathology model, in relation to their own practice. Here, the work of Kitzinger (1997) directs attention to the way that 'pro-child' discourses mirror media headlines about the 'theft' or 'violation' of childhood. If exploiting 'innocence' to incite public revulsion refutes a legacy of victim-blaming, it defines 'childhood' not in terms of age but as a romantic concept. This marketing of 'innocence' feeds the imagery of the erotic child as sexual object, stigmatises the 'knowing child', and denies children knowledge and power through an ideology of paternalistic control. Further, it is suggested that 'adult-centric' discourses can silence children by reconfiguring their resistance and survival strategies into symptoms of abuse: 'Such disease terminology obscures the child actively negotiating her way through the dangers of childhood. She is recast as a submissive object of victimization even by the process of intervention and treatment' (Kitzinger, 1997).

Lost for words? Sentencing, sickness and sin

In this final section we return to the institutional management of the 'child offender' whose stereotypical profile has become the totem of popular prejudice. Increasingly, treatment programmes have become a feature of penal custody and psychiatric care. Both authors have experience of working, with this client group, in high-security services in England (DM) and Canada (TS). In the former country, the serious sexual offender is likely to be sentenced to a term of imprisonment or, alternatively, to be detained for treatment in a Special Hospital under a section of the Mental Health Act (1983) on account of 'dangerous, violent and criminal propensities'. Under Canadian legislation a sexual offender will only serve his sentence in a hospital setting if found 'not fit to stand trial' or 'not criminally responsible'. After Remand Jail, depending on the conviction and length of the sentence, the offender is transferred to a Provincial or Federal Correctional Center. In each of these the inmate is typically placed in 'protective custody', on a Special Unit, and segregated from other offenders, akin to the Vulnerable Prisoner Units (VPU) in the British prison system.

A wealth of literature already exists in relation to the clinical effectiveness of treatment programmes in reducing recidivism, and the appropriateness of criminal justice or mental health disposals. In contrast we have chosen to access the 'narrative stories' of those charged with the responsibility to work in a custodial or clinical way with offenders, often a hybridised role which contains elements of the two models. Research in one maximum security hospital (Richman *et al.*, 1999; Mercer *et al.*, 1999) revealed the persistence of a concept of 'evil' as an obstacle to rehabilitative care planning and practice. In a taxonomic ordering, extreme offences such as adult–child sexual crime elicited responses outside of medical or psychiatric ideology. A similar exercise undertaken in the Canadian Correctional Service (TS) revealed similar discursive strands and conflicts in the language of security and forensic healthcare staff. Interview extracts, cited below, illustrate how these professional and lay constructs of the paedophile are interwoven in the institutional domain.

Prison officials responsible for security are more likely to consider the paedophile 'incomparable to other offenders' and 'mentally disordered' than staff involved in treatment initiatives. A label of 'mental illness' is seen as inappropriate, since they 'know what they are doing' and are 'accountable for their actions'. Indeed a diagnosis of 'mental disorder' was seen to 'excuse the offender from any criminal responsibility'. Others elaborated that 'all people have sexual desires, the paedophile simply does not control his', and that it is 'simply inappropriate behaviour control'. In contrast, those professionals operating rehabilitative programmes viewed the paedophile as a 'distinctive class of deviant'. Here, the 'affliction', as a 'very distorted thought process in relation to sex and children', was likened to 'the alcoholic', an 'individual also detected in the DSM(IV) [the diagnostic and statistical manual] but not perceived as mentally disordered'. Interestingly, though both groups of staff made reference to 'evil' existing in the world, this embraced, rather than condemned, the paedophile offender as 'a victim of abuse'.

Within correctional services the construction of the paedophile mirrored popular stereotypes but lacked any intense emotional reactions. This was explained in terms of an 'objective view' developed from working with this group of offenders, 'a non-permission to show disgust for the crimes', and a 'defence mechanism' to support continued therapeutic engagement. Prison officials were keen to stress 'recognition, advances and awareness' in relation to disposal and management: 'We now acknowledge that there is a problem, and to silence the paedophile would ensure that it never goes away'. The problem was expressed as a belief that 'most paedophiles are not motivated to change'. The label of paedophile was seen as an 'identity that people recognise' coupled to 'the recognition of responsibility' and 'essential to their safety and their treatment'. The value of listening to the 'stories' of the paedophile in relation to risk reduction was clearly linked to the degree of confidence that staff invested in efforts to rehabilitate the offender, recognising that 'being a paedophile is not a crime – only acting on it is'.

Security officials advocated a focus of control and surveillance within a secure environment: 'what else can we do, they won't change, lock them up forever'. Since one 'can't take the thought out of their head they should be kept away from the community'. This distinction echoed the rating of the paedophile within custodial cultures as the 'lowest on the pole' where 'the sex offender is even worse than a cell rat'. If forensic healthcare staff drew attention to the frustrations of a 'dilemma between care and custody', it was couched alongside the sobering observation that 'the system advances with the speed of a glacier'. Professionals working in forensic health asserted that the paedophile is 'already heavily burdened with his label; once labelled, there is no desire to hear'. The issue of sexuality was identified as an 'integral aspect to one's holistic health', a continuum of 'stimulants and behaviour' that increasingly held few surprises: 'We have heard it all, of tales from frocks to fowls'. It was only those acts of sexual conduct involving a partner incapable of offering consent that raised 'the red flags of concern', and any sexual act with a child was the 'hallmark division of non-consensus'. Given this, the voice of the paedophile became a repository of the 'demonic', where his fate could be 'no better than the witches of Salem'.

Conclusions

In a subject area as emotive and controversial as that covered briefly in this chapter it would be difficult, and probably ill-advised, to try and conclude with a 'checklist' of recommendations. Indeed, the territory is so divided that any such attempt would represent little more than a compromise of conflicting and discordant voices at best, a partisan polemic at worst. Rather, it remains to identify key themes and discourses from social policy, criminal justice, psychiatric practice and sexual difference in the construction of marginalised lives. Certainly we can discriminate between paedophile sexuality, paedophile politics and paedophile crime. And this, at least, is a beginning.

In the domain of mental disorder and sexual offending it has been noted that popular perceptions, based on confusion, ignorance and moral panic, increasingly demand retributive sanctions and social exclusion; an ironic appetite for both 'lurid description and prurient condemnation' (Grant, 1999). Sadly, guidelines for good practice in forensic care have been embarrassed by scandals and inquiries surrounding allegations of child abuse and pornography in 'controlled' rehabilitative environments (Porter, 1997). Within a range of residential and custodial settings attention has currently shifted from abusive regimes to a narrow focus on the 'detection' and 'control' of individuals labelled as 'career paedophiles' (Stanley *et al.*, 1999). Hopefully we have contributed in challenging the idea of simplistic solutions, fuelled by media outrage, and added to the broader sociological critique of sexual politics and power.

References

Bayer, R. (1981) *Homosexuality and American psychiatry: the politics of diagnosis*, New York: Basic Books.

Brame, G., Brame, W. and Jacobs, J. (1997) *Different loving: the world of sexual dominance and submission*, London: Century.

Brongersma, E. (1988) 'A defence of sexual liberty for all age groups', *The Howard Journal*, 27, 1: 32–43.

Bukowski, C. (1983) 'The fiend', in *The most beautiful woman in town and other stories*, San Francisco: City Lights.

Califia, P. (1994) *Doing it for Daddy*, Los Angeles: Alyson Books.

Cameron, D. and Frazer, E. (1987) *The lust to kill: a feminist investigation of sexual murder*, Cambridge: Polity Press.

Campaign Against Public Morals (CAPM) (1982) *Paedophilia and public morals*, London: CAPM.

Dines, G., Jensen, R. and Russo, A. (1998) *Pornography: the production and consumption of inequality*, New York: Routledge.

Dobash, R.P. and Dobash, R.E. (1992) *Women, violence and social change*, London: Routledge.

Doidge, N. (1999) 'Adult–child sex: Phaedrus to Foucault. The muddy waters of sexuality', *Comment, Canadian National Post*, January 20: 14–15.

Elliot, M. (1992) 'Images of Children in the Media: "Soft Kiddie Porn" ', in C. Itzin (ed.), *Pornography: women, violence and civil liberties*, Oxford: Oxford University Press.

Evans, D. (1993) *Sexual citizenship: the material construction of sexualities*, London: Routledge.

Evans, N. and Clarke, J. (2000) 'Addressing issues of sexuality', in C. Chaloner and M. Coffey (eds), *Forensic mental health nursing: current approaches*, Oxford: Blackwell Science.

Foucault, M. (1967) *Madness and civilisation: a history of insanity in the age of reason*, London: Tavistock.

—— (1977) *Discipline and punish: the birth of the prison*, Harmondsworth: Penguin.

—— (1981) *The history of sexuality: an introduction*, vol. 1, London: Pelican.

Goffman, E. (1961) *Asylums: essays on the social situation of mental patients and other inmates*, New York: Doubleday.

Grant, D. (1999) 'Multi-agency risk management of mentally disordered sexual offenders: a probation case study', in D. Webb and R. Harris (eds), *Mentally disordered offenders: managing people nobody owns*, London: Routledge.

Kellett, P. (1995) 'Acts of power, control and resistance', in R. Whilcock and D. Slayden (eds), *Hate speech*, London: Sage.

Kelly, L. (1992) 'Pornography and child sexual abuse', in C. Itzin (ed.), *Pornography: women, violence and civil liberties*, Oxford: Oxford University Press.

Kendall, G. and Wickham, G. (1999) *Using Foucault's methods*, London: Sage.

Kincaid, J. (1994) *Child-loving: the erotic child and Victorian culture*, New York: Routledge.

Kittrie, N. (1971) *The right to be different: deviance and enforced therapy*, London: Johns Hopkins University Press.

Kitzinger, J. (1997) 'Who are you kidding? Children, power and the struggle against sexual abuse', in A. James and A. Prout (eds), *Constructing and reconstructing childhood: contemporary issues in the sociological study of childhood*, second edn, London: Falmer Press.

Langevin, R., Lang, R., Wright, P. *et al.* (1988) 'Pornography and sexual offences', *Annals of sex research*, 1: 335–62.

Lee, R. (1988) 'Attitudes of sex offenders', in *Pornography and sexual violence: evidence of the links*, Minneapolis City Council Government Operations Committee, London: Everywoman.

Leifer, R. (1969) *In the name of mental health: the social functions of psychiatry*, New York: Science House.

McNair, B. (1996) *Mediated sex: pornography and postmodern culture*, London: Arnold.

Mercer, D., Mason, T. and Richman, J. (1999) 'Good and evil in the crusade of care: social constructions of mental disorders', *Journal of Psychosocial Nursing*, 37, 9: 13–17

Nabokov, V. (1955) *Lolita*, London: Weidenfeld and Nicolson.

O'Carroll, T. (1980) *Paedophilia: the radical case*, London: Peter Owen.

O'Connell-Davidson, J. and Layden, D. (1998) *Methods, sex and madness*, London: Routledge.

Paedophile Information Exchange (PIE) (1978) *Paedophilia: some questions and answers*, London: PIE.

Plummer, K. (1995) *Telling sexual stories: power, change and social worlds*, London: Routledge.

Porter, R. (1997) 'Ashworth "out of control"', *Nursing Times*, 93, 7: 5.

Prager, E. (1999) *Roger Fishbite*, London: Vintage.

Prendergast, W. (1991) *Treating sex offenders in correctional institutions and outpatient clinics: a guide to clinical practice*, London; Haworth Press.

Ray, R. (1998) *A certain age*, London: Penguin.

Richman, J., Mercer, D. and Mason, T. (1999) 'The social construction of evil in a forensic setting', *The Journal of Forensic Psychiatry*, 10, 2: 300–8.

Russell, D. (1993) *Against pornography: the evidence of harm*, California: Russell.

Scully, D. (1990) *Understanding sexual violence: a study of convicted rapists*, London: Unwin Hyman.

Simon, W. (1996) *Postmodern sexualities*, London: Routledge.

Spargo, T. (1999) *Foucault and queer theory*, Cambridge: Icon.

Stanley, N., Manthorpe, J. and Penhale, B. (1999) *Institutional abuse: perspectives across the life course*, London: Routledge.

Tate, T. (1990) *Child pornography: an investigation*, London: Methuen.

Wecht, C. and Bosworth, C. (1998) *Who killed JonBenet Ramsey?*, New York: Onyx.

Wyre, R. (1992) 'Pornography and sexual violence: working with sex offenders', in C. Itzin (ed.), *Pornography: women, violence and civil liberties*, Oxford: Oxford University Press.

17 Not in my back yard

Stigma from a personal perspective

Pete Shaughnessy

Introduction

In this chapter I would like to set out a personal view of the overlap between healthcare workers and the production of stigma through my interfacing with mental health services over a number of years. It is often the case that the social dynamics of such services are highly complex, yet through personal accounts the message that is communicated resonates with many people from all sides of the healthcare divide. This chapter is written from a personal perspective and is highly critical of mental health-care workers, or at least some of them. I will address issues relating to the stigma of employment, empowerment, mad culture and mad pride, for which I make no apologies.

Seven years ago I went to my GP after going on hunger strike outside the bus garage in Peckham, south-east London, where I then worked. The hunger strike was seen by some as totally out of character while I saw it clearly as a protest against privatisation: I did not want to work longer hours for shorter wages. Desperate measures were required for a desperate situation. Management had called my GP to see me at the garage the previous night, but I had already left before he arrived. When I did see my GP we talked about why I went on hunger strike, and then he asked 'Will you go to see a psychiatrist?' 'Yes', I replied. 'That's good,' he went on, 'you're lucky. I'm a psychiatrist. If you went to see one across the road, it would be on your medical file and it would affect any employment you went for in the future. As I'm your GP it doesn't have to go on your file.' This was an early indication of the tension between 'formal' and 'informal' approaches to the creation of stigma by healthcare professionals.

Collusion: the root cause of stigma

Unfortunately for me, five weeks later I was hospitalised in Ireland and my career as a lifelong user of mental health services was launched. Looking back at that chat with my GP, I often feel that there lies stigma's root cause: a form of collusion. Ostensibly for my own benefit, the GP was willing to say, 'This event never happened'. I had come close to a scrape with a 'shrink', but my well-meaning GP had prevented it so that my medical record remained 'shrink-free'. Why this collusion? Lots of well-meaning professionals collude because they anticipate society's prejudices, fears and discrimination. This is all very well but, in my view, until we cease this collusion the prejudices will merely be perpetuated because they are not challenged. It appears that few will stand up to be counted, possibly for fear of being attacked or discriminated against, and this collusion reaches ridiculous proportions – as the following example illustrates. Having recently moved to a new area a doctor's receptionist rang up to ask if I was home. 'No', said my partner. 'Can I take a message?' The receptionist hesitated, then said 'No'. My partner, sensing the hesitancy of a health worker, asked, 'is it anything to do with his manic depression?' 'Ah,' said the receptionist, 'now you have said that, I can tell you he's got an appointment with a doctor on Monday.' When I got home my partner said there had been a weird phone call and explained that the receptionist was trying to be discreet, no doubt, but far from helping me, had merely stigmatised me even more.

However, this well-meaning discretion in the leaving of messages is not so 'well-meaning' when it comes to that all-important area of boundaries, as the following examples show. The first highlights not-so-subtle strategies of establishing demarcation lines within healthcare settings. In my early days as a day hospital 'client' (who invented the term 'client'? Not a user of mental health services, I'll bet), there was a smoking room where 'clients' and staff would congregate for a cigarette. One day I wanted to see a member of staff and walked into the room where the staff was sitting. A member of staff told me firmly that I was not allowed in this room because it was 'the staff room'. I felt like I was back at school. Although this creation of a false boundary can be understood in terms of territoriality, what is not readily acknowledged is that it also perpetuates the feeling of social exclusion and increases the stigma of 'contamination'.

The second example identifies similar boundary divisions *outside* the healthcare domain. Another member of staff at the same day hospital was very friendly; he would often chat with the 'clients', eat at the same table as us, and generally show a great deal of interest – for instance in how our weekend had gone. One day he mentioned that he was playing football on Sunday, on his day off, at the local park. At this time I was at a low ebb, and decided it would be good to get out of bed and make an effort because this member of staff was 'a nice bloke'. I watched the game from the sidelines and chatted with the other spectators. After the game, I went over to him to say 'well done', only to be shunned. I had obviously crossed his boundaries. Being a 'nice guy', it appears, stops at the end of the shift. Needless to say, I went home deflated, confused and wishing I had never got out of bed. I was also left with the horrible feeling that these people are only 'nice' to me because they're paid to be. Perhaps 'client' is a truly appropriate word after all. More importantly, if the message going out to society or communities is 'Care for people in your professional time, but ignore people with mental health problems in your free time', it is a bad message with sophisticated and sinister connotations.

I am the first to agree that appropriate boundaries are needed. However, I always find it ironic that I would sometimes go for a drink in the pub with the directors of the NHS Trust following a meeting we had all attended, and this was seen as mutually beneficial and productive. Yet the manager of the day centre where I attended went for a drink with other members of staff after duty and sat in the opposite corner of the pub from where we, the users, were sitting, justifying it the next day by saying that the rules said we shouldn't socialise together! Users tend to have a low self-esteem, are isolated, vulnerable and may be openly ostracised. Therefore, to feel shunned in our social life just reinforces the exclusion that we feel from the wider society. The maxim that 'charity begins at home' is a good one to apply to health service staff, who appear quite happy to blame society, the media, and indeed anyone except themselves for initiating and maintaining stigmatising processes.

Employment

To be unemployed is a deeply stigmatising situation. Bearing in mind that apparently 85 per cent of people with severe and enduring mental health problems are unemployed, it is amazing that only one Trust, as far as I know, has made an active effort to employ users. To have a mental health problem and to be unemployed is a double stigma. Filling in an employment form puts you in a Catch-22 situation. It is difficult to decide whether to lie about one's mental health in the distant hope of achieving employment status, or to be truthful with the severely diminished chance of an interview. This is a dilemma every user has to face, gambling on whether the interviewer will have a stereotypical jaundiced view of mental health or be genuinely open-minded. It is this un/employment marginalisation process which probably explains why the Pathfinder (South West London and St George's) NHS Trust's policy aims to actively recruit 10 per cent of users to its workforce – which must be applauded.

In terms of this Pathfinder initiative, first, users can apply to the Trust, knowing that they will not be discriminated against, and second, the initiative states to the wider community that the Trust is confident about employing people with mental health problems (with support if need be). Other organisations now have a model to look to and ask how this can be achieved. If health organisations are barring users from working for them, this raises the question as to what sort of role model they present to society? It also raises the very thorny question: 'If the NHS won't employ these people, and they should know mental health best, why should we?'

Empowerment

To practise true user empowerment, meaningful employment has to be given and meaningful remuneration received. Another example will illuminate this point. In 1999 I was part of Lewisham and Guys' MH Trust team of staff and users which won the Gold Award in the NHS Equality Awards for User Empowerment. We were paid £20 an hour for going to meetings with staff. The financial aspect apparently impressed the judges, and when Lewisham and Guys' was asked what they would do with the prize money, they said they would invest it in paying users. I have spoken with staff at other Trusts, and they, too, will espouse the virtues of user empowerment, but when I ask if their users are paid to go to joint meetings, the answer is a resounding 'No'. In fact, one Trust employee told me: 'If the meeting is really important, we will pay the user's expenses but not their time.' I wonder whether we have got 'mugs' written on our foreheads! Let's imagine my toilet is overflowing: I ring up a plumber and I say 'It's really important for you to fix my toilet, so I'll pay your expenses'. Now, do you think the plumber will come? No! So why do they expect the user to turn up to 'important meetings' under the same terms?

Further questions to emerge from this relate to whether staff attend these important meetings in their own time? I considered that being paid £20 an hour for meetings at Lewisham and Guys' was completely normal practice for my consultancy, and I also considered that staff and users might have a drink together afterwards – and that that would also be normal. However, with experience I now realise that this is more akin to being considered unique. The reality is that most Trusts would find the Lewisham and Guys' model too pioneering, too futuristic and too enlightened. But it was we, as users, who won the award!

Without wanting to sound politically correct, the NHS, in my view, is Institutionally Mentalist and has a lot of soul-searching to do in the new millennium. While the police receive criticism for their 'canteen culture', the health service must look to its 'office culture' to begin to address the issues of prejudice. I conclude this section with a small anecdote. I was having a drink with a friend of mine in a pub when a 'liberal' social worker came in. She was going to sit down next to my friend, but recognised me as a user, finished her drink and quickly left. The next time she saw my friend she asked her if she, too, was a user. Why? Does it matter? When the stigma is applied by those very professionals who aspire to eradicate it, it raises the thorny issue of whether the prejudice against those with mental health problems can ever be truly demolished.

Mad culture

Why use the term 'mad'? The answer is that the alternative, preferred term 'user' is a meaningless, bureaucratic word. It has as much value as saying

'I'm a user of trains'. Just as a passenger has no control over the train they ride on, so the mental healthcare user has no control over their healthcare. Telling people 'I am mad' is taking some degree of control: 'I am taking control of my madness and accepting it'. The most painful moment of my career as a mental healthcare user was being told that I would be taking psychiatric drugs for the rest of my life. I was condemned, and could see no escape. So, by reclaiming language, I engage in a process of turning my prison into a fortress. A position of weakness, in society's eyes, is now my strength. I take on the role of underdog, chipping away at prejudice.

The group 'Reclaim Bedlam', with hindsight, was the inevitable consequence of being involved in the process of attempting to reform the Mental Health services. The reform of user involvement would mean that one might be invited to meetings with the Trust's Directors. Ironically, in my experience the most important Director, the Medical Director, was noticeable by his (it is always a man) absence. Or, if he did turn up, it was to have a nap before a (to him) more important meeting. However, despite the many meetings at the coalface on the acute wards, little was ever changed. The frustration at this led to direct action: Reclaim Bedlam.

It all started for me when the Maudsley and Bethlem Mental Health Trust decided to 'celebrate' 750 years of mental healthcare. The Bedlam Hospital was the first institution to open with the remit of 'caring' for those considered to be 'mad'. I had two personal grievances with their decision: celebration was not a word synonymous with mental health; and the Trust was really celebrating the institution, while the users were tacked on as an afterthought. To cap it all, the Trust organised a Thanksgiving Service at St Paul's Cathedral in London, which really upset users, since until recently suicide has been considered both a sin and a crime. We took the problem to the media, with an article published in *The Big Issue* and a feature on BBC2's 'From The Edge' programme. We saw it as commemoration service versus celebration service: a time to remember the unmarked graves; those who had taken their own lives; and those who were victims of people that had been ill.

It was time to take the debate out of the walls of the asylum and into society. Direct action was a springboard to get our undiluted voice out there. Reclaim Bedlam has gone on to do four more direct action events. The last was a march on SANE's HQ, as part of our opposition to compulsory treatment. On this occasion around 200 people gathered to march. Again we were covered by BBC2 and *The Big Issue*. What was significant was that Marjorie Wallace, SANE's Chief Executive, came out to talk to us. Some cynics say that she saw the cameras and decided to make an appearance. However, she has to be given some respect as she had to face 200 angry people. Many were expressing their anger because Wallace is seen as the only spokesperson on mental health, and she ignores their views. However, since the march, her tone is more conciliatory and hopefully we have got our point across to her.

We made sure the media were involved in our protest; we were striving for that 'oxygen of publicity'. When Reclaim Bedlam as a movement began, I believed that there would be a massive shift in attitudes, almost like an avalanche. However, in reality, it's like sitting in a cell and chipping away at the wall with a nail file. Working with Mental Health media over the last three years, I've given numerous interviews to journalists, hoping that it would have a cumulative effect. I'm one part of a small stone rolling down a hill, with the vision, and hope, that it will grow into a snowball. The downside of all this is that there is a personal cost to direct action, which has resulted in me being hospitalised following two of the five actions. This is a huge personal price to pay for my convictions as I am vulnerable to stress; therefore, in the future I will be looking at alternative ways to get the MAD message across.

Mad Pride

Involvement with 'mad pride' has offered a different way of taking the message out to society. Mad Pride grew out of Reclaim Bedlam, and is less overtly political, less confrontational and more about entertainment. The idea is similar to Gay Pride or Rock Against Racism. So far, we have staged gigs, putting on punk bands, and attracting their followers and users. We have gone for the anarchic feel. In a way, anarchy and madness are similar – both are about not conforming to society's norms. Citizen Fish, a well-known punk band, was attracted to our ethos because of our opposition to compulsory treatment orders and the proposed bill to deal with severe personality disorders. Mad Pride is about developing networks, and our aim is to encourage sufficient sponsorship to enable us to put on a one-day festival in London.

Ironically, while we are developing interest outside of the user population, within it there is a conflict of views. Many of the silent majority do not like the term 'Mad Pride', finding it offensive and merely pandering to society's prejudices. Maybe they see reform as the way forward by employing terms such as 'mental distress'. However, Rachel Perkins (1999) writes:

> Distress is a beautifully inclusive word. Something everyone can relate to. By adopting the term 'distress', we bridge 'them and us' and the 'sane' divide. We conjure a continuum: everyone gets distressed, some people get more distressed and for longer periods than others. We are all the same really. If that which has been excluded as madness can be reclaimed under an inclusive distress banner, then everything will be alright.

She goes on:

> … when faced with the enormity of oppression it may be tempting to minimise difference via the ostensibly inclusive language of distress. But the inclusion achieved by such linguistic gymnastics is illusory. We have much to learn from black and lesbian/gay politics, where acting 'white', passing as 'straight', are recognised for what they are – perpetuating oppression.

Passing as sane is no different. As she says, the denial of difference – 'they are just the same as us except for the colour of their skin, who they choose to sleep with, the extent of their distress' – does not foster inclusive communities.

> Real inclusion can only be achieved via the celebration of difference and diversity. The problem is not that difference exists, but the value attached to that difference – when black, gay, mad, mean 'less than', with all the denial of rights that this entails. So let's dispense with notions of distress, and embrace Mad Pride.
>
> (Perkins, 1999)

Respect for mad people has been a long time coming (Shaughnessy, 1998). Only in the last year of the twentieth century have mad people been given official voting rights. For the bulk of our history we have been locked away in institutions, 'out of sight, out of mind'. The fact that we live in the community has to be put into perspective; it is a recent phenomenon. However, it is vital that we learn from the past and from other civil rights movements. To collude, put our heads in the sand, and lie, just makes life worse in the long term. For me, it's healthier to be honest: as the Steel Pulse song 'Don't Give In' goes, 'Let faith be my shield, Let truth be my sword' (Steel Pulse, 1985).

There are times when I am rejected for what I believe, more so by fellow users than anybody else. I carry on, proving the rejections are wrong, and I know I will emerge stronger from the experience. yet the ultimate stigma is rejection: rejection from work and from relationships. When I lost my job at London Transport, I lost my friends and my social life too. I entered social isolation, became a social 'leper' at the most vulnerable time of my life. The irony was that when I needed friends they were nowhere to be found. Now that I no longer need them, they are everywhere. I'm fortunate to have a partner that I can talk to about anything that is going on in my head. Her acceptance is like a safety net. She is not a mad person, but she is on my side. I feel that we are working together. Quite simply, she is truly non-judgemental.

With support I feel strong enough to stand up to the discrimination, prejudice and ignorance, and to say it is wrong – even if I am a lone voice at times. Bearing in mind the disability of my madness, it takes an incredible amount of courage. I feel it to be a fight against the odds. My most proud direct action moments have been when I am on my own in Community Halls, advocating rights in the hostile community; or when I'm somewhere like Windsor Coroner's Court where I took the stand on behalf of Broadmoor's Patients' Council. One can only imagine the hostile atmosphere that I encountered there; but I felt there was a truth that had to be told. For me, the most important line I said in the Coroner's Court was 'The Council wishes to express sympathy to the family of the dead person.' The person had hanged himself in Broadmoor. Maybe it was a small line, but the context of the statement meant a lot to the man's family.

A good example of challenging stigma is *The Big Issue*, which gives homeless people an opportunity to sell a magazine and make some money for themselves. Opportunities are also provided for employment, or help with housing or health issues. However, no-one is forced into participation, and they only sell when and what they can. It is positive that when a buyer gets a copy of *The Big Issue*, they know that the person selling it is homeless. The point is to de-stigmatise homeless people and to express that they have a value and are not reduced to mere begging and thieving.

Similarly, we need projects that involve mad people without apologising or merely getting the sympathy vote. We need empathy. Until mad people stand up and feel self-respect, why should society respect us? Respect and value begin at home, so mad people need to learn self-respect. We have to prove society wrong in their low opinion of us; not necessarily to win them over, but to get them to respect us. Only when we are respected will we really be listened to. We can then have a meaningful dialogue in which our hopes and needs are taken into account. Most important of all, one day we will control the agenda. In the not too distant future we mad people will run our own asylum. There are doctors, nurses, receptionists, chefs and cleaners who are diagnosed as 'mentally ill'. Therefore, why should we not have our own space? In a conversation with Marjorie Wallace, Chief Executive of SANE, she talked about how, only 20 years ago, cancer victims were stigmatised. Now it has completely changed. The same should happen to mental health, she said. Well, I hope so, and I hope it happens in less than twenty years! One year is one too many.

In conclusion, in Autumn 1999 there was an exhibition called 'Cons to Icons' mounted in London by Nick Reynolds, the son of Great Train Robber, Bruce Reynolds. It featured pictures of 'Mad' Frankie Fraser, infamous gang enforcer nicknamed 'The Dentist', along with other notorious gangsters. The purpose of the exhibition was 'to explore how men whom society found morally repugnant were being turned into folk and media heroes'. Well, all I can say, now that they have had their 15 minutes of (in)fame, what about us truly 'mad' people? By the way, we're much nicer.

References

Perkins, R. (1999) 'Madness, distress and the language of inclusion', *Open Mind*, July/August, 98.

Shaughnessy, P. (1998) 'Media madness', *Mental Health Care*, 1, 11: 367.

Steel Pulse (1985) '*Let Faith be your Shield*', Reggae Greats Album, Island Records.

18 Smackheads, crackheads and other junkies

Dimensions of the stigma of drug use

Neil Hunt and Jon Derricott

Introduction

We write this chapter with two types of reader in mind: the first will encounter drug users because they have a formal intervention role relating to problems associated with someone's drug use. Most obviously, this might be a person working within a community drug team, although we recognise that interventions increasingly occur in criminal justice settings, general practice, or within services for young people. If this is you, we expect that you are largely empathic with the people you meet and hope that the chapter will assist with your existing, reflective approach concerning aspects of your relationship with drug users.

The second type of reader will become aware of someone's drug use either accidentally, or through a screening, assessment or surveillance process. Your role regarding the person's drug use is more likely to be one of referring or directing the drug user towards available services – when this is necessary and appropriate. The number of people fulfilling this role is rapidly expanding, but you may be a casualty or school nurse, teacher, general practitioner, occupational health worker, or work in the police or prison service. You may similarly empathise with the drug-related difficulties people experience. However, you may sometimes find drug use a perplexing or even an irritating aspect of your work. We hope that this chapter will be useful to you in providing information that counters many misleading stereotypes, that it will be helpful in making more sense of drug use and drug users and, ultimately, that it may in a small way help to reduce the stigma attached to drug use.

As we will show in this chapter, drug use/misuse can be discussed with reference to the same dimensions as other sources of stigma. We follow the model described by Jones *et al.* (1984) and consider this in terms of concealability, course and disruptiveness. However, drug use and misuse is a stigmatised activity that differs from others discussed in this book in one vital way, it is illegal. Although it can be argued that having a free choice to pursue intoxication using whatever substance a person prefers is a human right (Szasz, 1992; Friedman and Szasz, 1992; Nadelmann, 1997), the stigma attached to drug use is nevertheless 'government sanctioned' through its illegal status.

At the beginning of the third millennium it is widely regarded as incorrect to stigmatise people with schizophrenia, a physical disability, epilepsy, or who are lesbian, gay, black or Asian. By contrast, the illicit nature of a range of commonly consumed drugs creates greater ambiguity about the status of people who use them. After all, it is 'official': through legislation the state says drug use is a crime and is therefore bad; *ipso facto*, drug users are bad and rightly stigmatised. We suggest that this is a cardinal difference between the stigma attached to drug use and many of the other stigmatising phenomena discussed in this book, and one that must constantly be borne in mind when considering the stigma experienced by drug users.

The stigma of drug use

A range of research provides evidence of the way that drug users are stigmatised and the effects of this. For example, a study of American undergraduates reveals that a hypothetical HIV-positive man – 'Dan' – was much more stigmatised when he was described as homosexual or an IV drug user rather than as having been infected through blood products or as a result of healthcare work. Similarly, supposed infection with the illnesses AIDS and hepatitis resulted in higher levels of stigma than with paraplegia or flu (Crandall, 1991). Type of substance and level of dependence also affect expectations concerning treatment outcome.

Cunningham, Sobell and Chow (1993) compared attitudes to hypothetical people who used either tobacco, alcohol or cocaine and were described as having high or low substance dependence. Substance type affected whether self-change was seen as appropriate when compared to formal treatment, and was seen as more appropriate for smokers than people using cocaine or alcohol. Similarly, non-abstinent recovery was greeted more sceptically for people using alcohol and cocaine. In each case these assessments do not correspond with what is known about the pathways to recovery, in which self-change plays a prominent role for problem drinkers and a number of people achieve non-abstinent recovery.

It also appears that stigma can have enduring detrimental effects on well-being that persist long after more immediate substance misuse and mental health problems have been resolved (Link *et al.*, 1997). This study of people with a dual diagnosis of mental illness and substance 'abuse' found that, at one-year follow-up, psychiatric symptoms had largely resolved and drug-taking had generally stopped. Nevertheless people still perceived themselves as stigmatised, were actively using coping strategies to deal with this, and had residual levels of depression associated with its continuation.

Attitudes to substance misusers presenting to casualty departments have been illustrated in Jeffery's classic paper 'Normal Rubbish: Deviant Patients In Casualty Departments' (1979). Although focusing primarily on attitudes to 'drunks', Jeffery shows how these people (among others, such as drug addicts – seen to be trying to obtain drugs by blackmailing the doctor into prescribing more drugs – or people who intentionally overdose) are regarded as a nuisance to clinicians and seen as second-class patients of little clinical or social value. These groups break two 'rules': they are seen to be responsible for their illness, and to be difficult to treat as there is no straightforward answer to their problems. Some perception of rule-breaking regarding claims to the sick role[1] by people with substance misuse problems is a common feature of attitudes to drug users across the helping agencies and contributes to the stigma they experience. Referring specifically to injecting drug users – a group at high risk of experiencing serious health problems – and their relationships with primary health services, Grund (1993) says the following:

> Dissatisfaction with or fear of medical services has a ... negative effect on drug users health ... 'Addictophobia' is something all drug users may be subjected to but, having more health risks and being more easily identified as illegal drug users, something to which (unskilled) injectors are particularly susceptible. It does not take much intuition to understand the role which being identified as a member of an, if not hated, at least not cherished minority plays in presenting for treatment, or health status in itself.

Beyond explanations in terms of the sick role, there is also a wider political explanation that has been offered to account for the stigmatising of drug users. Friedman (1998) argues that drug users provide convenient scapegoats for social problems at times in the trade cycle when economic growth falters. He provides a historical analysis of the parallels between declining growth and increased scapegoating of drug users by governments. A public discourse that attributes responsibility for wider social problems to drug users through the mass media can readily be understood as a mechanism by which stigma may be increased.

What's in a word?

Before we proceed further, it is first necessary to address some specific points concerning the language used in this chapter. Deliberate use of language is one means by which stigma can be reduced. We try to contribute to a project of reducing the stigma of drug use and misuse here by an explanation of the terms we will use and those we will not.

Avoiding and challenging the use of terms that have become pejorative or connote unwelcome meanings is a commonplace strategy for tackling stigma. For example, we no longer generally discuss 'lunatics' or the 'mentally subnormal'. 'Queers' and 'faggots' have become 'gay' – though the reclaiming of the word 'queer' is a welcome indication of the increased confidence of those once marginalised by the term. If a white person uses the word 'nigger' today, this would often provoke more shock than their use of any sexual swear word. In recent history, a society for people with cerebral palsy included the medical term 'spastic' in its title, subsequently dropping it as the meaning gradually moved from one of neutrality to become a term of playground abuse. The list of such stigmatising labels could be extended considerably.

The Standing Conference on Drug Abuse – SCODA (1997) (which, ironically, has taken a lead in sensitising practitioners to a more precise and less stigmatising use of language) – has only recently managed to drop the term 'abuse' from its name, because of its merger with the Institute for the Study of Drug Dependence, into one organisation called DrugScope. Here, in keeping with terminology promoted by the Health Advisory Service and SCODA (Health Advisory Service, 1996; SCODA/CLC, 1999) we use the terms 'drug use' and 'misuse' and not 'drug abuse' or 'addiction'. Drug 'use' is defined as 'the consumption of a drug ... when the term "use" is contrasted with "misuse", "use" means the consumption of a drug that does not cause any perceptible immediate harm – even though it may carry some risk of harm'. Drug misuse is 'use of a drug or combination of substances, that harms health or social functioning – either dependent use (physical or psychological) *or* use that is part of a wider spectrum of problematic or harmful behaviour'.

According to the Concise Oxford Dictionary, the prefix 'mis' denotes the wrong or improper use of something. 'Abuse' is far stronger and implies corrupt or perverted practice. It has obvious resonances with physical or sexual abuse and is therefore a term to be avoided by those who wish to avoid stigmatising language. Many people who use drugs – problematically or otherwise – will immediately be alienated if addressed or described as drug or alcohol 'abusers'. To emphasise the point, the use of cars similarly involves risk to the driver, other road users and pedestrians. Consider your likely feelings if society arbitrarily decided to refer to drivers not as car users, but as 'car abusers'.

The term 'addiction' is associated with the medical diagnosis of a disease. Technically, 'addiction' has now been subsumed within the 'dependence syndrome' (World Health Organisation, 1992). However, the medical entity of addiction remains disputed and the extent to which it is socially constructed, rather than signifying some 'real' phenomenon, remains unclear. For a particularly lucid critique of the concept of addiction see Davies (1992). A glance at the boom in addictive 'diseases' in the USA – the 'holisms' such as those that afflict alcoholics, shopaholics, chocaholics, workaholics, etc. – gives an indication of the extent to which 'addiction' may be socially constructed. Historically, the medicalising of drug use through the disease model is nevertheless one way in which stigma has been countered. The 'British system' is regarded as an early and important model of a more humanitarian approach to the management of people with drug misuse problems – for example, see Stimson and Oppenheimer's (1982) account. Arguably, it is better to be ill than bad. By categorising people in this way it became possible to promote a more humane treatment approach instead of punishment. However, as is evident elsewhere in this book, being identified as *diseased* can be a source of stigma in itself. Consequently, although we do not contest the occurrence of many of the subjective experiences that currently constitute the 'dependence syndrome', we resist using the term ourselves, and urge the reader to look critically at the way that people are constructed as addicted or dependent.

Having considered some basic issues concerning the language currently used to discuss drug taking we now move on to examine drug use in terms of the underlying dimensions of stigma.

Concealability

The illegality of drug use causes it to be a widely concealed activity and makes much drug use invisible. The fact that the global illicit drug industry is estimated by the United Nations to comprise 8 per cent of all international trade (UNDCP, 1997: 124) – more than the global international trade in iron and steel and motor vehicles combined – coupled with the relative invisibility of drug use, indicates just how well it is concealed. This level of economic activity also gives a clue as to just how unproblematic much drug use probably is. Because of this concealment, services are more likely to encounter knowingly only people who self-identify with drug misuse problems. Seeking advice, treatment or care for problems associated with drug use makes it necessary to disclose this stigmatised behaviour in order to claim services. However, many more people attending health, social care and criminal justice agencies (and sometimes those who work in them) and who intermittently or regularly use drugs recreationally, never reveal this fact. This skews both professional and societal perceptions of drug use and drug users. To appreciate this, think how you might view drinking alcohol if you only met people who attend alcohol treatment services and never encountered people socialising in a pub in the evening or sharing a bottle of wine with a meal. The corresponding 'moderate' group of drug users is largely invisible.

There is a widespread and largely mistaken idea that drug use is easily spotted if you know what signs and symptoms to watch for. Consider the range of leaflets and media articles suggesting 'how to tell if your kids are on drugs'. In practice, drug use is easily concealed from friends, relatives, employers and even partners. Intoxication is not necessarily visible or externally evident. This also selectively results in problem drug use often being the only pattern visible.

There is, however, a growing readiness to subject the population to 'psychotropic scrutiny' through methods such as workplace drug screening, mandatory drug testing in prisons, testing for 'drug driving' and current proposals for legislation in Britain that would enable almost all arrestees to be tested for drugs (Home Office, 2000). Within the USA, drug screening of school children is now offered (on the Internet[2]) and has been contemplated within the UK. Testing technologies are increasing in their sophistication. For example, hair analysis can now give a lengthy drug history (McPhillips *et al.*, 1998). Such developments will increase the extent to which drug use is identified within a range of settings such as occupational health, in schools and in criminal justice systems. The move from voluntary self-identification of problem drug use towards identification through detection means that, although more drug users will become visible, a diminishing proportion will actually have drug problems – other than those arising from identification and labelling.

It will be increasingly important for people who encounter drug users within their work to appreciate that an understanding of drug use as inevitably problematic does not necessarily correspond with the perceptions or experiences of the person in front of them. Even among people who present with drug-related problems, it will be useful to be circumspect about the actual problems that the drug user may experience and the extent to which these conform to preconceived ideas.

Course

For someone who bears a stigmatising mark, its course has a bearing on their treatment. People who use illicit drugs are rarely physically marked by their drug use. However, the mark arising from bearing the deviant label 'drug abuser', 'addict' or similar is real in its effect on interactions between the drug user and others. This label includes a range of representations involving: the 'strung out', emaciated heroin user; the 'junkie' stealing to pay for their habit; the AIDS-infected injector; the ecstasy user on a life support machine; and the pop or sports celebrity in the private clinic.[3] These misleadingly imply a course that ends inevitably in physical or moral decay and possibly death.

A range of evidence contradicts these views. For example, it now appears that drug use has increased throughout the 1990s such that approaching half of all young people in England now experiment with drugs (Ramsay and Partridge, 1999). More than 90 per cent of 'clubbers' use drugs (Release, 1997; Winstock, 2000), yet very few of these people seek treatment for drug problems. Strikingly, in a rare longitudinal study of drug consumption patterns, Shedler and Block (1990) followed people from the age of 3 to 18 and compared the characteristics of abstainers, experimenters and frequent drug users. They found that experimenters were best adjusted and had received the highest quality parenting, as measured by a wide range of measures. This suggests that relative to abstinence or frequent use, drug experimentation should be understood not as an indicator of parental failure but as a reassuring phenomenon for parents, and one that is associated with healthy development and well-being.

In general, the course of illicit drug use careers can be summarised as follows:

- Substantial numbers of young people in the UK now try drugs experimentally.
- Some use them recreationally for a while; most then stop using drugs or integrate them into their lifestyle in a relatively adaptive way.
- Of the large number of people who try drugs, a comparatively small minority of people develop drug misuse problems.

Even when we examine the course of 'hard' drug careers, we find that this is far from predictable. This is most evident within research among 470 US soldiers returning from Vietnam (Robins, 1974). Heroin use was very high among soldiers in Vietnam. During 1971, approaching half (44 per cent) of all soldiers reported trying one or more 'narcotic', opiate drugs (mostly heroin or opium) during their tour of duty and a fifth considered themselves to 'have been addicted'. However, on follow-up in the USA between eight and twelve months after their return, only 9.5 per cent reported having used any 'narcotic' since their return and only 7 per cent considered that they were 'addicted'. The implications are that:

- Experimental or recreational use of heroin can occur.
- The course of a drug career is far from certain.
- Even in the case of heroin, one of the most demonised drugs in society, 'addiction' is far from inevitable.

For people encountering drug users the cautions are obvious. Many of the commonplace views of the course of illicit drug use – an inevitable path towards decline or death – are grossly misleading. Of course, this is not to deny that problems associated with drug use occur or that they may be severe – they can and sometimes are. Nevertheless, for many people, drug use has no problematic consequences and is managed in a way that does not result in harm. Many drug users are competent in the way that they use drugs and do so without producing adverse consequences in their health or social functioning. Even among people using the drugs that elicit the most anxiety within society – heroin and cocaine – a proportion of people consume these without developing problems.

Disruptiveness

Sources of stigma can be considered in terms of the capacity to disrupt the relationship between the 'marked' and the 'marker'. In contrast to people with a source of stigma, such as facial disfigurement, the drug user is not generally physically marked by their drug use, other than perhaps by injection marks which – again and in contradiction to the stereotypical image of the track-marked junkie – are usually easily concealed. Behaviourally, intoxication can be visible and a source of disruption if the drug user is either sedated or hyper-aroused. Nevertheless, drug use is often conducted in a way that does not interfere with ordinary social intercourse. A walk through any large town centre is likely to involve obliviously walking past people who are using heroin, methadone or amphetamine; yet stopping to ask many of these the time would not necessarily leave the enquirer with any awareness that they had been talking to a drug user.

An important source of disruption can nevertheless be the way that the label 'drug user' affects the interaction between a practitioner and someone who uses drugs. Deviance theory distinguishes primary and secondary deviance. In this example, primary deviance is the original act of taking drugs, upon which attention is focused by the 'marker'. Labelling someone as a drug abuser or addict produces secondary deviance. 'Secondary deviation is deviant behavior or social roles based upon it, which become a means of defense, attack or adaptation to the overt and covert problems created by the societal reaction to a primary deviation' (Lemert, 1967: 17). In other words, being labelled shapes the person's self-identify and the social roles available to them. In this way, labelling produces something of a self-fulfilling prophecy as people react to the 'deviant' person in ways that further channel them towards continued 'deviance'. Treating people in a certain way increases their propensity to behave in accordance with expectations. So, if we operate from a view that drug users are likely to be criminals (despite the fact that the best available evidence suggests that, even among people whose drug use has become highly problematic, half of all drug users do not steal to fund their drug use (Gossop *et al.*, 1998)), we increasingly nudge people towards criminality as a component of a drug-user identity – a process captured in the saying 'I might as well be hung for a sheep as a lamb'.

This process has been clearly illustrated in a qualitative study of the interactions between drug users and pharmacists (Matheson, 1998). Stigmatising treatment by pharmacists was discussed as something that would provoke a negative reaction from the drug user. Conversely, being treated like a normal customer engendered respect from the drug user and reduced the risk of activities such as shoplifting:

> ... it's like my chemist, that is where I get my stuff, they are good to me so I am good to them basically. It would be different if it was like

[pharmacy name] and things like that ... lowering their nose at you so like, you lower them even more, so like you maybe steal from them and laugh at them.

(Woman, aged 22)

Reducing the stigma of drug misuse problems

Despite the illicit nature of drug use it is now recognised, in the health service at least, that drug users have the same entitlements as other patients. This is a central principle of the guidelines on clinical management for drug misuse and dependence (Department of Health, 1999). As an expression of the basic human rights of drug users, this is also a valuable reference point for the way that drug users should be regarded within any public sector service. The stigma attached to drug use is a continuing impediment to this entitlement. Consequently it is important to reduce stigma if this principle is to be anything more than a worthy but unfulfilled aspirational statement. The final section discusses a range of ways in which the accomplishment of this aspiration can be assisted.

Questioning stereotypes

This chapter has discussed a range of factors that distort the understanding of drug use and sustain a range of demonstrably flawed stereotypes of drug users. The prohibition of drug use and its subsequent concealment can be seen to distort lay and professional understandings of the course of drug-use careers. Inevitably, some individuals who conform to stereotypes exist. However, the existence of a minority of such people has little bearing on the larger number of drug users who do not fit such images; images that nevertheless dominate the public perception of drug use. Indeed, by imposing stereotyped ideas and expectations on drug users we help produce the very reactions we would wish to avoid. A basic counter to much of the stigma of drug use is, therefore, continually to critically question the applicability of such stereotypes to individual drug users encountered in health, social and other care settings, and, if we use them at all, to employ widely-used ideas and terminology such as 'addiction' with great caution. Recognising that drug users generally have similar aspirations, morals and concerns as anyone else, along with similar expectations – indeed rights – to being treated with respect when encountering public services, and treating them accordingly, can be transformative in the relations between drug users and the agencies that encounter them.

Language

As we have already discussed, the careful and deliberate use of language is an established device for countering stigma. Not labelling people as 'abusers', 'addicts' or using blatantly derogatory terms such as 'junkie' is a simple and effective way by which stigma can be diminished. The first two of these terms remain widely used in professional circles and, although it may sometimes be appropriate to talk of addiction in a precise, technical sense, it is often used in a careless or imprecise way. Such language often persists in a way that is institutionalised; for example, highly regarded academic journals such as *Addiction* retain such titles even though they are an imprecise summary of their content – dealing, as they do, with a far wider consideration of drug taking and the corresponding social response.

Linked to this discussion of language, we want to suggest one simple question that can be useful when taking drug use histories – a common process in many encounters between drug users and services of all descriptions. A basic question to open this topic up productively can be to ask 'Do you use any drugs for pleasure?' rather than perhaps 'What drugs have you been abusing?' or something similar. The question conveys a recognition that drug use is not necessarily problematic, and may be perceived as a legitimate lifestyle choice by the drug-taker, albeit one that incurs risks.[4] Naturally, this works best if the rest of the conversation is undertaken in a way that is coherent with this basic position. It does not imply, however, that the practitioner should be uncritical and need not challenge the person's behaviour. If it is revealed that the drug-taking is in some way problematic to the individual or those around them, it will be valuable to identify this in order to investigate any available way to work effectively with them to minimise risk and harm. This is unlikely ever to become possible if the language employed by the worker immediately conveys that they lack a basic appreciation of the values surrounding drug-taking and have a monochromatic view of drug-taking as being necessarily problematic and requiring their intervention – often it isn't and won't.

Clarifying and communicating expectations, rights and responsibilities

Regardless of how well-trained staff in a service are, what anti-discriminatory training they may have received regarding the treatment of drug users and what the underlying values and ethos of a service may be, it remains the case that many drug users will approach services with an expectation that they will be treated in a prejudicial way. In some cases, services themselves will be unclear how to respond to drug users in important areas. For example, when a mother is using drugs, at what point might this become a child protection issue? Lack of clarity on this point is a major impediment to obtaining treatment or advice for many women who use drugs. Yet, in respect of drug-related behaviour, local Child Protection Committees often fail to clarify the criteria used to determine critical concepts such as 'significant harm' or 'neglect'. The bounded nature of confidentiality within services is another area that may not be clearly defined or communicated.

Alternatively, what are the obligations upon a service to report or act on Misuse of Drugs Act offences or other crimes that become known? The 'Wintercomfort' case, where the unfortunate managers of the eponymous homeless hostel in Cambridge were jailed, brings some of these issues into sharp relief. Where the management of a service is unclear on these issues, workers are not properly supported and the consequent uncertainties increase the risk of stigmatising treatment and poor care. To illustrate, it is arguable that a mother who occasionally uses cannabis socially while her partner is caring for her child, does not cause her child significant harm. However, where there is no local clarity, a practitioner might wrongly initiate child protection proceedings and cause substantial harm. Similarly, someone who has difficulties such as a serious threat to their safety associated with involvement in drug dealing may have anxieties about whether disclosure of this will result in police involvement.

Allied to an understanding of the rights and responsibilities of both services and drug users is the question of how these are communicated. Wherever information is made available about services, it will be useful to clarify such matters in order to improve the accessibility of the service by informing service users of the treatment that they have a right to expect, the expectations of them (clear messages about behaviour that is unacceptable to the service, such as dealing on the premises) and any limitations to the relationship regarding confidentiality. Such information should be clearly displayed in public areas. It may be particularly beneficial to adopt and display a charter of service users' rights within services. SCODA have developed a general statement of drug users' rights which can readily be adopted for use within services (SCODA, 1997). More specific examples also exist that clarify the stance of a service towards, say, parents who use drugs. For example, in Hammersmith and Fulham, health centres, social services and reception centres display a statement that says: 'It is the policy of Hammersmith and Fulham not to consider the children of people who misuse substances as being at risk of abuse or neglect by virtue solely of the fact that a parent is a drug user.'

Such statements are calculated to reassure people concerning unrealistic expectations, such as an automatic assumption that parental drug use will be reported to child protection services.

Involving drug users

It is increasingly possible to involve drug users directly in commenting on, guiding, and even delivery of non-stigmatising services. This is possible in a range of ways including the use of satisfaction questionnaires, local surveys, the employment of ex-drug users and user-representation within planning groups.

While useful and to be encouraged, such approaches also have identifiable limitations. Questionnaires and surveys do not necessarily enable the concerns of drug users to be clearly heard. Their terms are set by the initiating agency and they may fail to examine aspects of a service that are salient for users. They also have limited capacity to capture the views of people with poor literacy or for whom English is not their first language.

When user-representatives are invited on to planning groups, unless considerable care is taken regarding the way this process is managed there is the potential for the result to be unsatisfactory. Careful attention is generally necessary to the induction, training and support (including financial compensation for their time and effort) given to user-representatives for the process to work well.

Ex-users often have a valuable insight into the concerns of drug users and can contribute invaluably to services. Many effective drug workers draw on their personal history within their work, and drug users frequently feel that someone who has used drugs themselves is better placed to help them. However, the concerns of ex-users can also vary from those of current users and there are limitations to their ability to speak on behalf of drug users (Balian and White, 1998).

Fortunately, opportunities for effectively involving drug users are now greatly enhanced through the development of an umbrella National Drug Users Development Agency,[5] which supports the development of national and local drug user groups and provides training for services and drug users. Thus, groups like the Methadone Alliance,[6] the Dance Drugs Alliance or the Respect User's Union can now provide guidance regarding the concerns of drug users and the way that services can best be responsive to these. They provide a framework within which local drug users can be better supported, and are able to share good practice and lobby to reduce stigmatising treatment of drug users. By consulting, involving and supporting the developing drug user movement through these channels, and supporting the development of local user groups, services may be best able to act in a way that avoids some of the problems inherent in other methods of user-involvement and most effectively works to reduce stigma.

Training

Finally, we turn to the role of training in reducing stigma. To non-drug users, drug use can be a bewildering and perplexing activity and one where it is unclear what might constitute the best response – or, indeed, whether there is one. Working with drug users without proper training can be a source of stress and there is a shortfall of brief training courses appropriate to a range of practitioners, such as GPs, for whom dealing with drug problems is a common occurrence (Martin, 1996; Teijlingen and Porter, 1997). When people do not possess a good knowledge of basic aspects of drug use, the concerns of drug users, the responsibilities and opportunities for intervention and what constitutes good practice, they inevitably work from their lay understanding. When these are largely informed by a sensationalist press and popular but misleading stereotypes, the pre-conditions for stigmatising practice result.

Training can reduce negative feelings towards drug users, increase confidence, and provide the basis for improving practice (Preston and Campion-Smith, 1997), all of which enables the provision of less stigmatising services that better meet the needs of drug users. However, Martin (1996) highlights the shortage of appropriate training that meets the needs of the generalist in terms of content, accessibility and brevity. There is a growing number of training courses available at certificate, diploma and graduate level, many of which will increase understanding and reduce stigma. However, although some exist, there remains an urgent need for the development of shorter training courses that are tailored to the needs of the wider range of practitioners who now find dealing with drug use to be part of their work, yet for whom working with drug users is just one of a range of activities undertaken.

Conclusion

The stigma attaching to illicit drug use is, at least in part, both created and sustained by illegality. The language used to describe drug use and drug users is frequently informed by moral disapprobation of drug use. There is often an understandable desire to warn of the risks associated with drug use; however, where risk is not presented in context and extreme cases are presented as the norm, important information on risk reduction will be unheard or ignored. Use of stigmatising language and over-inflation of risks serve to hinder development of effective relationships between services and drug users. To work in a non-stigmatising way, people working with drug users need to have:

- Open and accepting attitudes.
- An awareness of the limitations of many stereotyped images of drug use.
- Sensitivity to the language used to describe drug use.
- Accurate and up-to-date knowledge.
- An appropriate framework within which to assess drug use and misuse – this will differ according to the context and whether the practitioner is more generic or specialised.
- Training in the use of interventions that are suited to their needs.
- A workplace where the rights and responsibilities of workers and drug users are clear, and where drug users are given a voice in the way services are provided.
- Confidence, engendered by possession of the above to know *when* and *what* to challenge and confront in drug using clients.

It is important to recognise that drug users commonly experience discriminatory treatment and that there is a corresponding need to cultivate anti-discriminatory practice, in line with that which benefits other marginalised groups.

Disclaimer: The views expressed in this chapter are those of the authors and not necessarily those of any organisation with which they are associated.

Notes

1 The 'sick role' has been elaborated by the sociologist Talcott Parsons as an account of the way that exemption from normal social responsibilities and claims on care are legitimised; see *The social system* (1951), New York: Free Press.
2 At the time of writing: http://www.drug-test.com/
3 Peril is another dimension of stigma that Jones *et al.* (1984) discuss. Although we shall not expand on it at length here, these images suggest the parallel perils that the stereotypes generate. These include the risks of theft from 'junkies' who are compelled to steal to feed their habit, the possibility of contamination from AIDS and hepatitis, drug-induced sexual depravity – seen historically in films such as 'Reefer Madness' (1937) and currently in the portrayal of crack cocaine as a drug that is so compelling that people will sell their bodies to obtain it. For parents, there is also the peril evident in representations of predatory drug pushers loitering at school gates to seduce unwilling children into drug use (rarely occurring in practice but sensationally reported from time to time). Similarly, drug users are generally viewed as pressuring their innocent peers to join them in their corrupt activity. This view prevails despite the criticisms of the research base in this area and the way that the role of peer pressure has been challenged as a valid explanation of the process by which young people come to use drugs (Coggans and McKellar, 1994).
4 Of course, in this sense drug-taking is no different to many other risk-laden activities such as just about any physical sport (but particularly activities such as rock climbing, motor racing or boxing), driving a car, motorcycling, riding a bicycle, using legal drugs (for example, alcohol and tobacco), having sex, doing the gardening or DIY – all of which activities annually result in a degree of morbidity and mortality that is generally seen as an acceptable individual or social cost for the corollary benefits.
5 Address: National Drug User Development, P.O. Box 33539, London E9 77N; tel: 020 8986 5475; fax: 020 8525 0199.
6 Methadone Alliance; tel: 020 8374 4395.

References

Balian, R. and White, C. (1998) 'Defining the drug user', *The International Journal of Drug Policy*, 9, 1: 391–6.
Coggans, N. and McKellar, S. (1994) 'Drug use among peers: peer pressure or peer preference?', *Drugs: Education, Prevention and Policy*, 1, 1: 15–26.
Crandall, C.S. (1991) 'Multiple stigma and AIDS: illness stigma and attitudes towards homosexuals and IV drug users in AIDS-related stigmatization', *Journal of Community and Applied Social Psychology*, 1: 165–72.

Cunningham, J.A., Sobell, L.C. and Chow, V.M.C. (1993) 'What's in a label? The effects of substance types and labels on treatment considerations and stigma', *Journal of Studies on Alcohol*, 54: 693–9.

Davies, J.B. (1992) *The myth of addiction*, Reading: Harwood Academic.

Department of Health (1999) *Drug misuse and dependence: guidelines on clinical management*, London: Stationery Office.

Friedman, M. and Szasz, T. (1992) 'On liberty and drugs: essays on the free market and prohibition', in A. Trebach and K. Zeese (eds), *Friedman and Szasz on liberty and drugs*, Washington DC: The Drug Policy Foundation Press.

Friedman, S.R. (1998) 'The political economy of drug-user scapegoating – and the philosophy and politics of resistance', *Drugs: Education, Prevention and Policy*, 5, 1: 15–32.

Gossop, M., Marsden, J. and Stewart, D. (1998) *NTORS at one year. The National Treatment Outcome Study: changes in substance use, health and criminal behaviour one year after intake*, London: Department of Health.

Grund, J.P. (1993) *Drug use as a social ritual: functionality, symbolism and determinants of self regulation*, Rotterdam: Instituut voor Verslavingsonderzoek (IVO).

Health Advisory Service (1996) *The substance of young needs – communicating and providing services for children and young people who use and misuse substances*, London: HMSO.

Home Office (2000) *Criminal Justice and Court Services Bill*, www.parliament.the-stationeryoffice.co.uk/pa/cm199900/cmbills/091/2000091.htm

Jeffrey, R. (1979) 'Normal rubbish: deviant patients in casualty departments', *Sociology of Health and Illness*, 1, 1: 90–107.

Jones, E.E., Farina, A. and Hastorf, A.H. (1984) *Social stigma: the psychology of marked relationships*, New York: W.H. Freeman and Company.

Lemert, E.M. (1967) *Human deviance, social problems and social control*, Englewood Cliffs, NJ: Prentice Hall.

Link, B.G., Struening, E.L. and Rahav, M. (1997) 'On stigma and its consequences: evidence from a longitudinal study of men with dual diagnoses of mental illness and substance abuse', *Journal of Health and Social Behavior*, 38: 177–90.

Local Government Drugs Forum & SCODA (1997) *Drug-using parents: policy guidelines for inter-agency working*, London: Local Government Association.

McPhillips, M.A., Strang, J. and Barnes, T.R.E. (1998) 'Hair analysis – new laboratory ability to test for substance use', *British Journal of Psychiatry*, 173: 287–90.

Martin, E. (1996) 'Training in substance abuse is lacking for GPs', *British Medical Journal*, 12: 186.

Matheson, C. (1998) 'Views of illicit drug users on their treatment and behaviour in Scottish community pharmacies', *Health Education Journal*, 57, 1: 31–41.

Nadelmann, E. (1997) 'The end of the epoch of prohibition', in L. Boellinger (ed.), *Cannabis science: from prohibition to human right*, Frankfurt am Main: Peter Lang.

Preston, A. and Campion-Smith, C. (1997) 'Education may make general practitioners feel more confident', *British Medical Journal*, 315: 601–2.

Ramsay, M. and Partridge, S. (1999) 'Drug misuse declared in 1998: results from the British Crime Survey', London: Home Office.

Release (1997) *Release drugs and dance survey*, London: Release.

Robins, L.N. (1974) *The Vietnam drug user returns.* Special Action Office Monograph, Series A, No. 2, Washington DC: US Government Printing Office.

Shedler, J. and Block, J. (1990) 'Adolescent drug use and psychological health', *American Psychologist,* 45 (5): 612–30.

Standing Conference on Drug Abuse (SCODA) (1997) *Getting drug users involved: good practice in local treatment and planning,* London: SCODA.

Standing Conference on Drug Abuse and Children's Legal Centre (SCODA/CLC) (1999) *Young people and drugs: policy guidance for drug interventions,* London: SCODA.

Stimson, G.V. and Oppenheimer, E. (1982) *Heroin addiction: treatment and control in Britain,* London: Tavistock.

Szasz, T. (1992) *Our right to drugs: the case for a free market,* New York: Praeger.

Teijlingen, E.V. and Porter, M. (1997) 'General practitioners' attitudes towards treatment of opiate users: study in Lothian confirms findings', *British Medical Journal,* 315: 601.

United Nations Drug Control Programme (1997) *World Drug Report,* Oxford: Oxford University Press.

Winstock, A. (2000) 'Mixmag Drug Survey', *Mixmag,* February.

World Health Organisation (1992) *The ICD-10 Classification of Mental and Behavioural Disorders,* Geneva: World Health Organisation.

Part II

Applications to practice

Section III: Dilemmas

19 Rosa's story

The burden of ill health when homeless

Clare Croft-White and Georgie Parry-Crooke

Stigma, derived from the five marks left on Christ's body by the Crucifixion known as the stigmata, can be regarded as a sign of beatification or a mark of shame. Among homeless people, the meaning is often all too clear – the mark of disgrace which leads them to be discredited and distrusted. Take Rosa's story, with her five personal stigmata.

On arrival at the local health centre, Rosa knew that she needed medical treatment but that she may well never receive help. Would the reception staff react to the style of her clothes – the old coat and tatty trainers, topped with a broad-brimmed boater – all she could find in a pile discarded outside the charity shop (*1 Aspect of physical appearance*) or that frightened look in her eye? She knew about this because other people had either obscurely or overtly made it plain that her comportment was not the norm (*2 Behaviour*). It had taken months for her to get to the door of the health centre, this potential entry into a new and better life. But even now, if she did manage the next step, one look and she would be discredited forever. She knew what they would see and what their gut reaction would be: a deviation from their expectations – a set of assumptions which begin in physical difference, course their way rapidly through such platitudes as 'she can't communicate with us' (*3 Language and communication*), 'look at those cuts to her face – fighting of course' (*4 Physical marking*) and 'she's only after the drugs', to culminate in that most derogatory, if unspoken, of all, 'she does not deserve our service'. She is already deemed unworthy (*5 The whole: the hole under the heart*) before being given the chance to speak or to explain. This is stigmatisation.

Sadly, this is not an uncommon set of events for homeless people when they try to gain access to a range of statutory health services – primary care, mental health and Accident and Emergency departments. 'It's a disgrace', we might say in response, yet this is often what the very professionals will say of the homeless people who turn to them. Who are these homeless people, and what kind of health problems do they experience? What is it that interrupts that first and crucial moment of communication? Where do these 'primitive responses'

(Jones *et al.*, 1984) come from and what can be done to overcome them? How does the individual lose the marks of stigma and gain entry to these essential services? And then, how can that relationship be sustained?

Taking each of these questions, we will argue that, while many services and the individual professionals within them have worked to ameliorate the worst of practices and attitudes, there is more to be done to address these issues. For homeless people this can and does result in poor access to health services, inadequate provision, and an experience that serves to keep people away rather than to invite them in.

Who are these homeless people, and what kinds of health problems do they experience?

For the purposes of this discussion, homeless people include those who have slept on the streets, been in hostels or short-term accommodation, and those living in other types of temporary situations. Many of these people are single, and an increasing number are asylum seekers and refugees. In London (and this is likely to be mirrored in other large cities), some 'types' of homeless people experience more prejudice than others within the healthcare system (Pleace and Quilgars, 1996). This particularly affects those sleeping rough and those who are mobile in a city where health services are provided on a geographical basis. Their health is often worse than others', and they are more likely to experience greater severity of symptoms and a higher prevalence of physical health problems. Indeed, it is now well known that nine of the most common health complaints are more prevalent in homeless people than in the rest of the population,[1] with the incidence of 'wounds, skin ulcers and other skin complaints' being two, if not three, times higher (Bines, 1994).

Mental ill health is also widespread, with well in excess of a quarter of hostel dwellers and people staying in bed and breakfast accommodation having a mental health problem (Scott, 1993). Current figures suggest that over 50 per cent of people using temporary hostels and sleeping rough experience severe mental health problems, and for many homeless people their mental ill health is exacerbated by accompanying alcohol or illicit drug misuse (O'Leary, 1997). Treatment is often hampered by lack of services for people with this 'dual diagnosis', typified by mental health workers feeling unable to treat someone who continues to drink (or take drugs), and substance misuse workers feeling unsupported and untrained to address the mental health treatment needs.

Given all of the above, it is hardly surprising that the life expectancy of someone sleeping rough is 42 years (compared with 74 for a man and 79 for a woman), and that the average age of death by natural causes is 46 years (Grenier, 1996).

What is it that interrupts that first and crucial moment of communication?

The Royal College of General Practitioners (RCGP) has a supporting Statement on Homelessness and General Practice, which says that 'homelessness and poor or inappropriate housing are major indicators and causes of ill-health and mental stress; work with homeless people therefore forms an important part of all general practitioners' work' (RCGP, 1993). However, this is not necessarily the experience of many. Where individuals do manage to take the step of locating and opening the door of a primary care service, the first encounter – and therefore that first moment of communication – is crucial to how a relationship between the homeless person and the service can develop. The interruptions to this early encounter are varied and can broadly be seen as encompassing two positions: those which are concerned with the provider; and those which are affected by homeless people's lack of confidence in using services effectively.

From the perspective of the provider, there is a growing body of evidence which demonstrates that homeless people are frequently stereotyped by medical staff. Such staff are concerned that homeless people may be time-consuming for a number of reasons. Longer consultation periods are required, with extra time needed to develop a relationship of trust with the homeless patient, to take a case history because no medical records are available, and to address the 'shopping list' of symptoms that they have stored up during their years of neglect (Craft, Croft-White and England, 2000). They disrupt the running of the surgery by failing to keep appointments or by turning up at a time that suits them. The time spent with them is perceived as wasted because they are seen as incapable of following through a treatment plan – a particular concern since there is evidence of an increase in communicable diseases such as TB and hepatitis B and C among homeless people (Rushdy and O'Mahony, 1998).

Homeless people are also seen to present a (real or imaginary) risk of violence, due to their presumed drug or alcohol use. Whether or not this is the case is not at issue here. More important is that staff feel the risk exists and are not always sufficiently confident or supported to work with homeless people where this arises. An added barrier is the notion that the homeless person's primary interest is not the medical treatment *per se* but access to drugs, or to medical letters in support of their housing claim.

Almost before these assumptions come into play, staff are concerned to protect other patients' rights, and the homeless person may well feel unwelcome by receptionists and other frontline staff in the service.

From the viewpoint of the homeless patient, equally important as a barrier to a profitable relationship developing between themselves and the medical staff is their own lack of confidence. Many homeless people have low self-esteem which is linked with an assumption that they will be refused help. Past experience of unsympathetic treatment and refusal by a GP practice is projected forward as an expectation of future contacts. However, it is more likely to be fear, rather than actual experience, of an abusive and excluding reaction from healthcare staff that may discourage people from seeking help. At the same time, some will experience embarrassment due to low standards of personal hygiene and dirty clothes which may make them shun seeking a service which requires them to undress. According to Pleace and Quilgars (1996), the lack of social skills has been attributed in some cases to low levels of literacy among homeless people, further marginalising them and increasing their difficulties when dealing with large organisations.

Where do these 'primitive responses' come from?

As to the origins of these 'primitive responses' and what can be done to overcome them, there is no need to look further than research studies designed to explore and understand the complex relationship between homelessness and access to healthcare. This impacts not only on the homeless people themselves and on medical staff, but also those working in homelessness agencies who may be unaware of their clients' rights to healthcare. There are important – simple – ways in which this situation can be ameliorated. These can be initiated by those who directly help homeless people to access services and those who support staff to work with a group they may find difficult to engage with.

For homeless people, health centres and Accident and Emergency departments could provide directories and information files on sources of advice as well as a store of replacement clean clothes. This could make a significant difference to their use of health provision, their self-esteem and therefore to their health and well-being. For homelessness agencies, an appropriate role for staff is to support homeless people to be more assertive, confident and informed when dealing with 'authority'. However, to be effective in this manner, they need to be 'up to speed' with information about their clients' right to healthcare, sources of primary healthcare and the benefits of health promotion.

The inadequate attention to health promotion for homeless people stems from a number of factors. These include their limited contact with health services; a lack of interest in the health needs of homeless people; poor inter-agency working; the absence of national and local strategies; and negative attitudes (Power *et al.*, 1999). Research into the needs of homeless people recommends that health promotion services should take a more proactive role in this area; that health authorities should adopt flexible interpretations of the 'Our Healthier Nation' targets and encourage GPs to permanently register homeless people; and that homelessness agencies should work with health services to develop local strategies (Hinton, 1999). Health promotion should therefore become a priority for both homelessness agencies and health service providers.

In the case of health service providers, an apparent sense of elitism on the part of *qualified* medical staff towards *unqualified* homelessness agency staff who may be acting as advocates could be broken down through awareness-raising, making use of a variety of strategies, including joint training, shadowing, and indeed, just talking and communicating about patients in common. Meanwhile, easier access to patients' notes to enable a check on past history would directly affect the way in which people are treated.

In essence, there is a need to raise awareness among medical staff of their responsibilities towards homeless people. The RCGP (1993) 'urges its members to practise equity in its registration policy. Homeless people should be registered permanently wherever possible and integrated into all health profile and promotion activity within the practice. A permanent address is not necessary for registration.'

How does the individual lose the marks of stigma and gain entry to these essential services?

Improved access to information on rights and the availability of services, more joint working that breaks down the professional barriers, and greater awareness of the health needs and priorities of homeless people, are important achievable goals to strive for. But how far can they ensure that Rosa – and others – can lose the marks of stigma and gain entry to these essential services to which they have a right?

One strategy to promote the availability of healthcare is the provision of specialist services within projects working with homeless people. The range of primary care services on offer in such projects varies. Larger projects receive regular visits from local primary healthcare workers – a local GP, psychiatrist, senior registrar or psychologist, a nurse or a CPN. Some also benefit through visits from a dentist, chiropodist and optician. Referrals are made to secondary and other specialist services where necessary, and support is also offered to protect staff in dealing with clients with physical or psychiatric problems. Such 'on-site' services are usually the first choice for homeless people (Pleace, Jones and England, 2000), but their lack of availability out of hours (i.e. when primary care workers are not present at the project) delays treatment and attention to health problems which may subsequently become more acute.

Many homelessness projects have elected to designate a team member with responsibility for healthcare issues; in others the responsibility is shared amongst team members. They may or may not be medically trained, but hands-on experience of working with this client group and participation in training make them amply qualified for the role of improving health awareness within both the staff team and the service user group. They can encourage clients to use visiting medical services, act as advocate on behalf of their clients, and liaise between external medical services and the client group.

A number of building-based medical centres that target single homeless people also exist around the country. One of the largest is Great Chapel

Street Medical Centre in London, established in 1978. It provides a daily primary care medical service in central London through sessional inputs from a GP, a psychiatrist, a dentist, a CPN, a drug and alcohol specialist, a social worker, and an occupational therapist. The specialised supportive environment makes it more accessible to people who, typically, lead a chaotic lifestyle and are unable or unwilling to use appointment systems.

Dedicated primary healthcare teams serve areas where there is a high prevalence of homeless people. While they may have a static base where clients and patients can be seen by medical staff, a major aspect of their function is to provide outreach work and sessions in settings that are frequented by homeless people. This might typically include weekly sessions in drop-in centres or lunch clubs; visits to short-stay hostels and cold weather shelters (in season). Services include medical care, health advice and information, advocacy, support and referral to mainstream, specialist and secondary services. The teams are also instrumental in encouraging local GPs to register homeless people by offering support to the patient – and the surgery staff – in using the service appropriately. Their smaller-than-average caseloads allow them to undertake holistic assessments that include the identification of needs around welfare benefits, housing issues, social care and education. This can be followed through by liaison with local authority departments to monitor and improve the living and environmental conditions for homeless people. And finally, many have a training role with a commitment to provide tailor-made training sessions and materials for primary care and other staff working with homeless people.

Many of these primary care teams make contact with homeless people with mental health problems and specialist teams (funded by the Department of Health under the Homeless Mentally Ill Initiative). The aim of these multi-disciplinary outreach teams is to 'identify clients not in touch with statutory services, make an assessment of their needs, provide medical and social interventions and refer them to statutory services as appropriate' (Craig *et al.*, 1995).

The Health Act (1999) has brought new roles, responsibilities and opportunities for nurses in meeting the primary healthcare needs of homeless people. A number of the Personal Medical Services (PMS) pilot schemes have focused on improving the access and acceptability of services to deprived and 'hard to reach communities' and, by March 2000, 129 pilot schemes (48 per cent) had identified their commitment to different communities, including the homeless.

A feature of some of these pilot schemes is the central role of the nursing staff, working alongside the salaried GP. Preliminary research of PMS pilots indicates that the nurse practitioners provide an instrumental role, working with the homeless patient throughout their contact with the surgery. They facilitate the registration process and encourage continuing attendance to follow through a course of treatment. They ensure that the homeless patient receives the new-patient (and other) routine health checks. They allocate sufficient 'consultation' time to develop a trust relationship with the patient and to explore the psycho-social issues that may impact on their health and well-being. They act as advocates for the patient where onward referral is required. And, where necessary, they take the primary care service to the individuals, through visits to hostels, day centres and other venues where homeless people congregate.

The pilots have identified two key success factors in de-stigmatising the homeless patient. The first is the need to adopt a non-discriminative, non-judgemental approach. This includes a degree of tolerance towards certain behaviour in the waiting area, without compromising the rights of other patients. The second is a multidisciplinary approach that transforms the surgery into an entry point to a wide range of other support mechanisms that will slowly break down barriers. This demands not only an appropriate skills mix and access to help within the surgery, but also robust links with the local voluntary homelessness agencies, social services and housing departments.

The establishment of NHS Direct presents another opportunity for nurses to be in the front line. But can it become a life saver to Rosa, who no longer has to worry about her appearance, smell or lack of a medical 'past'? Not if she does not have easy access to a telephone or the wherewithal to pay for the call. An experimental project to test the acceptability of the service to homeless people began in early 1999. Dedicated phone lines were installed in two homelessness projects in South London – one of which offered accommodation linked with training opportunities and the other being a day centre. They are located in a discrete, quiet location within the project, are free of charge, and are routed to a call handler who is able to provide advice and information that is appropriate to the caller. Only a sustained period of provision will reveal whether this anonymised source of help will be the first step towards the homeless person's release from stigma, or will simply be another way of enabling the health professions to avert their eyes.[2]

The NHS Walk-in Centres, the first of which opened in 2000, offer another opportunity for homeless people to by-pass the inflexibility presented by the appointment system. Their extended 'walk-in-off-the-street' operation might just tip the balance for Rosa.

Where next for Rosa?

This brief chapter has highlighted the barriers and circumstances that prevent Rosa and others from accessing the facilities to meet their health-care needs. It suggests a few simple solutions to break down some of these barriers, and describes some recent initiatives that aim to tackle health inequalities. But the questions still remain. Are services designed to respond to the often complex needs and stigmatisation of the transient homeless person? Will using these services be any different from attending the local

A & E when the need becomes too great? Will the attitudes of the staff be any less judgemental than those often encountered by homeless people? Will they be able to advocate on their behalf and open other doors? Will they encourage joint working with the other professional groups with an interest in and responsibility for this group of patients?

Or will they continue to be a sticking plaster to cover only temporarily the wounds of stigmata? Time will tell.

Notes

1 The illnesses are chronic chest or breathing problems, heart problems, wounds and skin ulcers, musculo–skeletal problems, fits or loss of consciousness, digestive problems, frequent headaches, and mental ill health.
2 The NHS Direct Homelessness Line is to be evaluated by the Immediate Access Project, Guy's, King's and St Thomas' School of Medicine, concluding in 2001. NHS Direct is a free telephone helpline staffed by qualified and experienced nurses who provide advice and information about health and illness over the phone on a 24-hour basis. After piloting, it became a national service at the end of 2000.

References

Bines, W. (1994) *The health of single homeless people*, University of York, Centre for Housing Policy.

Craft, M., Croft-White, C. and England, J. (2000) *Research priorities in primary care: homeless people, refugees and asylum seekers*, 3 Boroughs Primary Health Care Team, Lambeth Southwark and Lewisham Health Authority.

Craig, T., Bayliss, E., Klein, O. *et al.* (1995) *The homeless mentally ill initiative: an evaluation of four clinical teams*, London: Department of Health.

Grenier, P. (1996) *Still dying for a home*, London: Crisis.

Hinton, T. (1999) *The icing on the cake*, Health Action for Homeless People, Brent and Harrow Health Authority, Queen Mary and Westfield College.

Jones, E.E., Farina, A., Hastorf, A.H. *et al.* (1984) *Social stigma, the psychology of marked relationships*, New York: W.H. Freeman.

O'Leary, J. (1997) *Beyond help?*, London: National Homeless Alliance.

Pleace, N. and Quilgars, D. (1996) *Health and homelessness in London*, London: The King's Fund.

Pleace, N., Jones, A. and England, E. (2000) *Access to general practice for people sleeping rough*, York: Centre for Housing Policy.

Power, R., French, R. and Connelly, J. (1999) *Promoting the health of homeless people: setting a research agenda*, London: Health Education Authority.

RCGP (1993) *Statement on homelessness and general practice*, London: Council of the Royal College of General Practitioners.

Riley, A. (2000) Private correspondence on Personal Medical Services. Department of General Practice and Primary Care, Queen Mary and Westfield College, University of London.

Rushdy, A. and O'Mahony, M. (1998) *PHLS Overview of Communicable Diseases Committee*, Disease Report, November, vol. 8, supp. 5.

Scott, J. (1993) 'Homelessness and ill health', *British Journal of Psychiatry*, 162: 314–24.

20 Involuntary childlessness and stigma

Eric Blyth and Ruth Moore

Introduction

Involuntary childlessness can be seen as a life crisis that evokes a series of cultural, emotional, social and psychological responses (Daly, 1999). It is frequently unanticipated, may be unexplained, may last for an indeterminate length of time, and can affect both individuals and relationships (Whiteford and Gonzalez, 1995). In pronatalist societies, i.e. virtually all known cultures, married couples are expected both to want and to have children, and motherhood is seen as a defining characteristic of women. Those who deviate from these cultural norms, such as the involuntarily childless, are consequently likely to be stigmatised (see, for example, Veevers, 1980; Miall, 1986, 1994; Daly, 1999).

Historically, involuntary childlessness was met with a mixture of fatalism and reliance on divine intervention (Pfeffer, 1993), while the latter part of the twentieth century saw the rise of technological developments aimed at helping individuals to achieve parenthood.

This chapter explores two dimensions of stigma in this realm – concealability and course – by focusing the discussion on the treatment process and the outcomes of treatment. Throughout this discussion the authors indicate how healthcare policies and health workers may contribute to the stigmatising process, before considering how the social stigma of involuntary childlessness can be ameliorated.

It is axiomatic that any attempt to determine the prevalence of a given phenomenon is contingent upon its definition. We consider here two terms, 'infertility' and our preferred term 'involuntary childlessness'. Couples are considered to have primary infertility if they have been unable to conceive after one year of engaging in sexual intercourse without contraception and if conception has not previously occurred. Couples are considered to have secondary infertility if they fail to conceive following one or more births, or following conception, or fail to carry a pregnancy to term (McFalls, 1979). However, this reading of 'infertility' includes only those conditions ascribed medical legitimacy, and fails to take into account individuals who may have no medically diagnosed reproductive impairment, but who are nevertheless 'involuntarily childless'. Involuntary childlessness may also result from sexual orientation and/or lack of an opposite-sex partner: factors which, themselves, may well increase individuals' exposure to stigma. Involuntary childlessness, therefore, encapsulates both medical and social phenomena, taking fuller account of the social and psychological implications for those who have been unable to realise their wish to become a parent.

In broadening the definition beyond that which is restricted to medical contingencies, the task of determining the prevalence of our chosen phenomena is made that much more difficult. Even so, estimates of the prevalence of 'infertility' alone are likely only to have ballpark accuracy. Various studies have reported prevalence rates in the range one in five couples to one in ten couples (Miall, 1986). It is generally estimated that up to one in seven couples, including those wanting a second pregnancy, seek specialist (i.e. medical) help because of a problem in conceiving (Human Fertilisation and Embryology Authority, n.d.). This would represent an unknown underestimate if a wider social definition of involuntary childlessness is utilised. Perceptions of sharing a problem with vast numbers of other people do not, however, characterise the experience of the involuntarily childless: 'I feel sometimes like we're the only ones in the world who have this' (Daly, 1999: 19).

Involuntary childlessness and stigma

Negative cultural representations of involuntary childlessness are reflected in everyday language. *Roget's Thesaurus*, for example, places 'infertile' in the company of terms such as 'barren', 'fruitless', 'impotent', 'incompetent', 'sexless', 'unproductive', 'waste', 'withered'. In the media, childless women are frequently portrayed as 'obsessed' or 'desperate' (Pfeffer, 1987; Franklin, 1990). Small wonder, then, that the reported experiences of involuntarily childless individuals include those of alienation, failure, guilt, inadequacy and isolation (see, for example, Pfeffer and Woollett, 1983; Miall, 1986; Whiteford and Gonzalez, 1995; Daly, 1999).

The source of the stigma and social disapproval experienced by the involuntarily childless is considered to lie in their violation of traditional cultural norms in pronatalist societies: that motherhood is 'the only real path to self-realization and normality for women' (Sandelowski, 1986: 446) and that all married couples should produce children (Veevers, 1980; Miall, 1986).

Evidence indicates that involuntary childless women and men may experience differential levels and types of stigma. On the one hand, given the presumed centrality of childbearing and motherhood for women, the inability to reproduce challenges a woman's femininity and 'strikes at the very essence of one's being' (infertile woman, cited by Miall, 1985: 272). While fatherhood is considered less central to the identity of men than motherhood is to women, fertility difficulties in men are viewed more negatively, tending to be associated with impotence or a lack of virility (Humphrey, 1969; Owens, 1982; Miall, 1994). Consequently, a female partner of a man with fertility difficulties may well pretend or allow others to assume that she has a fertility difficulty in order to protect the man from the even greater stigma associated with male sexual dysfunction.

The career trajectory and information management

Involuntary childlessness may be anticipated by some individuals, such as those with known inherited disorders likely to affect fertility, or those whose lifestyle or sexual orientation generally preclude heterosexual relationships. However, for most heterosexual couples the possibility of a fertility difficulty only emerges following failure to achieve a pregnancy despite unprotected sexual intercourse. Whether or not couples initially conceal the fact that they are trying to conceive, the absence of a desired child becomes an obvious public blemish distinguishing them from the child-rearing population, about which family and friends may begin to express interest or concern, while the personal knowledge that they are unsuccessfully attempting to conceive reinforces internalised perceptions of difference and deficiency (Whiteford and Gonzalez, 1995) – factors that are likely to create the motivation to seek professional (i.e. medical) assistance.

Diagnosis of a fertility difficulty is infrequently a defining event, but is more likely to be a lengthy, potentially indeterminate process in which the possibility of achieving conception – with or without medical help – is rarely excluded absolutely (Greil *et al.*, 1988): 'In some ways the seeds of hope [are] nourished by the soil of uncertainty' (Daly, 1999: 21).

While, historically, the involuntarily childless had few options for ameliorating their condition, medical expertise and technological advances now appear to offer 'new' choices. However, the medicalisation of involuntary childlessness comes at a cost. It reinforces biological constructions of women (Patrick Steptoe, cited in Stanworth, 1987: 15), thus making the choice of *not* pursuing medical intervention illusory (Sandelowski, 1986). Despite the hope offered by the apparently limitless capacity of technology, as a result of which neither age nor seriously malfunctioning reproductive systems any longer represent insurmountable barriers to successful conception, embarking on treatment imposes pressures to 'try everything possible', even beyond what is reasonably likely to be helpful. Some possible options may themselves attract further social disapproval, such as surrogacy or seeking treatment as a post-menopausal woman.

Rothman claims that the range of reproductive options has created 'a new burden for the infertile – the burden of not trying hard enough' (Rothman, 1984: 31). Given that most couples entering treatment will remain childless, the hope and lure of success offered by technology are infrequently fulfilled in the lived reality experienced by the involuntarily childless: 'The very process of medical intervention further stigmatizes women and devalues them for any accomplishments outside of reproduction. Once into the process of medical intervention, the woman's identity as a person is all too often determined by the outcome of the medical intervention, her ability to reproduce' (Whiteford and Gonzalez, 1995: 36).

Unsurprisingly, individuals are reluctant to accept the label 'childless', not only because of its stigmatising attributes, but also because it is tantamount to accepting defeat, preferring instead to regard themselves as 'not-yet-pregnant' (Greil, 1991) or as 'parents in waiting' (Meerabeau, 1994). Meerabeau also cites unwillingness to accept the status of 'childless' as a reason for the failure of most couples in her study to join potentially useful self-help groups. Daly (1999) notes that conventional linear models of adaptation to loss and bereavement do not apply in involuntary childlessness, where the 'process is much messier', observing that few couples in his study referred to anything resembling 'closure'. Frequently, the end of treatment – and hence of the quest for parenthood – will result from the cessation of funding rather than from an independent clinical judgement made by doctors about the likely success of continuing.

As involuntary childlessness is not readily apparent, it may be conceptualised as a 'secret stigma' (Whiteford and Gonzalez, 1995), a discreditable or potentially stigmatising attribute (Goffman, 1963). Consequently, involuntary childlessness is amenable to relatively high levels of concealability. Evidence from a wide range of empirical studies indicates that the employment of different strategies of information management is influenced by key variables, including the passage of time.

At the outset, apprehension about the likely response of others and lack of a specific diagnosis mean that involuntarily childless individuals are likely to disclose little if anything about their fertility status. They are likely to avoid sensitive events or topics of conversation, or other people whom they consider might make them feel uncomfortable about their childlessness. Initial appointments with doctors or at specialist centres are likely to be kept secret, although, at this stage, some form of selective disclosure, even if only to professionals whose assistance is sought, will become inevitable. A further strategy of partial disclosure ('therapeutic disclosure'), which allows for 'renegotiation of the negative meanings attached to infertility' (Miall, 1986: 266) may be made, especially to family, close friends or other infertile people, to enhance the individual's self-esteem or to renegotiate personal perceptions of stigma. Miall identifies a further level of disclosure of discreditable attributes which attempts to influence others' actions or ideas about oneself, or about infertility in general. A frequently-used form of such 'preventive disclosure', intended to deflect blame directed towards the individual, is a medical disclaimer attributing responsibility for the fertility difficulty to a medical condition. 'Deviance avowal' is another mechanism used by involuntarily childless individuals. In one form of this, as we have seen, female partners of men with fertility difficulties falsely assume responsibility for the couple's child-lessness, on the basis that women with fertility difficulties are less likely than men to be stigmatised. In a second version, involuntary childlessness is specifically acknowledged in order to pre-empt the more stigmatising attribution of *voluntary* childlessness (Veevers, 1980; McAllister with Clarke, 1998).

Both Miall (1986) and Daly (1999) note that the wish for secrecy on the part of involuntarily childless individuals generally reduces over time. Such a move may be facilitated, on the one hand, by the practical difficulties of maintaining a consistent cover story over an extended period in the face of the pressure of increasingly inquisitive and suspicious significant others; and, on the other, by a reduction in initial feelings of shame and inade-quacy and by the acquisition of knowledge and a vocabulary for talking about their condition.

Disclosure of such sensitive personal information increases the indi-vidual's vulnerability to stigmatisation, as recounted by one man interviewed by Daly: 'When I first mentioned it at work I felt shunned – they say, "What the hell is that? Are you shooting blanks?" ' (Daly, 1999: 20).

However, disclosure also enables the involuntarily childless to moderate the experience of stigma, reassert control over their life, redefine their self-image and secure support both from their regular social networks and from others in a similar position: 'Infertile women use therapeutic disclo-sure as a strategy to relieve anxiety, to restore self-esteem, and to renegotiate personal perceptions of infertility as discreditable. Indeed, several respondents observed that the ability to reveal infertility at all was suggestive of the beginning of adjustment to the possession of a stigma-tizing attribute' (Miall, 1986: 266).

Male factor subfertility or infertility, especially where treatment options involve the use of third-party gametes or embryos, are further key vari-ables affecting disclosure. As previously discussed, there is widespread agreement that male infertility is seen and experienced as a greater stigma than female infertility. While much of the technological and pharmacolog-ical effort has been directed at improving the fertility of women and circumventing malfunctioning female reproductive systems, the medical treatment of male infertility has, until the recent development of intracyto-plasmic sperm injection (ICSI) which enables the sperm of subfertile men to be used for successful conception, been rudimentary. Prior to ICSI the conventional medical 'remedy' for male fertility difficulties was donor insemination (DI). DI was characterised by additional potentially stigma-tising attributes: the introduction of an anonymous donor as a quasi-adulterous intruder into the marriage relationship; the creation of a quasi-illegitimate child (in the UK the legal status of such children was not clarified until 1987), and recourse to masturbation for the production of sperm for insemination. Historically, even when this was successful – or perhaps even more so if it was successful – if individuals had never previously disclosed their involuntarily childless status, there seemed little purpose in doing so once they were no longer childless and could pass as 'normal' (Goffman, 1963). Indeed, continuing secrecy has been both advocated by professionals and practised by parents of children conceived following DI (Blyth, 1999): 'We just want to carry on as though nothing has happened' (DI recipient, cited in Snowden and Snowden, 1998: 46).

However, the extent to which people can 'carry on as though nothing has happened' has been challenged, primarily by 'donor offspring' (those born as a result of DI). Some parents of donor offspring have asserted that the maintenance of secrecy may be illusory and that family relationships may be seriously damaged by deception (see, for example, Donor Conception Support Group of Australia, 1997; Blyth *et al.*, 1998).

Countering the stigma of involuntary childlessness

The stigmatisation of involuntary childlessness is inherently bound up with culture-linked pronatalist assumptions. Despite concerns about global overpopulation, disquiet about decreasing fertility rates in the developed world means that simply calling for the abandonment of pronatalism as a means of countering the stigma of involuntary childlessness would be both naïve and futile.

Less radical, but potentially achievable, strategies would include the encouragement of wider political and educational initiatives to authenticate and legitimise adult roles that do not centre on the ability to produce and rear children. Specifically, this would include recognising elective non-parenthood as a socially valued lifestyle. If the choices of those who do not want children in the first place are respected and legitimised, then being 'childfree' at the end of unsuccessful fertility treatment is likely to be perceived as a less negative alternative.

Educational programmes in schools, for example as part of proposed citizenship education in the UK, should facilitate consideration of adult lifestyles that do not focus exclusively on parenting. At the same time, conventional sex education in schools, with its understandable emphasis on preventing involuntary conception, should be expanded to ensure both awareness of involuntary childlessness and preventive strategies to reduce the incidence of fertility difficulties. After all, the statistics enjoying current credence suggest that five children in every class of thirty students are likely to experience fertility difficulties in adulthood.

Healthcare provision should focus more on the availability of preventive services, hitherto comparatively neglected and under-resourced. At the same time there should be more equitable access to fertility treatment services, which currently depends to a large extent either on individuals' ability to pay for their own treatment or to what extent treatment is publicly funded by the health authority in whose areas they live. Arguably, such discrepancies contribute to the construction of 'desperateness' and stigma.

Stigmatisation is not infrequently compounded once the involuntarily childless enter into fertility treatment (Whiteford and Gonzales, 1995). This is especially so for women, whose reproductive system is the focus of most 'therapeutic' intervention, while men are more likely to be sidelined. Such experiences can be countered by policies and practice which focus on person-centred and holistic healthcare, promoting user participation and control to the potential benefit of both male and female users and of clinical staff (Shattuck and Schwarz, 1991). Solomon (1989), an involuntarily childless feminist, argues for the development of non-technical alternatives such as increased emotional and personal support to both involuntarily childless women and men.

The development of such models can also help to overcome a major barrier to changing the stigmatising culture surrounding involuntary childlessness – the extent to which the sole yardstick of treatment success, and the reputation of individual practitioners, is the 'take home baby' rate. This pressure is compounded by attempts to compare the performance of treatment centres. In reality, although in the UK information is regularly published as a means of improving the quality of information available to potential customers and hence to enhancing choice and decision-making (Human Fertilisation and Embryology Authority, n.d.), no way has yet been devised of adequately comparing the performance of different centres.

Given that most treatments have low success rates in terms of the 'take home baby' rate, this criterion is destined to set up for failure both professional staff and users. Consequently, it is in the best interests of fertility professionals and the involuntarily childless to reconsider the basis on which 'success' is judged. Effective holistic care, even if not accompanied by conception and birth, can result in individuals leaving treatment free to move on with positive expectations about a childless life, as illustrated by Kathy Baker when she writes about her aspirations at the end of 'unsuccessful' treatment:

> I have realised that if I have no child to leave to posterity, which is for most people their greatest life achievement, the need to achieve in other ways becomes even more of a priority.
>
> (Baker, 1999: 17)

References

Baker, K. (1999) 'Infertility and bereavement', *Journal of Fertility Counselling*, 6, 3: 15–17.

Blyth, E. (1999) 'Secrets and lies: barriers to the exchange of genetic origins information following donor assisted conception', *Adoption and Fostering*, 23, 1: 49–59.

Blyth, E., Crawshaw, M. and Speirs, J. (eds) (1998) *Truth and the child ten years on: information exchange in donor assisted conception*, Birmingham: British Association of Social Workers.

Daly, K. (1999) 'Crisis of genealogy: facing the challenges of infertility', in H. McCubbin, E. Thompson, A. Thompson and J. Futrell (eds), *The dynamics of resilient families*, Thousand Oaks: Sage.

Donor Conception Support Group of Australia (1997) *Let the offspring speak: discussions on donor conception*, Georges Hall, New South Wales: Donor Conception Support Group of Australia Inc.

Franklin, S. (1990) 'Deconstructing "desperateness": the social construction of infertility in popular representations of new reproductive technologies', in M. McNeil, I. Varcoe and S. Yearly (eds), *The new reproductive technologies*, London: Macmillan.

Goffman, E. (1963) *Stigma: notes on the management of spoiled identity*, London: Prentice Hall.

Greil, A.L. (1991) *Not yet pregnant: infertile couples in contemporary America*, New Brunswick: Rutgers University Press.

Greil, A., Leitko, T. and Porter, K. (1988) 'Infertility: his and hers', *Gender and Society*, 1: 172–9.

Human Fertilisation and Embryology Authority (n.d.) *The patients' guide to infertility and IVF clinics*, London: HFEA.

Humphrey, M. (1969) *The hostage seekers*, London: Longman.

McAllister, F. with Clarke, L. (1998) *Choosing childlessness*, London: Family Policy Studies Centre.

McFalls, J. (1979) *Psychopathology and sub-fecundity*, New York: Academic Press.

Meerabeau, L. (1994) 'Fertility and reproductive technology', in C. Webb (ed.), *Living sexuality issues for nursing and health*, London: Scutari Press.

Miall, C. (1985) 'Perceptions of informal sanctioning and the stigma of involuntary childlessness', *Deviant Behavior*, 6: 383–403.

—— (1986) 'The stigma of involuntary childlessness', *Social Problems*, 33: 268–82.

—— (1994) 'Community constructs of involuntary childlessness: sympathy, stigma and social support', *Canadian Review of Sociology and Anthropology*, 31: 392–421.

Owens, D. (1982) 'The desire to father: reproductive ideologies and involuntary childless men', in L. McKee and M. O'Brien (eds), *The father figure*, London: Tavistock.

Pfeffer, N. (1987) 'Artificial insemination, in vitro fertilisation and the stigma of infertility', in M. Stanworth (ed.), *Reproductive technologies: gender, motherhood and medicine*, Oxford: Basil Blackwell/Polity Press.

—— (1993) *The stork and the syringe: a political history of reproductive medicine*, Cambridge: Polity Press.

Pfeffer, N. and Woollett, A. (1983) *The experience of infertility*, London: Virago.

Rothman, B.K. (1984) 'The meaning of choice in reproductive technology', in R. Ardetti, R. Klein and S. Minden (eds), *Test-tube women: what future for motherhood?*, London: Pandora.

Sandelowski, M. (1986) 'Sophie's choice: a metaphor for infertility', *Health Care for Women International*, 7: 439–53.

Shattuck, J. and Schwarz, K. (1991) 'Walking the line between feminism and infertility: implications of nursing, medicine and patient care', *Health Care for Women International*, 12: 331–9.

Solomon, A. (1989) 'Infertility as crisis: coping, surviving – and thriving', in R. Klein (ed.), *Infertility: women speak out about their experiences of infertility*, London: Pandora.

Snowden, R. and Snowden, E. (1998) 'Families created through donor insemination', in K. Daniels and E. Haimes (eds), *Donor insemination: international social science perspectives*, Cambridge: Cambridge University Press.

Stanworth, M. (ed.) (1987) *Reproductive technologies: gender, motherhood and medicine*, Oxford: Basil Blackwell/Polity Press.

Veevers, J. (1980) *Childless by choice*, Toronto: Butterworth.

Whiteford, L. and Gonzalez, L. (1995) 'Stigma: the hidden burden of infertility', *Social Science and Medicine*, 40, 1: 27–36.

21 Teenage pregnancy, stigma and differential provision of healthcare

John Jacono and Brenda Jacono

Introduction

Teenage pregnancy has been identified as a major source of social, ethical and financial concern in most industrialised countries. The problem has been described as an epidemic by many, and its onset has been invariably attributed to the 'sexual revolution of the sixties'. An increased freedom extant from the proliferation of two-income families, the attendant increase in parental divorce/separation often leading to single parent families, the glorification in the mass media of unchecked sexuality, peer pressure, hormonally induced rebelliousness and, paradoxically, the availability of safe, easy birth control and abortion, have all been described at one time or another as the root cause of this problem (Romig and Thompson, 1988; *Behavior Today*, 1990; Chilman, 1990; Dusek, 1991; Rodriquez and Moore, 1995). More recently, the failure to impart 'adequate sexual education', and the low expectations for the future of teenagers in light of diminishing opportunities, have also been cited (The Social Exclusion Unit, 1999).

While many of these proposed precursors have been challenged, and these will be the subject of further discussion later in this chapter, the problem is unfettered in most if not all industrialised nations. The country with the dubious distinction of leading the pack of industrialised nations with this problem is the USA. More than half a million babies are born to teenage mothers every year in America (Vinovski, 1981; Hayes, 1987; Henshaw, 1993). This represents only about 60 per cent of all conceptions to this group. While the actual birth rate for this age group has declined in the last four years, the proportion of births to teenagers in relation to total births shows no sign of decrease (Vinovski, 1981). In western Europe, Britain has the highest rate of teenage pregnancy, with over 20 per 1000 teenagers giving birth annually, once again only representing approximately 60 per cent of all teenage conceptions (The Social Exclusion Unit, 1999). Factors leading to teenage pregnancy have already been alluded to; however, the ensuing results of teenage pregnancy are even more dramatic. In the USA, about a half of all teenage mothers go on welfare within one year of the birth of the baby, with a further 27 per cent joining their ranks within five years (*USA Today*, 1993). The picture in England is, if anything, worse – about 90 per cent of all teenage mothers receive income support (Davies *et al.*, 1996). The choice to go on social assistance often translates into a cycle of poverty, isolation and depression, which may be merely a continuation of the teenager's previous history, or the start of a new cycle of need (Furstenburg, 1991).

The socio-economic implications for the mother and, ultimately, her offspring are not the sole problem, however. Babies born to teenage mothers are also at an increased risk of a large number of immediate and long-term problems. Death rates, low birth-weights, and rates for other psycho-physiological dysfunction are higher in children of teenage mothers than in children of other older mothers (Grazi *et al.*, 1983; Kitzes, 1986; Children's Defense Fund, 1988; Jacono *et al.*, 1992). All of these risk factors translate into a substantial burden on national exchequers, with concomitant adverse reactions from the tax paying public and their elected representatives. Escalation in the costs for provision of healthcare and income support to teenage mothers and others has resulted, in the recent past, in several initiatives that have as their basic premise taxpayer relief from a drastic reduction in allocation of funds to this sector. These reductions have frequently been portrayed as an attempt to ensure fiscal responsibility, on the part of both the donor and the recipient. At a time when significant employment losses are being experienced due to restructuring, failures and mergers – at least in some industries – many of these cost-cutting initiatives have been well received by the general public. This has severely impacted an already onerous cycle of exclusion and scapegoating for disadvantaged groups like the pregnant teenage group. Sadly this is not a new phenomenon.

Putative origins of stigmatisation in teenage pregnancy

The origins of latter-day stigmatisation and social exclusion of pregnant teenagers may have their genesis in beliefs going back as far as the sixteenth century. It has been argued that some proportion of the success of the industrial revolution was buttressed by the predestination theology of John Calvin (1509–64). In short, this theology argued that Man was and continues to be depraved unless chosen by God. Such elevation or choice of an individual by God was an irresistible belief that impacted the thinking of many. It did not require a great leap of mind for people of this time period, and those who followed, to equate this belief with economic success. Those who 'made it' were, in this view, intrinsically better than those who didn't. The theses of Malthus, Smith, Ricardo, Mill and Darwin have all reflected this philosophy and resulted in what Kenneth Clark (Clark, 1974) termed the real reason for the Poor Laws of 1834. He argued, as have others, that these laws were not designed to abolish poverty, but to prevent the poor from becoming a nuisance.

Workhouses, so well described by Dickens, were mandated to extract a heavy price for the meagre shelter and sustenance they provided. Whether the conditions described then continue to be mimicked today has been the subject of much discussion. What is, however, less uncertain is the trend towards ensuring a more stringent form of quid pro quo from the recipients of social assistance. Moreover, the level of assistance has been steadily diminishing, and the requirements for accessing this assistance have been getting steadily more numerous. While some might argue that assistance is not decreasing, pointing to the yearly increased burden on national budgets for providing assistance, they do not counterbalance their argument with reference to increases in cost of living, fewer opportunities for income, and punitive deductions for those with the initiative to ameliorate their financial position. The result of all this stringency has been a continuing disempowerment of those who are least capable or willing (for a variety of valid reasons) to claim this support.

There is a variety of potential explanations for the failure of pregnant teenagers to utilise available resources. Some proportion can be attributed to the teenagers' inability (for any number of reasons including illiteracy, opportunity, cost, shame) to get to understand and use 'the system'. Some may actually prefer a modicum of disadvantage if this allows them to escape the scrutiny, constraints and labelling associated with receipt of assistance. Some teenagers indubitably do find themselves victims of less-than-conscientious civil servants, and some will want to prove to themselves and others that they have the capacity to 'make it on their own'. However, as we have pointed out earlier, more than 70 per cent in the US and more than 90 per cent in the UK ultimately apply for and receive social assistance. And it is the impact of the need for and acceptance of this assistance which should be of as much concern to society as the cost of the assistance itself. Becoming dependant on others for one's own and one's baby's existence is disempowering, especially since it comes at an age when personal autonomy is in its formative stage. Dependency, coming at this age, entrenches commonly held stigmatising beliefs in the teenagers themselves, and leads the teenagers to operationalise such beliefs in a way that results in social exclusion. Despite these facts, it should be doubtful that the teenager should bear the degree of responsibility resulting from teenage pregnancy that some would like them to shoulder.

In a *USA Today* health supplement (*USA Today*, 1999) dealing with the costs of teenage pregnancy in the United States, Democratic Representative Nita Lowey was quoted as saying 'I believe we have to give it the stigma it used to have – that it's not cute to have a child when you are 15 years old'. This hackneyed but still effective strategy of placing total responsibility directly on the victim, without consideration for other significant factors, continues to play well with a financially overtaxed public. It assumes, contrary to available evidence, that there are no penalties attached to having an early, out-of-wedlock baby. How are such perceptions about teenage pregnancy formed? Susan Sontag argues that the vaguer the aetiology of a condition, the more intractable its resolution and the more obdurate the stigma that is attached (Sontag, 1977). And these factors are certainly important to the degree of stigma attached to teenage pregnancy. Since there appear to be no social, religious, economic or cultural boundaries that it does not cross, it generates a great deal of fear in those who perceive themselves (or their loved ones) to be at risk for becoming part of the group.

Redressing the negative perception of pregnant teenagers

There is no disagreement that adolescence is a sometimes-turbulent transitional period leading from childhood to adulthood. This period places teenagers in the precarious position of being able to physically act like an adult, without having the necessary cognitive and psycho-social tools to judge and temper their actions. Kasen *et al.* (1998) however, in a study of 452 New York adolescents, found that while affiliation with deviant groups can elevate the risk for deviant behaviour, a nurturing educational system can and does favourably impact on outcome. Such a system can do so, even in the presence of pre-existing problems (for example, behavioural problems, lack of mental acuity and a disadvantaged socio-economic background) which would customarily be expected to attenuate the benefits of a nurturing environment. In addition, social learning theorists have argued that – whether they become parents or not – teenagers very often think and act in imitation of and from observation of others whom they perceive to be appropriate role models (Dusek, 1991). Rather than being irrational actors, victims of a hormonal storm over which they have no control, these theorists suggest that teenagers seek to conform, to belong, and to lay down a path for their future evolution as adults.

However, social learning theorists also note that the future that teenagers perceive for themselves is dependant on their history, and will influence their choices. If they come from an 'appropriate' background, they will engage in associations with temperate, approved, high achieving groups of peers, and society will consider them successful. But for many, both their familial history as well as their own personal attainments make such associations almost impossible. Since pregnant teenagers are most likely to come from disadvantaged groups, they make associations with such groups. When associating with these groups, who do no more than mirror (like the high achieving peer groups) a set of practised and tacitly approved mores of their society, society will call such pregnant teenagers deviant and stigmatise them.

The work of Kasen *et al.* (1998), previously mentioned, might alter this perception by society of pregnant teenagers, if it were widely known. For instance, they found that female teenagers were far less likely to have

committed or been convicted of committing a crime, to have been diagnosed with an antisocial personality disorder, or to have abused alcohol
than their male peers in the two years antecedent to their study. In addition, the male peers in Kasen *et al.*'s (1998) study were far less likely than
other teenagers to have been involved in a teenage conception. It is interesting to speculate on what perceptions might develop from knowledge of
results such as these. Based on these results, for instance, one could
conclude that the fathers of the babies of disadvantaged teenagers come
from the upper echelons of society, though this is not necessarily so. It may
be that many of the misconceptions associated with teenage pregnancy for
decades, if not longer, are just that: misconceptions. However, it is very
likely that these misconceptions (i.e. perceptions) are at least in part
responsible for much of the misery these young adults and their babies are
burdened with for much of their remaining lives.

More important, perhaps, to understanding the plight of pregnant
teenagers it is necessary to realise that pregnant teenagers are very often
seeking no more than continuity to their lives. By necessity, this continuity
reflects the prevailing personal/societal values of their social group, values
that very often are inimical to climbing to a higher socio-economic bracket.

Thus, teenagers from single parent families are more likely to end up in
single parent families themselves. Teenagers born to teenage mothers are
more likely to become teenage mothers themselves and teenagers from
poor families are more likely to continue the cycle of poverty in their own
lives. Teenagers who yearn for the love and guidance of an absent father
are more likely to seek a replacement even at the risk of sexual, mental or
physical abuse.

It is, we think, folly to assume that these individuals fail to recognise the
depredations of their existence, as we think it equally foolish to assume
that these persons are happy in their condition. The so-called information
age has made sure that we are all equally aware of the rewards of success
and the price of failure. It is also folly, we feel, to view these teenagers as
the victims of a genetic predisposition, or as somehow marked by an
unreasonable 'deity' as being less than deserving, in the way that previous
theses already presented would have one believe. Jones *et al.* argue that
responsibility for a person's stigmatising condition is very often difficult
for anyone to determine. Consequently we are impelled to act on our fears:
fear that our loved ones could be reduced to the same level of existence as
those we shun; fear that we have a responsibility to look after them
because we owe it to them; fear that, in looking after them, we may be
consciously or otherwise validating their existence and denying potential
resources to our more deserving offspring. When we decide that only the
person is the author of his or her own misfortune, we are quick to stigmatise and to shun (Jones *et al.*, 1984).

A more realistic picture of the pregnant teenager is beginning to emerge
from current research. In a recent study, Rodriquez and Moore propose

that 'the pregnant teen is usually described as outgoing and typically not rebellious, maladjusted or deviant' (Rodriguez and Moore, 1995). Moreover, as early as 1982, Roosa *et al.* reported that almost 90 per cent of their observed Mexican-American teenage mothers, in spite of having all of the risk factors for neglect, tended to assume responsibility for caring for their children (Roosa *et al.*, 1982). This was echoed very recently in the Social Exclusion Unit's (1999) report to the Prime Minister of Britain, which clearly identified teenage mothers' wish to look after their children and their aversion to placing their offspring for adoption or in foster care. More telling, perhaps, is the increasing realisation that a substantial proportion of conceptions in teenagers do not occur at the hands of teenage peers, but rather at the hands of older men. In addition, Olds *et al.* studied the long-term effects of home visits on dependence, child abuse, criminality and repeat pregnancy in at-risk families. They found that fifteen years after initiation of these home visits, families visited exhibited far fewer deviant characteristics than similar families left to fend for themselves (Olds *et al.*, 1997). The view of pregnant teenagers which emerges from these studies runs counter to the stereotypic view of pregnant teenagers. Nevertheless, reaction to the phenomenon is intractable and shows no evidence of changing in the foreseeable future. Despite this seemingly unchangeable attitude of many in society, the problem of teenage pregnancy does require urgent redress. The healthcare system has a significant role to play here.

Conclusion

A healthy self-esteem, engendered by familial or others' support, is necessary for the teenager to give appropriate care to her newborn infant. Fortunately for the teenage mother, there is evidence that health professionals can give that support. Kissman and Shapiro found that the presence of a trusted professional greatly attenuated the crises associated with the early parenthood of adolescents. This finding was further echoed in a later study by Burke and Liston, who found that the intervention of home-visiting nurses was termed 'very helpful' by adolescent mothers (Kissman and Shapiro, 1990; Burke and Liston, 1994). Unfortunately not all pregnant teenagers can avail themselves of similar personal attention. Many, in fact, experience obstacles and rejection – including by health professionals – who could be of such assistance. The teenage mother then reacts predictably by becoming introspective, ashamed, isolated or depressed, and as events become more unmanageable she enacts the self-fulfilling stigmatising prophecy.

Prenatal care is the first filter of care, since it includes disclosure (diagnosis) of pregnancy and the appropriate periodic monitoring to ensure a healthy pregnancy. Many present for antenatal care far too late in their pregnancy. This has been variously attributed to fear of disclosing pregnancy, with a concomitant absence of an intimate relationship between the teenager and her mother; the fear of being 'ill treated' by professionals staffing antenatal care centres, the difficulty in accessing service, or – as previously suggested – the personal choice of not wanting to be labelled (and sometimes sequestered) by the system (Picard *et al.*, 1998). Nevertheless, it is apparent that either those who feel unwell as a result of their pregnancy or those with the support and the will to rear their baby, will find their way to antenatal care early in their pregnancy. This fact does them credit, as there is clear research evidence to show that medical and paramedical health providers tend to have and display a low opinion of 'working-class' clients (MacIntyre and Porter, 1989). Provision of a more 'culturally' sensitive and holistic approach to the diagnosis of pregnancy and antenatal care is clearly needed. Care delivered in a 'local' setting by medical and paramedical providers who are nearer to the age of the teenagers might be one strategy which would have a beneficial effect.

As previously mentioned, the provision of a 'trustworthy' individual (often *in loco parentis*) has been shown to greatly enhance self-esteem, motivation and an actual improvement in lifestyle as much as fifteen years after initiation of contact (Burke and Liston, 1994). Clearly society cannot legislate that the teenager should have healthy relationships with either her parent(s) or the putative father. In addition, although society can legislate some form of accountability for the putative father, in a highly mobile society this will be at best difficult to enforce. However, society can make provision to train, retain and support healthcare workers to initiate and hopefully maintain long-term relationships with pregnant teenagers. Healthcare workers dedicated to such a service may be less likely to exhibit what has been termed 'courtesy stigma', i.e. the fear of being labelled by association with the labelled (the pregnant teenager). Previous research has shown that this phenomenon is unlikely to happen when the worker is giving professional assistance (Jones *et al.*, 1984). If we agree that, to a substantial degree, pregnant teenagers are not the ogres that we have grown to believe, then they may also constitute a substantial pool of potential recruits as support persons to other pregnant teenagers. To a healthcare delivery system that values 'experienced reflective practitioners' rather than book-trained practitioners, such teenagers should be a valued resource.

References

Behavior Today (1990) *Sexuality: sexual activity and contraception rise dramatically among teenage women*, 19 November, 21: 47.

Burke, P. and Liston, W. (1994) 'Adolescent mothers' perceptions of social support and the impact of parenting on their lives', *Pediatric Nursing*, 20: 593–9.

Children's Defense Fund (1988) *Teenage pregnancy: an advocate's guide to the numbers*, Washington D.C.: Adolescent Pregnancy Prevention Clearing House.

Chilman, C.S. (1990) 'Promoting healthy adolescent sexuality', *Family Relations*, 39: 121–31.

Clark, K. (1974) *Civilization*, Rugby, Warwickshire: Jolly and Barber.

Davies, C., Downey, A. and Murphy, H. (1996) *School age mothers: access to education*, London: Save the Children Fund.

Dusek, J.B. (1991) *Adolescent development and behaviour*, second edn, Englewood Cliffs, N.J.: Prentice Hall.

Furstenburg, F.F. Jr. (1991) 'As the pendulum swings: teenage childbearing and social concerns', *Family Relations*, 40: 127–38.

Grazi, R., Redheendran, R., Madalian, N. and Bannerman, R. (1983) 'Offspring of teenage mothers – congenital malformations, low birth-weight and other findings', *Journal of Reproductive Medicine*, 27, 2: 89–96.

Hayes, C.D. (1987) *Risking the future: adolescent sexuality, pregnancy, and childbearing*, Washington, D.C.: National Academy Press.

Henshaw, S. (1993) 'Teenage abortions, births and pregnancy statistics by state 1988', *Family Planning Perspectives*, 25: 122–6.

Jacono, J., Jacono, B., St Onge, M. *et al.* (1992) 'Teenage pregnancy: a reconsideration', *Canadian Journal of Public Health*, 83, 3: 196–9.

Jones, E.E., Farina, A., Hastorf, A.H. *et al.* (1984) *Social stigma: the psychology of marked relationships*, New York: W.H. Freeman and Company.

Kasen, S., Cohen, P. and Brook, J.S. (1998) 'Adolescent school experiences and dropout, adolescent pregnancy, and young adult deviant behavior', *Journal of Adolescent Research*, 13, 1: 49–72.

Kissman, K. and Shapiro, J. (1990) 'The composites of social support and well being and parenting attitude among teen mothers', *International Journal of Adolescence and Youth*, 1: 247–55.

Kitzes, J. (1986) 'Having a baby under 16', *Emergency Medicine*, 18, 3: 28–44.

MacIntyre, S. and Porter, M. (1989) 'Problems and prospects in promoting effective care at the local health level', in M. Enkin, M. Keirse and I. Chalmers (eds), *Effective care in pregnancy and childbirth*, Oxford: Oxford University Press.

Olds, D., Eckenrode, J., Henderson, C. *et al.* (1997) 'Long-term effects of home visitation on maternal life course and child abuse and neglect', *Journal of the American Medical Association*, 278: 637–43.

Picard, L., Jacono, J., Pitblado, R. *et al.* (1998) *The influence of health beliefs on health behaviors and birth outcomes in pregnant adolescents*, Canada: Report to the National Health Research and Development Programme.

Rodriquez, C. Jr. and Moore, N.B. (1995) 'Perceptions of pregnant/parenting teens: re-framing issues for an integrated approach to pregnancy problems', *Adolescence*, 30, 119: 686–7.

Romig, C.A. and Thompson, J.G. (1988) 'Teenage pregnancy: a family systems approach', *American Journal of Family Therapy*, 16: 1.

Roosa, M., Fitzgerald, H.E. and Casson, N.A. (1982) 'Teenage parenting and child development: a literature review', *Infant Mental Health Journal*, 3: 4–18.

Sontag, S. (1977) *Illness as metaphor*, New York: Allen Lane.

The Social Exclusion Unit (1999) *Teenage pregnancy: the Social Exclusion Unit's remit to the Prime Minister*, London: Office of the Prime Minister.

USA Today (1993) *Face up to sex education*, 8 June.

—— (1999) *Teen pregnancy bill*, 2 February.

Vinovski, M.A. (1981) 'An "epidemic" of adolescent pregnancy? Some historical considerations', *Journal of Family History*, 6: 205–25.

22 The stigmatisation of breastfeeding

Mary Smale

Stop breast-feeding, pub tells mum.

(*Yorkshire Post*, 2000)

Introduction

In almost any public place in Britain today it is possible that a mother is being ushered to a toilet to continue breastfeeding. A recent survey in a town in the north of England showed ten cafés that allowed breastfeeding. Another suggested a mother bring bottled breastmilk. Yet another forbade breastfeeding, declaring it to be 'like having sex on the table'. A Royal College of Midwives survey found that, although only 9 per cent of respondents would complain or leave, 93 per cent of people disagreed with women breastfeeding anywhere they chose. Provided no complaint was made, 79 per cent of restaurants said they would allow breastfeeding (*Modern Midwife*, 1993).

The word 'allow' reveals stigmatisation of breastfeeding as an entrenched reaction. A difficulty for women is that the conditions for cultural unease with public breastfeeding are unclear. Defence or apology may be needed at any time, as it becomes 'a public boob' (Welford, 1990: 32). In the government's quinquennial survey, 40 per cent of breastfeeding women reported having problems finding somewhere to feed in public, compared with 24 per cent of bottle-feeders. Half the breastfeeding women had never tried feeding away from home (Foster *et al.*, 1997). Such surveys do not inquire how often a mother rushed home or to the nearest ladies' lavatory with a distressed baby rather than risk feeding in public.

It is not only in the public arena that women meet difficulties. A study of inner-city mothers in Glasgow revealed sanctions against breastfeeding even within the home (McIntosh, 1985). Typically a respondent named the lavatory as the only place in her multiple occupancy home she could use for breastfeeding.

The stigmatisation of the delivery of a fluid so clearly validated both by the medical establishment and by society at large may surprise some health professionals, especially any who have breastfed themselves without disapproval. It may seem outrageous that it should be relegated to areas set aside for the elimination of waste products. Health professionals may contribute to the negative experience of women by refusing to acknowledge the reality of hesitations about feeding. A professional's confidence may not help a woman in considering her options. On the other hand, health professionals and voluntary agencies have sometimes been expected to pass on social mores. 'The woman who sits with her breast openly exposed in a public restaurant will be intruding on the sensibilities of many people who certainly do not see this as acceptable dinner-time behaviour' (Field, 1984: 80).

I shall draw on the concepts of 'origin' and 'peril' in Jones *et al.*'s examination to suggest ways in which breastfeeding as constructed in our culture, while not 'disfiguring' a woman's body, may be transformed into a 'degrading affliction' (1984: 58). In considering this 'woman's issue', the places and times in which breastfeeding is seen as especially threatening, and the language and images used when describing it, will be examined. The final part of the chapter makes suggestions for health professionals' contributions towards women's undisturbed breastfeeding.

Cultural differences

In most parts of Africa and Asia and in much of Scandinavia breastfeeding is not stigmatised as in Britain. 'In Norway we breastfeed in most all situations and no one raises an eyebrow any more when baby gets served too' (Nylander, 1994). In England, breastfeeding appears to be less tolerated the further from London one moves. The survey commissioned for the Royal College of Midwives, already referred to, showed the highest rate for objections was in the Granada TV region (*Modern Midwife*, 1993). Salt suggests that the different rates of prevalence in two similar cities results from such cultural differences (Salt *et al.*, 1995).

The dimension of 'origin'

How might 'the mark' of breastfeeding be said to 'develop' (Jones *et al.*, 1984: 56)? Whereas in some conditions the sign of the bearer is constantly visible, for a breastfeeding woman the most literal of all revelations of her state are the damp stains from her nipples and the possibility of a related smell. Millions of breastpads are sold in this country to manage this. More powerful streams of milk arching from her breasts if a baby stops feeding while letdown is at its height may embarrass her (see Figure 22.1).

Noises – gulping – betraying the passage of body fluid from one person to another, are an audible signal, although even silent or discreet breast-feeding may provoke reaction in particular contexts.

The bearer's responsibility for their 'condition' is seen as influential in the degree of stigmatisation experienced (Jones *et al.*, 1984: 57). One

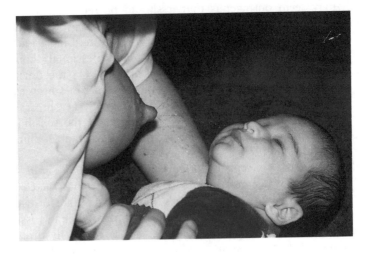

Figure 22.1 Letdown: with thanks to Hilary English

aspect of the stigmatisation of breastfeeding which may seem particularly unjust is that women are urged, for the sake of their baby's and their own health, to opt for breastfeeding, yet some feel driven to apologise for the repercussions of the decision. Breastfeeding mothers must be discreet, never 'blatant' (Knight, 2000).

Having chosen this route, women may restrain themselves complaining about difficulties, since as in other stigmatised conditions there can be an element of reaping one's deserts (Jones *et al.*, 1984: 60). Jones *et al.* suggest that conditions may seem to be the result of some earlier sin. In breastfeeding, any difficulties can be seen as an inevitable element of the style in which breastfeeding is undertaken, especially in relation to so-called demand feeding: women are frequently told that by feeding the baby whenever he or she demands it they are 'making a rod for their own backs'. 'Our survey shows a large number of men have personal difficulty in accepting that hungry babes cannot wait for feeding until a private home is available' (RCM, 1993).

The dimension of peril

There is probably little perceived physical danger to someone sitting near the breastfeeding mother: she is surely less likely than most to attack strangers, and it is unlikely that a theoretical fear of contamination by milk bearing hepatitis drives the stigmatisation. Nevertheless I suggest that breastfeeding is constructed culturally as a threat to order. Managing the transfer process discreetly may be particularly difficult for women with twins or large breasts, for example.

Breastmilk as food and eating out

Breastmilk, seen as pure and wholesome for a baby, nevertheless is positioned ambiguously between cooked and raw food. Disgust is exemplified in the reluctance of many women to taste their own milk. Jokes about putting it in food or drink indicate disquiet with this body fluid. Caution about expressing reveals it as a worrying product (Gauden, 1990). I suggest it is milk flowing from the nipple which presents the most perilous aspect of breastfeeding. As containers, breasts are less reliable than bottles.

Murcott (1993) writes about two-way *cordons sanitaires* erected around a mother and baby for the delivery of semi-solid food. However, the peril seems more than simply a matter of controlling messiness. Douglas (1975: 214) writes of the need for rules 'whenever the organic erupts into the social'. One anthropologist's examination of breastfeeding on the west coast of Northern Ireland links a universal failure of breastfeeding with 'a rigid vigilance of what goes into and what comes out of the body', as well as the woman's sexual shame even in front of her husband (Scheper-Hughes, 1979: 122). Visser describes babies as 'not quite human' and 'feeding off their mothers like cannibals' (Visser, 1991: 39 and 41). Debrette's *New Guide to Etiquette and Modern Manners* is even clearer: it is bad manners to expel any liquid from any orifice in public, especially during breastfeeding which is 'revolting' (Morgan, 1996).

Closeness to other forms of eating provokes particularly strong reactions betraying a sense of 'peril'. For example, a businessman complained of his lunch being 'spoilt when three apparently well-educated young ladies sat at the table next to us with their babies in tow and within five minutes of sitting down proceeded to breastfeed them' (*Sunday Times*, 5 February 1999).

To imagine how the escape of such fluid might feel without having experienced breastfeeding gives an onlooker a limited understanding. This can apply to health professionals as well as to the general public. It may be that working where hygiene is valued may make this yet more difficult (Lawler, 1991).

Breasts and nipples

Breasts are the most obvious signifiers of female gender and in Britain they make breastfeeding seem rude to children (Gregg, 1989). Nipples in particular, the most hidden part of the breast, are revealed only accidentally or provocatively. Erect and moist tissue near a mouth alarms onlookers, even if seen only in a Department of Health poster considered to be 'too sexy'. One journalist writes that 'Breastfeeding in public is the female equivalent of flashing' and describes asking for the right to breastfeed in the House of Commons 'grotesque' (Littlejohn, 2000). This mirrors some objections to public breastfeeding raised by the respondents to the Royal College of Midwives' survey mentioned above, as a form of 'exhibitionism' which 'draws attention' (RCM, 1993). Breastmilk threatens, the visible nipple affronts, and the combination of them in breastfeeding in certain contexts is overwhelming. Stigmatisation may be worse if the observer feels trapped or surprised by seeing breastfeeding outside a family context (Hoddinott and Pill, 1999).

Here Jones *et al.*'s examination of peril suggests that, because there is difficulty coping with breastfeeding, there may be a need to consider the needs of a breastfeeding mother, placing a 'burden of intervention and rescue' on us as others shun their company (Jones *et al.*, 1984: 66). The helplessness of onlookers may have a bearing on their feelings. There is also the possibility that, having felt sympathy for the person who must take their baby everywhere with them and feed frequently, there may be some disturbance in finding delight in this inability to share care: 'such people challenge our whole view of the world' (Jones *et al.*, 1984: 65). A relaxed breastfeeding woman challenges someone who may not have been able to pursue this act either for cultural or medical reasons. A lack of imaginative understanding may lie at the root of some of the most destructive ideas about breastfeeding. The influential doctor Truby King, whose work began influencing feeding practices before the Second World War, felt that men would not be willing to feed their children more than five times daily – so neither, of course, should mothers.

The key dimension of peril in relation to breastfeeding is especially dynamic through time. The trajectory of breastfeeding means that it may be more difficult to guarantee milk containment initially, through the inexperience of both parties. Later, a baby may be distracted. Feelings about offering the breast to babies with teeth or speech, signs of autonomy, are not based on biological but cultural objections. Social support for the breastfeeding mother changes to toleration, then, via indifference, to active encouragement for, and 'social coercion' towards, weaning (Morse and Harrison, 1987: 205). Pressure to wean may relate to an imagined attribution of enjoying breastfeeding too much, too long or too often for 'transparently self-serving reasons' (Jones *et al.*, 1984: 59). The merely aberrant becomes the 'abhorrent', and the mother needs to evolve strategies to help herself. (Jones *et al.*, 1984: 61; Wrigley and Hutchinson, 1990).

Jones *et al.*'s useful exploration of empathy brings us near to psycho-dynamic understandings of breastfeeding as a relationship. Onlookers may be appalled by the insatiability of the baby, seeing it as an unimaginable burden. Seeing a baby instantly gratified may anger those with needs which are not similarly met. A young child seeing a breastfeeding mother may think she is being eaten; adults, too, may harbour fantasies about breastfeeding being depleting.

Other difficult places

In church I was once asked 'Can I sit with you – someone was breast-feeding and I don't want anyone to think I'm with them'. The time when a lactating woman might resume church attendance was once determined according to papal advice (Bede, in Knowles, 1910). The intrusion of breastfeeding into forbidden areas has been examined in a recent discussion on breastfeeding in Parliamentary Committee rooms (*Nursing Standard*, 2000). This may be considered to exemplify the perilous juxtaposition of the irrational needs of a baby with adult behaviour. One journalist's diatribe against demand feeding blamed the American defeat in the Vietnam War on lax breastfeeding style (Waugh, 1994).

The work context

Our culture separates work and mothering as mutually exclusive tasks. Rodgers' examination of an earlier scandal in the House of Commons concludes that breastfeeding reveals the woman in her essence and so worries not only men whose territory is invaded but also women, since 'a woman who is visibly pregnant or known to be breastfeeding is at her most explicitly female', engendering fears in other women of being revealed by association as being 'out of place' (Rodgers, 1981).

Language and silence

The unspoken nature of breastfeeding is indicated by euphemism, in which the breastfeeding mother is said to be 'feeding the baby herself' (Holder, 1989). Journalists have compared public breastfeeding to siting urinals in bars or vomitaria in restaurants, and to self-medication ('shooting up') by diabetics (Littlejohn, 1991; Birchill, 1990). These powerful parallels reveal powerful meanings, just as the action of an irate shopkeeper – throwing dirty water over a mother and baby as they breastfed outside his shop – recalls that of someone separating copulating dogs.

Breastfeeding is not simply the potential leakage of a body fluid from the mother via a 'rude' place, it also symbolises the incontinence of the baby's needs. The use of 'demand' to describe feeding in which the baby determines the timing and duration of breastfeeds reveals social concern around such behaviour, however rational that behaviour's biological basis (RCM, 1991). A recent American commentator writes that 'respectable mothers must also manage the child's desires' (Blum, 1999: 133). Breastfeeding provides a powerful example of how 'women's bodies when unsupervised can generate chaos' (Smart, 1992: 173).

Feminist scholars have argued that the insistence on exclusive hetero-sexual availability in Western culture limits responses to other forms of intimacy (Carter, 1994). Fears around incest emerge as children become sensually aware. Breastfeeding may be seen to threaten the mother–father tie 'by invoking the generational tie in which eroticism is taboo' (Blum, 1999: 128). Associations are demonstrated well in one newspaper's reaction to an episode of Channel 4 TV's 'Brookside', in which public breastfeeding was dealt with positively. The writer locates public breastfeeding firmly in the problematic area of life, comparing this with earlier coverage in the soap opera of date rape, euthanasia and incest (*Daily Mail*, 10 February 1999).

While it is hard to see breastfeeding mothers as blemished, neither are they considered normal. While two in three women begin by breastfeeding their babies, the decline in numbers is quick thereafter and, combined with its privacy, this tends to make it hidden from view other than in the family. The enlarged and/or leaking breasts of a lactating woman render her deviant in our society with its comparatively low childbirth rates. Breastfeeding can be constructed as a refusal of the woman to make the expected rite of passage back to the pre-pregnant state, extending a dangerous or liminal state. Oakley suggests that women's lives are more 'medicalised, and so are some of their transitions' (Oakley, 1987: 32). Breastfeeding is often subject to more surveillance than formula feeding, which may be seen to be more reliable. However well understood the biological process of breastfeeding may be, it is possible for the medical profession to feel it is an area in which they must carry out the wider social task of 'tidying up, ensuring that the order in external physical events conforms to the structure of ideas' (Douglas, 1975: 53). The restraints on breastfeeding can be seen as an extension of the need to manage birth, similarly disruptive yet celebrated, where ambiguity and uncontrollability threaten (Lomas, 1966). This may explain a new spate of books emphasising the need for babies to have scheduled feeds and lives, to which women turn partly to avoid stigmatisation of being 'caught short' (Birchill, 1990; Ford, 1999).

Another solution for stigmatisation is serial or contemporaneous feeding by breast and bottle. Women may bottle-feed in public, either with expressed breastmilk or formula, while they continue to breastfeed at home, or, increasingly, let their partners share in feeding the baby with expressed milk. Health professionals need to be aware of the ramifications of these patterns on the long-term outcome for breastfeeding and be ready to explain these to women.

Breastfeeding has recently been described as 'the only remaining truly women centred activity' which was 'initially the most difficult area for the medical profession to control' (Taylor and Littlewood, 1994: 1). However, signs of an increasing sense of responsibility for breastfeeding may indicate the re-medicalisation of breastfeeding as a necessarily taught skill enabled only by experts.

Using Swedish research, one of the UNICEF Babyfriendly steps enjoins hospitals to allow women and babies skin-to-skin contact immediately after birth, ideally until the baby comes to feed in his own time (WHO/UNICEF, 1989). Many mothers are delighted to do this and it may provide an unhurried and non-stigmatising environment in which breast-feeding can begin. One mother compared it with a previous experience when she was mocked for putting her baby to the breast and asked, 'you at that already?'

Every health professional has been fed as a baby, and stories or silences carry cultural messages. Knowing the value of breastmilk does not auto-matically translate into an ease in the presence of breastfeeding. This exploration of the stigmatisation of breastfeeding, however brief, indicates the need for health professionals to enter imaginatively the personal and social world of each mother in order to help her sustain her chosen feeding relationship with her baby.

Suggestions for helping women to destigmatise breastfeeding

- See breastfeeding as a relationship, not a procedure to be managed – medicalisation may not help society to see breastfeeding as socially acceptable.
- Avoid acting upon women – women need to be confident in their skills to withstand stigmatisation.
- Consider it irresponsible to argue women into breastfeeding as a health act without some help with the self-defence they may need.
- Be informed about how breastfeeding works (Renfrew *et al.*, 2000; RCM, 1991). Information, offered at appropriate times, can act as useful self-defence strategies for mothers and help them apply princi-ples to any compromises for breastfeeding in an unsupportive relationship.
- Use words sensitively in tune with the mother – avoiding euphemisms.
- Avoid rushing to offer tissues if the mother leaks. Be aware of other body language, e.g. reaction to sudden letdown. Think of meanings of what is said or done, e.g. curtain drawing. Ask women what they want.
- Give sound information, e.g. the possible health dangers of formula (UNICEF/BFI), remaining non-judgemental of the person and under-standing the social pressures against breastfeeding – health arguments may exacerbate defensiveness by those stigmatising.
- Encourage open discussion from the antenatal period onwards about the interpersonal aspects of breastfeeding – a woman who cannot imagine ever feeding anywhere but in the bedroom may gradually extend her boundaries.
- Offer practical ideas for life outside the clinical setting – seeing what breastfeeding really looks like in a mirror, using loose tops, waistcoats, patterns.

- Involve others who have experienced or feared stigmatisation.
- Don't hide your own breastfeeding, although it should not be the main focus of the conversation.
- Offer discreet feeding as only one of a series of responses, including rehearsing assertiveness, excursions in pairs, saying '*we* have decided that …', offering alternatives, e.g. 'if I do not feed my baby now she will become very noisy,' asking to see the manager, or to have sight of a policy (many public places do have policies supporting breast-feeding, but employees do not always know this).
- Get involved in policies – does your setting have a non-stigmatising breastfeeding policy and is everyone aware of it? Are health profes-sionals themselves able to express somewhere private?
- Consider the initiation of schemes whereby premises are designated as safe areas for women to breastfeed.

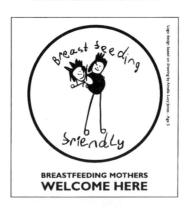

Figure 22.2 Breastfeeding-friendly leaflet

- Work *sensitively* in schools. Seeing breastfeeding away from a friendly context may put children off (Hoddinott and Pill, 1999). Attacking the chosen feeding methods of parents may be counter-productive. It may be better to speak to someone they know e.g. their teacher – if not stigmatising – or another person who is culturally acceptable, such as voluntary or peer supporters.
- Respect women's long-term intentions – don't assume a baby's age means it is time to stop, since mastitis in the mother and diarrhoea in

the baby are best treated by continuing breastfeeding. Decisions about stopping are not best made in crisis.

- Avoid separation in wards where another child, mother or baby are admitted.
- Avoid the justification of a cultural preference by pseudo-medical arguments such as the comparative ineffectiveness of breastmilk. Breastmilk continues to provide a source of immune responses triggered by those diseases encountered by the mother for as long as she feeds (Woolridge and Baum, 1993).
- Consider the boundaries around your own comfort with breastfeeding. It is not easy to say which aspects of stigmatisation will be operating for any one person, and it may well be that a mixture of the feelings lie behind any adverse reaction to breastfeeding. Talk with someone you trust about how your own experience may affect your care.
- Hear distress for regret over bottle feeding, avoiding rescue by refusing to acknowledge guilt. Exoneration implies the right to blame. Reflecting the mother's words usually leads her to admit how little choice she had.
- Accept (i.e. be prepared to hear and reflect) the position of those in your own profession who stigmatise breastfeeding. This prolongs the conversation in an adult-to-adult encounter. Agreeing or disagreeing curtails it.

References

Birchill, J. (1990) 'Feeding on the milk of human grossness', *Mail on Sunday*, 27 May.

Blum, L. (1999) *At the breast: ideologies of breastfeeding and motherhood in the contemporary United States*, Boston: Beacon Press.

Carter, P. (1994) 'Breastfeeding and the social construction of heterosexuality, or "What breasts are really for" ', *Conference of the British Sociological Association*, 28–31 March.

Daily Mail (1999) 'Breastfeeding mother breaks a soap taboo', 10 February.

Douglas, M. (1975) *Implicit meanings*, London: Routledge and Kegan Paul.

Field, P.A. (1984) 'Breastfeeding at work and nursing facilities in public places', contribution to *Breastfeeding: a Challenge for Midwives*, seminar and workshop, Imperial College, London, quoted by P. Van Esterik in S.F. Murray, *Baby friendly mother friendly*, London: Mosby.

Ford, G. (1999) *The contented little baby book*, London: Vermilion.

Foster, K., Lader, D. and Cheesbrough, S. (1997) *Infant Feeding 1995*, London: Office of National Statistics.

Gauden, C. (1990) 'Furtive expression', *New Generation*, Dec.

Gregg, J.E.M. (1989) 'Attitudes of teenagers in Liverpool to breastfeeding', *British Medical Journal*, 299: 147–8.

Hoddinott, P. and Pill, R. (1999) 'Qualitative study of decisions about infant feeding among women in East End of London', *British Medical Journal*, 318: 30–4.

Holder, R.W. (1989) *Dictionary of euphemisms*, London: Faber and Faber.

Jones, E., Farina, A., Hastorf, A. *et al.* (1984) *Social stigma, the psychology of marked relationships*, New York: W.H. Freeman.

Knight, I. (2000) 'It's mad mother season', *Sunday Times*, 23 July.

Knowles, D. (ed.) (1910) *Ecclesiastical history of the English nation*, London: J.M. Dent and Sons.

Lawler, J. (1991) *Behind the screens: nursing, somology, and the problem of the body*, London: Churchill Livingstone.

Littlejohn, R. (1991) 'Who gives a monkey's: a look at modern life', *Punch*, February, 20–26.

—— (2000) 'Do your blouse up for the lads', *The Sun*, 12 May.

Lomas, P. (1966) 'Ritualistic elements in the management of childbirth', *British Journal of Medical Psychology*, 39: 207–13.

McIntosh, J. (1985) 'Barriers to breast feeding: choice of feeding method in a sample of working class primaparae', *Midwifery*, 1: 213–24.

Modern Midwife (1993) 'Men's attitudes to breastfeeding', November–December, 7.

Morgan, J. (1996) *Debrette's new guide to etiquette and modern manners*, London: Headline.

Morse, J.M. and Harrison, M. (1987) 'Social coercion for weaning', *Journal of Nurse-Midwifery*, 32: 205–10.

Murcott, A. (1993) 'Purity and pollution: body management and the social place of infancy', in S. Scott and D. Morgan (eds), *Body matters; essays on the sociology of the body*, London: Falmer Press.

Murray, S.F. (ed.) (1994) *Baby friendly mother friendly*, London: Mosby.

Nursing Standard (2000) 'Midwives plan protest over breastfeeding ban', 17 May.

Nylander, G. (1994) 'Breast is Best', video: Health-Info, Video Vital AS, PO Box 5058 Majorstua, N-0301 Oslo, Norway.

Oakley, A. (1987) 'Gender and generation: the life and times of Adam and Eve', in P. Allat, T. Keil and B. Bytheway (eds), *Women and the life cycle: transitions and turning points*, London: Macmillan.

Renfrew, M.J., Fisher, C. and Arms, S. (2000) *Bestfeeding*, second edn, Berkeley: Celestial Arts.

Rodgers, S. (1981) 'Women's space in a men's house', in S. Ardener (ed.), *Women and space: ground rules and social maps*, London: Croom Helm.

Royal College of Midwives (1991) *Successful breastfeeding*, London: Royal College of Midwives.

—— (1993) *Men's attitudes to breastfeeding*, news release, 5 November.

Salt, M.J., Law, C.M., Bull, A.R. and Osmond, C. (1995) 'Determinants of breast-feeding in Salisbury and Durham', *Journal of Public Health Medicine*, 16, 3: 291–5.

Scheper-Hughes, N. (1979) *Saints, scholars and schizophrenics: mental illness in rural Ireland*, Berkeley: University of California Press.

Smart, C. (1992) *Regulating womanhood: historical essays on marriage, mother-hood and sexuality*, London: Routledge.

Sunday Times (1999) 'Winner's Dinners', page letter to 'Style' magazine, 14 February.

Taylor, L. and Littlewood, J. (1994) *The breastfeeding experiences of mothers of premature and full-term infants*, report prepared for the National Childbirth

Trust by Women and Welfare Research, Department of Social Sciences, Loughborough University.

UNICEF/BFI (1999) *Delivery room practices*, http:/www.babyfriendly.org.uk; UNICEF/BFI, PO Box 29050, London WC2H 9TA.

Visser, M. (1991) *The rituals of dinner*, Harmondsworth: Penguin.

Waugh, A. (1994) 'Stop this breast feeding', *Daily Telegraph*, 18 May.

Welford, H. (1990) 'Breastfeeding – a public boob?', *Parents*, December.

WHO/UNICEF (1989) *Protecting, promoting and supporting breastfeeding: the special role of maternity services*, joint statement by WHO/UNICEF, Geneva: World Health Organisation.

Woolridge, M.W. and Baum, J.D. (1993) 'Recent advances in breast feeding', *Acta Paediatrica Japonica*, 35: 1–12.

Wrigley, E.A. and Hutchinson, S.A. (1990) 'Long term breastfeeding, the secret bond', *Journal of Nurse-Midwifery*, January–February, 35: 1, 35–41.

Yorkshire Post (2000) 'Stop breast-feeding, pub tells mum', 6 May.

23 The stigma of terminal cancer

Tom Donovan

> It evokes many of the deepest fears of mankind. It can spread throughout the body. It can also spread into social and emotional domains, drastically disrupting families and challenging the very values that make life worth living.
>
> (Weisman, 1979)

Although there are many illnesses that could be described as 'terminal', cancer merits particular consideration.

Cancer is a major global health problem. In the UK, cancer is second only to cardiovascular disease as a cause of death. Every year one in every 250 men and one in 300 women are diagnosed with cancer (Souhami and Tobias, 1998).

Remarkable achievements in medical technology, diagnosis and treatment have made many previously incurable cancers amenable to cure and have improved both longevity and quality of life for those living with the disease. It appears that over recent years the status of cancer has changed from a terminal to a chronic illness, characterised by periods of remission and recurrence. Many people with cancer today are cured. However, a significant number remain for whom the diagnosis equates with prolonged periods of illness, unpleasant treatment and, ultimately, death.

Until recently, cancer was discussed in hushed terms. The word itself carried a powerful emotional message, promoting feelings of anxiety, fear and dread. If fear lies at the root of the stigmatisation of cancer, then cancer is a fearful disease. Cancer is a mysterious, silent killer; its origin is unknown, and the few facts available are both ominous and terrifying. Cancer challenges not only a person's resilience to withstand disabling and invasive disease and disruptive and disagreeable treatment, but also confronts an individual with their tenuous hold upon life itself. Cancer forces us to look into the face of death against our reflexive instinct to look away.

At the beginning of the twentieth century, cancer and tuberculosis formed a sinister alliance as two of the most feared and reviled diseases. 'A diagnosis of either ... was a death sentence and caused the person to be stigmatised, isolated and humiliated, a fate similar to that of persons with leprosy or syphilis' (Holland and Rowland, 1990).

Sontag (1978) describes an intertwining of tuberculosis and cancer that both confused and confirmed the meaning of cancer in the public's perception: 'Any disease that is treated as a mystery and acutely enough feared will be felt to be morally, if not literally, contagious. Thus, a surprisingly large number of people with cancer find themselves shunned by relatives and friends and the object of practices of decontamination by members of the household, as if cancer, like TB, were an infectious disease.'

When tumours were visible, the similarity of their appearance to syphilitic lesions led to the mistaken perception that cancer was also a sexually transmitted disease. This close association of terminal disease with fear of contagion is a problem that persists today.

The impact of the stigma was such that the diagnosis, until recently, was rarely disclosed to patients, and then rarely shared with friends or even close family members. Indeed, in some instances it was common practice to withhold the diagnosis from the patient in the belief that 'the truth will be intolerable to all but exceptionally mature and intelligent patients' (Sontag, 1978).

Until the advent of chemotherapy and radiotherapy, surgery provided the only possible hope of cure for many people with cancer. Often radical, surgery frequently involved the resection or amputation of organs or limbs. Mutilating surgical procedures, such as abdomino–perineal resection for rectal cancer or radical mastectomy for breast cancer, provided a lasting cure but left patients with physical and emotional scarring.

The emotional impact of breast cancer, and mastectomy in particular, was so profound that it generated a wealth of psycho-oncological studies that form a foundation for practice today. Consistency in the findings of concerns following mastectomy underpins the perception of mastectomy as a mutilating and alienating procedure. Findings demonstrate negative body image, a diminished sense of femininity, a decrease in sexual attractiveness and function, and shame and guilt.

In contemporary breast cancer management, breast conservation is of paramount consideration. The decision to remove the breast is taken only when medical or hormonal treatment is considered not to be efficacious (Holland and Rowland, 1990).

Early radiation treatment for cancer, although increasingly successful, did little to alleviate the associated stigma. Radiation itself, especially in the period following the Second World War, came to be regarded as equally frightening as the disease it sought to cure. Radioactivity posed a new threat in the post-war period. The aftermath of Hiroshima engendered powerful associations with cancer. The possible disadvantages from the drive for nuclear energy also produced new concerns in the mind of the public.

Until more sophisticated administration techniques evolved, patients undergoing this form of therapy frequently experienced disfiguring burns and scarring, adding considerably to the burden of poor self-image. Consequently, many cancer patients withdrew socially and isolation became the norm for many in this group. An additional fear of 'being radioactive' served to strengthen the sense of alienation and *otherness* that people experienced.

The dilemma of radiotherapy is that, in order to treat an internal organ with an external source of radiation, damage must accrue to the healthy structures through which the beam passes. Consequently, many people continue to experience discomfort and scarring long after treatment has ceased. In several instances, damage from radiotherapy is not apparent until many years after treatment. The extent of the damage ranges from superficial scarring to severe fibrosis, fistulae and the development of further cancers.

By the 1950s, chemotherapy and radiotherapy began to offer more than palliation. For the first time a cure became a distinct possibility for some cancers. This, coupled with the emergence of hard evidence linking tobacco smoking as a possible cause, significantly raised the public profile of cancer. In the early 1960s, the language of cancer began to enter the public domain.

As the aetiology of cancer becomes clearer, so too grows the perception of cancer as a preventable disease. Popular lifestyle pursuits, such as smoking, alcohol consumption and sunbathing, necessitate a degree of responsibility to prevent self-harm. Consequently, self-blame and guilt become part of the emotional burden. In Iain Banks's (1993) novel, *Complicity*, the hero gets his 'just deserts' after a lifetime of risky behaviour.

> And so you sit on Salisbury Crags, remembering that still-present darkness and looking out over the city, feeling sorry for yourself and cursing your own stupidity and the institutional thoughtlessness, the sanctioned legal, lethal greed of the companies, the governments, the shareholders; all of them. A tennis ball. They say it's the size of a tennis ball.
>
> (Banks, 1993)

The concept of individual responsibility for healthy life practices has been the foundation for disease prevention initiatives in recent years. The notion that individuals might cease their 'dangerous' habits, adjust their diet and claim ownership of their health, shifts the burden of responsibility from the healthcare providers to individuals. The difficulty with this somewhat simplistic concept is that it assumes that harmful practices are freely chosen and therefore avoidable. This ignores the social and cultural pressures that shape behaviour and attitudes.

Self-blame for illness is commonplace. The consequence could be the accumulation of guilt and shame to an already physically and emotionally onerous condition. Some writers suggest that this degree of self-blame can lead to guilt, self-recrimination and depression. This may also impact upon patients' adjustment to their illness by leading them to focus upon ways in which their disease could have been prevented (Taylor, 1995).

There is extensive research into the emotional impact of a cancer diagnosis. The issues outlined in the preceding paragraphs give an indication of the psychological and emotional burdens this illness places upon individuals. The overwhelming emotional response to cancer is fear. Sometimes irrational, but always understandable, this fear fuels the perception of stigmatisation and exclusion.

The language of cancer, until recently, was one of obfuscation and metaphor. In an erroneous attempt to protect patients from the dreaded word, a vocabulary emerged which served to mislead and confuse.

Health professionals became adept at describing cancers as 'little ulcers', 'areas of inflammation' or 'small growths'. Although often well intentioned, the practice of misleading patients with euphemistic diagnoses and over-optimistic prognoses engendered mistrust and impaired professional–patient relationships. Another common practice, and one which persists, is the collusion of health professionals and relatives to withhold information from patients. The situation tends to occur when professionals consult carers before speaking to patients, or when carers coerce professionals to withhold the truth from the patient, in the mistaken belief that it is kinder to protect the patient from psychological harm. The consequences of this action further segregate the cancer patient, and place an additional burden of secrecy on the carer.

> It has long been acknowledged that communicating effectively with terminally ill cancer patients, although challenging, lessens stress and promotes stronger interpersonal relationships. Simply talking about a problem often makes it easier to bear.
>
> (Buckman, 1988)

To deny dying patients the opportunity to express their feelings and to adapt to the certainty of approaching death adds to their isolation. In a confusing world in which they cannot reconcile the optimistic entreaties of their carers with the reality of their own failing health, patients invariably become withdrawn and depressed. A further consequence of collusion results in added difficulties for carers, after the death of the patient and during the subsequent bereavement period. Typically, because the dying patient's wishes were unknown before death and, therefore, were unfulfilled, bereaved carers have to cope with 'unfinished business' which often manifests as feelings of guilt (Faulkener, 1995).

Far from enhancing communication at this crucial time, collusion creates a barrier to communication that isolates patients and compromises both patient autonomy and professional trust.

Communicating with dying patients is difficult. Until recently, health professionals were not educated in effective communication skills. Consequently, communication techniques were acquired through often bitter experience, resulting in professionals avoiding their patients rather than engaging with them. Acknowledged as a difficult area of practice, many professionals report that talking about death and dying challenges the professional ideation of competence and generates feelings of distress for the practitioner.

Kaye (1995) recognises this dilemma, and identifies factors that also contribute to the situation. These include:

- Not having enough time.
- Not having the appropriate skills.
- Fear of the patient becoming distressed.
- Fear of being unable to handle difficult emotions.
- Doing more harm than good.

Buckman (1992) also describes several professional 'fears' that impede effective communication. These include:

- Fear of being blamed

'Blaming the messenger' is a familiar human trait. When faced with a dying cancer patient, health professionals frequently find themselves in the invidious position of feeling powerless to help those in most need, despite possessing a wealth of professional knowledge. When medical science cannot offer a cure, the hapless professional is frequently reduced to offering sympathy and regret.

> Intellectually, humans find it very difficult to grasp and grapple with bad news when it arrives, and people have a great propensity to personify the bad news, to identify it with another person (usually the person who brings it) and thus to direct their sense of anger or outrage at that person.
>
> (Buckman, 1992)

- Fear of therapeutic failure

Patients respect health professionals for their knowledge and expertise. Advances in medical technology have raised expectations in the public perception to such a degree that patients sometimes act with disbelief or anger when a poor prognosis is given. Training in the health professions emphasises the potential benefits of modern practice and leaves little room to develop the skills required to support patients when treatment fails. Consequently, many health professionals are unprepared to cope with feelings of 'therapeutic impotence'. This is compounded by the increasing threat of litigation when treatment is unsuccessful. As a corollary of society's high expectations of success, therapeutic failure now incorporates the ever-present risk of culpability.

• Fear of eliciting a reaction

The emotional burden of the dying patient is immense. For the healthy individual, it is almost impossible to comprehend the range of emotions and depth of despair that many terminally ill people face. It has long been recognised that expressing feelings and sharing concerns has a therapeutic effect that enables people to adapt and cope with appalling difficulties. Yet often the health professional places barriers in the way of the therapeutic process. There remain some health professionals who believe it is wrong to 'upset' patients by talking about painful emotional issues. More often, though, health professionals feel uncomfortable and helpless when faced with a distressed patient. The discomfort may be due to a lack of confidence or skill in dealing with difficult emotional issues, or the patient's reaction may generate painful feelings for the health professional. Health professionals often cope by adopting an objective stance, demarcating the boundaries of the patient–professional relationship. There are advantages for maintaining this position. Suspending emotions allows professionals to remain calm and make objective judgements. It also reinforces the expected demeanour of the health professional, which is to remain calm and evoke a sense of assured competence.

Unfortunately, the stance of the emotionless professional will sometimes impede the most basic expression of sympathy and support.

The deliberate avoidance of dying patients was also recognised by Maguire (1985), who describes several 'blocking' behaviours used by professionals which seek to prevent dying patients disclosing their feelings and engaging in meaningful and therapeutic dialogue. Health practitioners adopt sophisticated strategies that prevent discussion of emotional issues. Typically, blocking behaviours include focusing on physical symptoms, ignoring emotional 'cues', changing the subject and giving false or premature reassurance.

Good communication lies at the heart of effective care for dying patients. Good communication can 'make or mar' a person's experience of illness (Wilkinson, 1999). Fortunately, the emergence of effective educational programmes and training in communication skills has made a significant impact upon the competence and confidence of professionals to deal with the emotional needs of dying people (Maguire and Faulkener, 1988; Wilkinson, 1999).

Most people in the UK die in hospital or other institutions, rather than in their own homes. There is considerable debate about the appropriate care setting for the terminally ill. Several factors, including patient choice, the physical and emotional health of carers, and access to resources, all have a considerable role in deciding where end-stage care occurs. Home care for dying patients, although often desirable, requires planning and coordination of professional and lay support networks. Herd (1990) identified that 74 per cent of carers in this situation reported emotional strain and 51 per cent physical strain. Effective home care is more likely to be achieved where there is one or more resident carers, and both patient and carer desire home care. Younger, married patients are also more likely to be cared for in their home setting (Cantwell *et al.*, 2000).

Hospice and palliative care services have grown exponentially in the UK since the early 1980s. A considerable body of knowledge and expertise exists which seeks to ensure that patients achieve a death free from distressing symptoms, and that they and their carers are supported emotionally and spiritually.

Modern palliative care grew out of the early pioneering work of the founders of the modern hospice movement. Recognising the distress of dying cancer patients and acknowledging that general medical services were unable to meet the special needs of these patients, small hospice in-patient and home care services evolved throughout the country. The majority of these institutions developed within the independent charitable sector and, as such, were less constrained by the political, economic and legislative factors that enmeshed the NHS. Despite its undoubted success the hospice movement has not been without its detractors. Although generally free from national regulatory frameworks, many hospices developed individual policies and philosophies which may not have accounted for local or national strategic planning or the health needs of their local populations. It could be argued that, in developing palliative care away from mainstream care provision, dying patients are further marginalised and separated from the wider care setting.

Some critics argued that the proliferation of small specialist units could not meet the huge demand for palliative care and that, in some instances, hospices were highly selective in the patients they chose to help (Douglas, 1992; Addington-Hall *et al.*, 1998). Particular groups of dying patients singled out for exclusion from hospice care include patients with non-cancerous conditions, the very elderly, and those with dementia (Addington-Hall *et al.*, 1998)

The growth in palliative care services over the last ten years is remarkable. Most areas of the UK have access to in-patient, day care and home support palliative care services. There are now over 3,000 in-patient beds and significant developments in the provision of specialist nursing and home support services (Hospice Information Service, 1998). This growth is expected to continue. Many health authorities have prioritised palliative care development and instigated novel and innovative approaches to coordinate and improve the care of dying patients in a variety of care settings.

The National Council for Hospice and Palliative Care seeks to represent the interests of palliative care services. This crucial initiative, representing hospices, the NHS, charitable and professional organisations, considers a range of professional and ethical issues that impact upon the care of dying patients. The Council provides advice and recommendations to palliative care services to promote best practice in palliative care.

An increase in the availability educational courses, from Certificate to Master's-level degree programmes, has further invigorated interest in this speciality and helped to raise the profile of palliative care in non-specialist settings.

It is vital that educational and policy initiatives such as those outlined above are allowed to develop and flourish within the structures of contemporary healthcare. An increasingly elderly population will undoubtedly result in an increase in the incidence of chronic illnesses, including cancer. The need for palliative care has never been greater. The sterling work developed by hospices and other palliative care providers must be widened to become a routine part of health service planning, so as to provide equitable access to care for people with cancer and advanced and terminal illness.

Palliative care developed from the recognition of the abysmal neglect of a susceptible and marginalised group. The pioneering work of Dame Cicely Saunders and other nurses and physicians bequeaths a legacy which health services are morally bound to embrace if the needs of this most vulnerable group are to be valued and addressed.

References

Addington-Hall, J., Fakhoury, W. and McCarthy, M. (1998) 'Specialist palliative care in non-malignant diseases', *Palliative Medicine*, 12: 417–27.

Banks, I. (1993) *Complicity*, London: Abacus.

Buckman, R. (1988) *I don't know what to say*, London: Macmillan.

—— (1992) *How to break bad news*, London: Pan.

Cantwell, P., Turco, S., Brenneis, C. *et al.* (2000) 'Predictors of home death in palliative care cancer patients', *Journal of Palliative Care*, Spring, 16, 1: 23–8.

Douglas, C. (1992) 'For all the saints', *British Medical Journal*, 304, 6826: 479.

Faulkener, A. (1995) *Working with bereaved people*, London: Churchill Livingstone.

Herd, E. (1990) 'Terminal care in a semi-rural area', *British Journal of General Practice*, 40: 248–51.

Holland, J. and Rowland, J. (1990) *Handbook of psychooncology*, Oxford: Oxford University Press.

Hospice Information Service (1998) *Directory of hospice and palliative care services*, London: St Christopher's Hospice.

Kaye, P. (1995) *Breaking bad news: a ten step approach*, Northampton: EPL.

Maguire, P. (1985) 'Barriers to psychological care of the dying', *British Medical Journal*, 291: 1711–13.

Maguire, P. and Faulkener, A. (1988) 'Improve the counselling skills of doctors and nurses in cancer care', *British Medical Journal*, 297: 847–9.

Sontag, S. (1978) *Illness as metaphor*, London: Allen Lane.

Souhami, R. and Tobias, J. (1998) *Cancer and its management*, third edn, Oxford: Blackwell Science.

Taylor, S. (1995) *Health psychology*, New York: McGraw-Hill.

Weisman, A. (1979) *Coping with cancer*, New York: McGraw-Hill.

Wilkinson, S. (1999) 'Communication: it makes a difference', *Cancer Nursing*, 22, 1: 17–20.

Wilkinson, S., Bailey, K., Aldridge, J. and Roberts, A. (1999) 'A longitudinal evaluation of a communication skills programme', *Palliative Medicine*, 13, 4: 341–8.

24 Stroke sufferer

Bernard Gibbon and Caroline Watkins

Introduction

Stroke is common, with an incidence of about 2–2.5 per 1000 per year and a prevalence of 6 per 1000 in the UK (Wade, 1992). The incidence appears to be declining, and yet it remains one of the most common causes of acute medical admission to hospital. This could be attributed to the combined effects of increased incidence of stroke with advancing age and increasing proportions of older people in the population. Approximately 20 per cent of the UK population is over the age of 65, which represents almost 11 million people. As nearly 80 per cent of strokes occur in those over the age of 65, it has been estimated that the numbers of new strokes per year will increase by 30 per cent in the forty years from 1983 to 2023 (Malmgren *et al.*, 1989).

The government now recognises that stroke care is an important issue as, even today, stroke contributes at least 6 per cent to the health bill and to the loss of an estimated 7.7 million working days each year (Secretary of State for Health, 1992). Reduction in stroke-related mortality has been included in the Health of the Nation objectives and has led to improvements in healthcare. However, it is becoming increasingly apparent that reducing stroke-related death alone is insufficient, as it is those who survive with disability (as reflected by increased prevalence rates) who arguably contribute most to the financial burden of stroke care. Currently, although a third of those who suffer a stroke will die in the first month and a third will recover with virtually no residual physical problems, the remaining survivors will have moderate to severe disability requiring help from others in their day-to-day lives (Bamford *et al.*, 1990).

The effects of stroke on the individual

While it may be possible to determine, medically and scientifically, that the stroke evolved over a period of time, perhaps as a result of identifiable risk factors, nevertheless – as the name 'stroke' implies – the person is suddenly struck down. Regardless of the enduring physical effects, the experience of the person is such that the stroke is an acute catastrophic event, and it is inevitable that their life will change forever. The stroke event is so catastrophic for some people (approximately 15 per cent of those hospitalised: Wealleans, 1998) that they experience post-traumatic stress disorder (PTSD), which has been more commonly associated with war veterans. PTSD and more familiar emotional problems (e.g. low mood and anxiety) are common following stroke (see, for example, House *et al.*, 1989). Stroke is known to have a devastating impact on an individual, mainly as a consequence of the physical, psychological and social sequelae (Burton, 1999).

It is also important to recognise that the needs of the stroke patient change as the stroke progresses. They require emergency assessment and intensive monitoring in the first three days to prevent worsening of the stroke and other complications; then 'life supporting' care in the sub-acute phase, with intensive rehabilitation and planning for discharge; and then long-term rehabilitation encouraging adjustment, adaptation and reintegration into an acceptable lifestyle.

Stroke and its origin

A stroke is 'characterised by a focal neurological deficit due to local disturbance in the blood supply to the brain: its onset is usually abrupt, but it may extend over a few hours or longer ... it persists for more than 24 hours' (World Health Organisation, 1971), a description which both defines stroke and provides some account of its origin. The causes of stroke include hypertension and heart disease, while the underlying risk factors for these disorders can be attributed to cigarette smoking (Marmot and Poulter, 1992) and/or alcohol and obesity. These findings, together with the lack of intervention as yet determined to treat stroke, have resulted in management strategies aimed at prevention rather than cure. While this is laudable, it can inadvertently give rise to stigma in the case of 'failures', i.e. when such strategies have failed to prevent stroke.

There is little doubt that effective strategies to stop people smoking would see a decrease in the number of strokes. However, to suggest that people should simply stop smoking is naïve, as this would not prevent strokes altogether. The association between smoking and stroke can result in healthcare professionals applying labels to individuals, considering them to have brought the illness upon themselves. In addition to smoking, it is noteworthy that hypertension, another risk factor for stroke, can be caused by excessive alcohol consumption. This, too, can give rise to suggestions that the person is in some way responsible for their own ill health. It is important to note that not all strokes are caused by smoking or other excesses, and that hypertension can be caused by many other factors.

Nevertheless, in investigating the cause of stroke, healthcare professionals are encouraged to identify possible risk factors. A staff member will ask the patient about their previous medical history and possible risk factors at an early stage, generally soon after arrival in the hospital casualty department. Healthcare professionals should be mindful that their questioning could give the appearance of attributing blame to the individual for their stroke.

Appearing to attribute blame to the person who has suffered the stroke can be inadvertently continued in the rehabilitation setting, where staff are encouraged to find ways of motivating people to participate in rehabilitation. It is generally agreed that rehabilitation should be patient-focused, and that individualised rehabilitation goals should be set with each patient. Furthermore, patients should be encouraged to take responsibility for their own recovery in order that they do not feel that rehabilitation is something that is done to them. Healthcare professionals must once again be mindful of achieving a balance between empowering the patient in their own recovery and allowing the patient to feel totally responsible for any failures to achieve the goals set.

Stroke and concealability

The symptoms and signs of the stroke will be dependant upon the area of the brain affected. While some strokes may cause changes in vision, perception, cognition, personality, mood and emotional expression, these may be less obvious, particularly to those who do not know the person well. However, more commonly, one side of the body is overtly affected, with the sufferer being unable to conceal the 'mark'. There may be complete paralysis (hemiplegia) or weakness (hemiparesis) which could involve the face, arms and/or legs, but by implication also involves abdominal and chest wall muscles. At rest these problems are apparent through their effects on the face (drooling, expression) as well as limb (dropped shoulder, arm hanging down) and trunk (lopsided) positions. Some of these problems can be concealed by careful positioning, but as the person attempts to use or move the affected parts, the full extent of the problem becomes glaringly obvious.

With regard to limbs, the person may have difficulty in standing up straight, maintaining balance once standing, or they may be unable to pull the affected leg in front of the other. Even if they can manage to walk, they may still need to recruit muscles not normally required in order to achieve forward motion, which contributes to an abnormal gait. With regard to the face, the person may have difficulty smiling or frowning, or may choke on attempting to swallow even their own saliva.

Other common problems include faecal and/or urinary incontinence, and communication difficulties, with some patients rendered unable to speak and others losing the capacity to understand what is being said. The nature and combination of these problems results in few people being unable to recognise a stroke victim.

Stroke and healthcare

To many healthcare professionals, stroke patients are viewed as 'heavy' (Kirkevold, 1990), physically demanding and requiring much care and assistance. Yet in examining this issue empirically it is clear that nearly a third of people who have a stroke recover quickly with no – or only minimal – deficit (Bamford *et al.*, 1990), require little physical nursing care, and will have only a short hospital stay. Furthermore, while pharmaceutical interventions to limit the effects of the ischaemic event have not proved effective, there is already an existing treatment which is 2–3 times as effective as streptokinase in myocardial infarction: that is, there is robust evidence, following a Cochrane Review (Stroke Unit Trialists' Collaboration, 1997), to demonstrate that managing people who have suffered a stroke in specialist stroke units (acute and rehabilitation), as opposed to general wards, confers significant advantages to patients in terms of survival and functional outcome. Despite this evidence, and although it is apparent that more stroke units are opening, the extent and pace with which stroke services are being reorganised is surprisingly low.

The general public and many healthcare professionals continue to regard stroke as untreatable and, while stroke should be regarded as an acute medical emergency, not all stroke patients are admitted to hospital. People continue to suggest that it is possible to provide stroke care in the community (Mulley and Arie, 1978; Wade and Langton-Hewer, 1985). While this is possibly the case for post-acute rehabilitation (Wade *et al.*, 1985; Young and Forster, 1992), there is no evidence to suggest that patients can be managed safely in the acute phase.

Organising designated, geographically defined units that cater for a single diagnostic group (particularly relevant due to the heterogeneity of stroke) confers many advantages on both patients and staff (Gibbon, 1993; O'Connor, 1996). Staff can be facilitated in developing expertise and effective team working to deliver:

- detailed assessment and monitoring;
- appropriate treatment and care to prevent stroke progression in the acute phase, and also the development of complications due to the effects of the stroke itself;
- comprehensive rehabilitation (functional, social and psychological);
- the initiation of secondary prevention.

At all stages, the services of the multi-professional team are required, as the patient has complex problems which cannot be met by any one professional group in isolation. Although physiotherapy and occupational therapy have been regarded as the mainstay of therapy for stroke patients, there is little evidence to support such assertions, and the impact of psychological factors is becoming increasingly apparent (see, e.g., Robinson *et al.*, 1984; Sinyor *et al.*, 1986; Watkins, 1999). Despite knowing the effects of mood on recovery, services have not been developed to respond to the psychological treatment needs of stroke patients. Somehow depression after stroke has been dismissed as an understandable psychological reaction (House *et al.*, 1991) requiring no treatment. Once again, healthcare services have not been developed in this area for people who have suffered a stroke, despite overwhelming evidence to suggest that it is desperately needed. It is imperative for those who provide and purchase healthcare to reflect on why this may be, in order to overcome what would seem to be prejudices. It is also apparent that the views of patients themselves should not be ignored. Recent evidence suggests that the expectations of people who have recently suffered a stroke, in terms of what they believe will help them adjust and what will happen to them in the future, regardless of its accuracy, predicts survival and physical and emotional recovery. Those with high expectations of what will help but low expectations of what will actually happen to them, are more likely to be dead, dependent or depressed at three and twelve months after their stroke (Watkins, 1999). Healthcare professionals must take this on board and develop services and care to allow patients' expectations of what will help to become a reality, in order to improve outcome.

Healthcare professionals must be aware of the impact of promoting their therapies as aimed at achieving 'normality of movement', as if movement which is not normal is unworthy. For example, physiotherapists commonly employ the Bobath Technique (Bobath, 1978), although there is increasing evidence that other physiotherapy approaches may be more effective. Bobath seeks to exploit the untapped potential of the affected side of the brain by inhibition of abnormal patterns of spasticity and by the facilitation and stimulation of normal (autonomic and voluntary) functional movements. Therapists feel strongly that this approach will improve the person's functional outcome and will minimise the overt nature of the physical manifestations of stroke, reducing the incidence of 'abnormal' contractions by placing the patient in 'normal' positions. Healthcare professionals should always take care not to dismiss the ideas or goals of the patient and their family. Watkins (1999) reports that a person with a stroke, when relating her ideas of what would help her get better, described how her daughter had brought in a soft ball for her to 'exercise the bad hand with', but the daughter had been told by the physiotherapist 'We don't use those these days ... as they encourage abnormal movements.'

Even the importance that hospitals place on rehabilitation is brought into question, when patients spend less than one hour in therapy a day while much of the remaining time is spent in inactivity or isolated disengagement (Tinson, 1989). Similar findings were reported by Gibbon and

Little (1995) in stroke patients cared for on general medical wards. It is suggested that therapeutic activity takes place when patients spend time with therapists being 'taught' independence skills, which is then reinforced by 'learning' from nurses how to be independent (Gibbon, 1999). However, it is important for staff to be aware of their approach to conveying what they believe to be efficacious.

The stigmatising process

In regard to the key dimensions of 'concealability' and 'origin' (Jones *et al.*, 1984), stroke is a stigmatising condition. Stroke is highly visible: its physical manifestations have been outlined above and it is unlikely that a person would not be recognised as having had a stroke. The paralysis of one side of the body causes the person to adopt a characteristic posture. The 'mark' can be made less obvious by adopting certain positions, such as sitting in a chair which supports the affected arm and head. But even this does not afford complete concealment, since facial features may be affected, the person may not be able to maintain the face in a symmetrical position with facial expressions, sitting balance may be poor, and the person may appear to be lopsided or uncomfortable in the chair. In addition, the person may not be able to speak clearly and coherently, or to understand questions put to them. As such, they cannot engage in normal social interaction and hence reveal themselves as someone with a 'condition'. Other manifestations, such as incontinence, may also emphasise the visibility of the condition. Even the best-managed patients may have tell-tale signs giving rise to visibility, such as the presence of (medical) equipment.

Difficulty in eating or swallowing, or the excessive production of saliva, may cause the person to opt out of eating in company and thus highlight the visibility of their condition. Other people may find these characteristics unsightly and ensure that they do not join the patient at the dining table, which also contributes to the visibility of the condition. Perceptual problems and problems concerning memory can act as overt markers of the condition. All of these factors have a negative affect on interpersonal relationships. They are also frequently apparent on first encounter, and hence may influence a relationship from the outset, giving rise to feelings of uncertainty and discomfort in both the stigmatised and the non-stigmatised parties.

The overt nature of the 'mark' in stroke does, of course, serve to alert the interactant to the existence and nature of the condition. This can offer some comfort to both parties, in that expectations will be modulated.

The origin of stroke as a stigmatising condition is an important dimension for consideration. The 'mark' is a consequence of altered pathology (either a blood clot or a bleed which prevented blood from reaching a part of the brain) which resulted in brain damage. The brain damage is such that paralysis and other manifestations ensued. As stated previously, stroke can occur at any age, but the incidence increases with age. The pathology changes over a considerable timescale, but the stroke itself is sudden. It is only when the stroke occurs that the underlying pathology is known.

The altered physiology is attributed to lifestyle factors such as smoking, obesity, stress and alcohol consumption. These are all common events in life, but they do not cause stroke in all people. It is also the case that other (medical) causes of stroke exist, such as heart disease and diabetes. Origin as a dimension of stigma, in Jones *et al.*'s (1984) model, concerns who is perceived to hold the responsibility for the onset of the condition (stroke). To the observer the cause of stroke is not obvious, and indeed until recently stroke was commonly known as a cerebro-vascular accident, a term which implies that a stroke is an accident, though that is clearly not the case in the normal meaning of this term.

It is likely that, if the stroke occurs in someone who is grossly obese, this will be viewed negatively and the person will be thought to have brought the condition upon themselves. This may also be the interpretation if the person is seen to be a smoker or a drinker, or if they are a 'workaholic' who has brought high levels of stress upon themselves. Those with other causes cannot be distinguished from these groups by the observer, and hence all stroke patients may be stigmatised.

Stroke can also be seen as a socially degrading condition, in that the survivor often requires the assistance of others in a range of basic functions, such as caring for hygiene and toileting needs. The negative views held by others towards stroke patients can also be exacerbated by the consequences of not recovering fully from the stroke. That is, the person can be blamed for causing the stroke through their lifestyle actions, and can be blamed for maintaining the consequences of the stroke by failing to gain independence through rehabilitation. The patient who appears not to have the will to seek independence, migrating towards dependence upon others, is likely to be held more responsible than the person who seeks independence.

Stigmatisation and healthcare professionals

In many cases the stroke patient asks the family doctor to visit them, or to be conveyed by ambulance to hospital. These actions can commence the stigmatising process. Most patients entering hospital are admitted to a ward which is identified by a hospital indexing system (e.g. M1 – Medical Ward 1) or named after a hospital benefactor (e.g. William Jones Ward), and these labels do not identify the diagnostic group of the client. Even wards that specialise in specific client groups (e.g. Gynaecology) do not go so far as to make the client's diagnosis evident. Yet the stroke patient is usually admitted to the 'Stroke Unit', which acts to label the patient and can exacerbate stigma. Units such as 'Stroke Unit' or 'Coronary Care Unit' act both to give 'special' status and to reveal the nature of the patient's condition.

The healthcare professional's previous experience of stroke is likely to evoke feelings which may or may not be positive. Staff attitudes towards stroke patients are at best neutral and at worst negative (Hamrin, 1982; Gibbon, 1991). Much of this view rests in the sense of therapeutic nihilism that healthcare professionals experience. Healthcare professionals feel that there is little they can do to improve the patients' outcome, but recent studies are demonstrating that their interventions do make a positive difference (Stroke Unit Trialists' Collaboration, 1997). An early study (Stockwell, 1972) provided some insights into the characteristics of unpopular patients, and many of these can be found in stroke patients. Examples include a protracted length of in-patient stay, uncooperativeness, difficult to talk to, and being unlikely to progress.

Overcoming the stigma

The advent of the Stroke Unit has gone a long way to address the stigmatising process. While the labelling of the ward in such a way can be viewed negatively, as we have seen, the fact that staff are dedicated to that unit, and have (largely) self-selected to work there, has led to the development of expertise and confidence among staff. This is also evidence that staff attitudes towards stroke patients can be improved (Gibbon and Little, 1995).

In a study by Gibbon (1999) the multi-professional team on a stroke unit was shown to develop better levels of integration than in disparate areas of the hospital. Teamwork was evident in the shared rehabilitation plans and was best exemplified by the team conferences where the team discussed and arrived at decisions concerning the rehabilitation plan for each patient in the unit. The core professionals at the centre of the stroke rehabilitation team appeared to have acquired specific roles at the team conference. The physiotherapist took on the role of 'proposer' of decisions, and the occupational therapist as 'seconder'. The doctor retained the role of 'sanctioner', in that this profession held responsibility for the admission and discharge of patients, and the nurse took on the role of actioning decisions (Gibbon, 1999). The team conference also acts to legitimise non-direct patient care activity and, as such, allows the team to develop a sense of collaboration.

References

Baker, A.C. (1993) 'The spouse's positive effect on the stroke patient's recovery', *Rehabilitation Nursing*, 18: 30–3.

Bamford, J., Sandercock, P., Dennis, M. and Warlow, C. (1990) 'A prospective study of acute cerebrovascular disease in the community: the Oxfordshire Community Stroke Project. 2. Incidence, case fatality rates and overall outcome at one year of cerebral infarction, primary intracerebral and subarachnoid haemorrhage', *Journal of Neurology, Neurosurgery and Psychiatry*, 53: 16–22.

Bobath, B. (1978) *Adult hemiplegia: evaluation and treatment*, London: William Heinemann.

Burton, C.R. (1999) 'An exploration of the stroke co-ordinator role', *Journal of Clinical Nursing*, 8: 535–41.

Doolittle, N. (1991) 'Clinical ethnography of lacunar stroke: implications for acute care', *Journal of Neuroscience Nursing*, 23: 235–40.

Folden, S.L. (1994) 'Managing the effects of a stroke: the first months', *Rehabilitation Nursing Research*, Fall, 79–85.

Gibbon, B. (1991) 'A reassessment of nurses' attitudes towards stroke patients in general medical wards', *Journal of Advanced Nursing*, 16, 11: 1336–42.

—— (1993) 'Implications for nurses in approaches to the management of stroke rehabilitation: a review of the literature', *International Journal of Nursing Studies*, 30, 2: 133–41.

—— (1999) 'An investigation of interprofessional collaboration in stroke rehabilitation conferences', *Journal of Clinical Nursing*, 8: 246–52.

Gibbon, B. and Little, V. (1995) 'Improving stroke care through action research', *Journal of Clinical Nursing*, 4: 93–100.

Haggstrom, T, Axelsson, K. and Norberg, A. (1994) 'The experience of living with stroke sequelae illuminated by means of stories and metaphors', *Qualitative Health Research*, 4: 321–37.

Hamrin, E. (1982) 'Attitudes of nursing staff in general medical wards towards activation of stroke patients', *Journal of Advanced Nursing*, 7: 33–42.

House, A., Dennis, M., Mogridge, L. *et al.* (1991) 'Mood disorders in the year after first stroke', *British Journal of Psychiatry*, 158: 83–92.

House, A., Dennis, M., Molyneux, A. *et al.* (1989) 'Emotionalism after stroke', *British Medical Journal*, 298: 991–4.

Jones, E.E., Farina, A., Hastorf, A.H. *et al.* (1984) *Social stigma: the psychology of marked relationships*, New York: W.H. Freeman.

Kirkevold, M. (1990) 'Caring for stroke patients: heavy or exciting?', *Image: Journal of Nursing Scholarship*, 22, 2: 79–83.

Malmgren, R., Bamford, J., Warlow, C. *et al.* (1989) 'Projecting the number of patients with first ever strokes and patients newly handicapped by stroke in England and Wales', *British Medical Journal*, 298: 656–60.

Marmot, M.G. and Poulter, N.R. (1992) 'Primary prevention of stroke', *Lancet*, 339: 344–7.

Mulley, G. and Arie, T. (1978) 'Treating stroke: home or hospital?', *British Medical Journal*, 278: 1321–2.

Mumma, C.M. (1986) 'Perceived losses following stroke', *Rehabilitation Nursing*, 11: 19–24.

O'Connor, S. (1996) 'Stroke units: centres of nursing innovation', *British Journal of Nursing*, 5: 105–9.

Robinson, R.G., Starr, L.B., Lipsey, J.R. *et al.* (1984) 'A two-year longitudinal study of post-stroke mood disorders: dynamic changes over the first 6 months of follow-up', *Stroke*, 15: 510–17.

Secretary of State for Health (1992) *The health of the nation: a strategy for health in England* (white paper), London: HMSO.

Sinyor, D., Amato, P., Kaloupek, G. *et al.* (1986) 'Post-stroke depression: relationship to functional impairment, coping strategies, and rehabilitation outcome', *Stroke*, 17: 1102–7.

Stockwell, F. (1972) *The unpopular patient*, London: Royal College of Nursing.

Stroke Unit Trialists' Collaboration (1997) *A systematic review of specialist multidisciplinary team (stroke unit) care for stroke inpatients*, The Cochrane Database of Systematic Reviews, issue 1 (CD Rom).

Tinson, D.J. (1989) 'How stroke patients spend their days', *International Disability Studies*, 11: 45–9.

Wade, D.T. (1992) 'Stroke rehabilitation and long term care', *Lancet*, 339, 8796: 791–3.

Wade, D.T. and Langton-Hewer, R. (1985) 'Hospital admission for acute stroke: who, for how long and to what effect?', *Journal of Epidemiology and Community Health*, 39: 347–52.

Wade D.T., Langton-Hewer, R., Skilbeck, C.E. *et al.* (1985) 'Controlled trial of a home care service for acute stroke patients', *Lancet*, 1: 323–6.

Watkins, C. (1999) *The effects of patients' expectations on the rehabilitation process*, PhD Thesis, University of Liverpool.

Wealleans, G. (1998) *Post traumatic stress disorder in survivors of stroke*, Doctoral Thesis in Clinical Psychology, University of Liverpool.

World Health Organisation (1971) *Cerebrovascular diseases: prevention treatment and rehabilitation*, Technical Report Series No. 469, Geneva: World Health Organisation.

Young, J.B. and Forster, A. (1992) 'The Bradford community stroke trial: results at six months', *British Medical Journal*, 304: 1085–8.

25 The older person

Caroline Watkins and Bernard Gibbon

Introduction

Particular attention has been drawn in recent years to the increasing proportion of older people within Western populations. We are repeatedly reminded that in the UK the proportion of people over the age of 60 will increase by more than 65 per cent by the year 2030, such that the current proportion of 20 per cent comprised of over-60s will increase to 33 per cent (e.g. Greengross *et al.*, 1997; Khaw, 1997). These increases are suggested to be the result of decreased mortality, and the consequent increased longevity is suggested to be due to a reduction in childhood illnesses and infectious diseases, and an increase in primary and secondary preventative health measures and improved nutrition (Office of National Statistics, 1996).

It is inevitable that there will be a subsequent increase in the prevalence of disability and chronic illness, particularly due to disorders associated with ageing. Therefore we are constantly challenged to improve the quality of those 'extra' years. We are charged with the task of not merely 'adding years to life' but legitimising this by demonstrating that we can 'add life to years'.

Inherent in this is the suggestion that, if older people are going to live longer, then the only acceptable, or even ethical, circumstances in which this can take place are those where the person has an active life which is free from disability. That is, that they need to still be seen to contribute to the family and to the community. They must also not be a physical, mental or social burden to society. These attitudes are apparent from the perspective that the costs of chronic disease and disability are regarded, which includes studies examining the increase in family burden from caring for people who are physically and/or mentally frail (see, e.g., Gray and Fenn, 1993; Max *et al.*, 1995), and also studies which examine how caring for or treating older people increases the costs of medical care (see, e.g., Ostir *et al.*, 1999). We are reminded that supporting older people is costly, and it is younger people who are working (and whose numbers are diminishing) who are expected to provide resources through taxation to support healthcare for older people.

Consequently it is no longer acceptable merely to demonstrate that interventions or treatments improve physical function or mental well-being, as they are also expected to improve the person's quality of life. Hence the measurement of quality of life has become a burning issue in determining the effectiveness – and also the cost-effectiveness – of interventions aimed at curing, stabilising or maintaining diseases or disorders, across the lifespan but particularly those targeting older people. Tools commonly used to justify the allocation of healthcare resources that claim to take account of quality of life, for example 'Quality Adjusted Life Years' (QALYs), discriminate against older people. They have been suggested to perpetuate commonly held views that younger people should receive care however costly, whereas older people are seen to have had their turn and therefore the costs cannot be justified (Williams, 1997). Tools used to allocate or deny services or treatments must in future take account of the heterogeneity of people at different ages.

The effects of ageing on the individual

Despite the fact that some older people may suffer from a range of problems, many are fit and well and others may only have but a single health problem. Furthermore, these problems may or may not be directly associated with ageing itself. As with people of all ages, some health problems may be hereditary, congenital or developmental, or they may be the result of the individual's lifestyle. Some of these problems may be seen to be controllable (diet, smoking, alcohol consumption) and others uncontrollable (heart defects, degenerative neurological disorders). Nevertheless the subsequent burden on society is frequently viewed as the result of the person's ability or inability successfully to cope with their own problems. The necessity for families, societies or the state to intervene is frequently viewed as a failure of the individual.

The range and nature of the problems to be coped with vary in their expected course and consequences. Problems may be:

- recoverable, or appear to be curable and to disappear with time and/or treatment (e.g. dermatological problems);
- progressively disabling, affecting physical or mental functioning (e.g. Parkinson's disease, or senile dementia of the Alzheimer's type);
- of sudden onset but chronically disabling (e.g. stroke or myocardial infarction).

There may even be an absence of any organic or functional problem.

None the less, older people may be the subject of social stigma. For example, they may be viewed as gullible or vulnerable even though they are cognitively normal. This may alter people's behaviour towards an older person because of their own misconceptions and poor attitudes, but the older person, despite noticing their altered behaviour, may not appreciate the origin of that behaviour. There may also be a visible or at least a noticeable problem that is obvious to others but not to the older person. Once again, the older person may notice altered behaviour but be unaware of the origin of the disdain. For example, those with cognitive or attentional problems may repeat information to others on several occasions, but be completely unaware of doing so. An older person may have an unpleasant odour but be unaware of it.

The stigma associated with such disorders may be a result of the blame seen to be attributable to the older person, or of the embarrassment caused by the physical and functional consequences of the resultant problems or features of the disorder. There is also the contrast between actual changes or features and the person's beliefs about those changes or features. These beliefs could be accurate or inaccurate.

The person's beliefs and those of others may affect the way a person is actually treated. That is, treatment may be aimed at modifying the social significance of the problem, e.g. using cognitive therapy or systematic motivational counselling. The alternative course of action may be to aim treatments, such as physiotherapy, at modifying the progression of the disorder.

The effects of ageing and disruptiveness

It may be that, if a problem is seen as irreparable, it is also seen as less acceptable. For example, relatives may tolerate incontinence in the acute stages of a disorder which affects the ability of the person to make it to the toilet in time. However, if the incontinence is seen as a permanent feature, then this may be viewed with disdain. Also, if the problem is visible and aesthetically displeasing or dangerous, then there can be an increased strain on interpersonal relationships. This can be compounded when the problem blocks or interferes with interpersonal communication. For example, following stroke, where there is gaze paresis, there is difficulty in gaining or maintaining eye contact; in the case of hearing difficulties, constant eye contact is necessary, with or without the need to talk at a louder level; these factors can increase interpersonal strain.

Where others perceive a given solution to a problem to be the only course of action, but the affected person is unwilling or unsure about addressing the problem in that way, then this, too, can cause tension and can potentially result in stigma. For example, in the case of an older person with hearing loss, others may perceive the only course of action to be for that person is to get a hearing aid, and they may despise the person if they do not do this. Also, after stroke in a known smoker, it may be felt that the person should stop smoking. If they do not, then people may feel an aversion, as the person is then viewed as unnecessarily draining health service resources.

The stigmatising process

It may be that the best course of action is to decrease the visibility of the problem in order to decrease the stigma. For example, incontinence can be managed by catheterisation or by the use of discrete pads. Unfortunately, the remedies themselves may increase stigma. For example, putting people with similar problems together is frequently thought to reduce stigma, but this is not necessarily the case (Comer and Piliavin, 1975). For example, younger people (or those who view themselves as being younger) may be unwilling to attend day centres, thought to be aimed mainly at older people.

Overcoming the stigma

So what can people do in an attempt to reduce their stigma? People may disavow or minimise the feature. For example, those with hearing loss may pretend that they can hear, while those with memory problems may make jokes to cover up instances where memory loss is apparent. If the feature is not clearly visible, e.g. melancholy, then the person may be able to choose whether or not to disclose that they are feeling bad. Although problems such as incontinence may be concealable in the short term, following long interaction it is almost inevitable that they will become apparent.

Although one may assume concealable problems are better, an obvious problem may sometimes be easier to address. However, no situation is clear-cut, as problems are rarely either obvious or concealable but are more often somewhere in between. The circumstances of interaction also have a bearing, in that something previously undetectable may become blatantly obvious with changing circumstances.

Ultimately the action taken, in terms of what the stigmatised person says or does, depends upon the characteristics of the problem and also of those interacting with them. The circumstances of the interaction must also be taken into account.

Addressing stigmatisation by healthcare professionals

Older person's hospital wards or day centres may provide a useful forum for older people to meet other people. This may afford older people the opportunity not only to socialise with others, but also to discuss their own problems with people who may share a similar perspective. However, it should be noted that the older person placed in such a situation may feel themselves to have been uprooted from a comfortable environment where normally they might not feel the need to disclose their problems.

Education about normal ageing and its associated problems may start at an early stage. Schools should be responsible for informing students about, for example, the normal bladder function, and the effects of ageing on pelvic floor muscles (particularly in women) and on the prostate gland in men. By appreciating the near-inevitable and universal nature of these problems, students will develop a more positive attitude to such things as incontinence in later life. This could form the basis for more specialist knowledge later. Healthcare professionals should be encouraged to review their knowledge of normal ageing, the effects of ageing, and those interventions and implications relevant to older people. It would be preferable for healthcare professionals specialising in such issues to learn by the use of multi-disciplinary, enquiry-based formats, which prompt reflection and critical review of problems from a variety of perspectives. The stigmatising processes, and how they may be avoided or addressed, may form an integral part of the debate.

Clear policies must be developed which ensure maximisation of the potential of older people, maintain their dignity and allow their contribution to society to be recognised – both in work and in social networks and family relationships.

References

Comer, R.C. and Piliavin, J.A. (1975) 'As others see us: attitudes of physically handicapped and normals toward own and other groups', *Rehabilitation Literature*, 36, 7: 206–21, 225.

Gray, A. and Fenn, P. (1993) 'Alzheimer's disease: the burden of the illness in England', *Health Trends*, 25, 1: 31–7.

Greengross, S., Murphy, E., Quam, L. *et al.* (1997) 'Ageing: a subject that must be top of the world agendas', *British Medical Journal*, 315: 1029–30.

Khaw, K. (1997) 'How many, how old, how soon?', *British Medical Journal*, 319: 1350–2.

Max, W., Webber, P. and Fox, P. (1995) 'Alzheimer's Disease: the unpaid burden of caring', *Journal of Ageing and Health*, 7, 2: 179–99.

Office of National Statistics (1996) *National Population Projections* (based upon 1994 data), ONS, London: The Stationery Office.

Ostir, G.V., Carlson, J.E., Black, S.A. *et al.* (1999) 'Disability in older adults. 1: Prevalence, causes, and consequences', *Behavioural Medicine*, 24, 4: 147–56.

Williams, A. (1997) 'The rationing of healthcare by age: the case for', *British Medical Journal*, 314: 820–2.

26 From stigma to the social exclusion of disabled people

Bob Sapey

The social construction of stigma

In her study of deafness on Martha's Vineyard, Groce (1985) describes how the birth of a deaf child was seen as 'a minor problem, rather than a major misfortune' (p. 53). What is remarkable about this is that it strikes at the heart of the debate about disability and normality.

It is possible to argue that we should try to view the world as being populated by a wide range of human diversity and that, as such, normality is essentially a social construct, derived predominantly from statistics which itself is a relatively new branch of mathematics. One counter to this is that there is an instinctual, rather than cultural, relationship in the way people view the wholeness of the body. For example, is it not quite natural for parents, at the point of birth, to enquire if their child is alright – complete, with ten fingers, ten toes and so forth? Indeed the joy of a new-born child is often soured by any detraction from this concept of whole or normal. What was supposed to be a natural process becomes a major medical event!

The situation on Martha's Vineyard in the eighteenth and nineteenth centuries was that, due to genetic factors, this relatively isolated population had a high incidence of deafness. As a result, a large proportion of the islanders had learnt to be bilingual, both speaking English and using sign language. As a further consequence of this, deafness did not result in any particular barriers and so the attitudes that were constructed towards deafness were not negative. Despite this level of enlightenment, Groce (1985) records that attitudes of the islanders towards other forms of impairment were no different to those elsewhere, thus reinforcing the notion that their attitude towards deafness was indeed socially constructed.

As a result of deafness being sufficiently common to change the attitudes of the islanders towards deaf people, the stigma attached to the condition was considerably reduced. Deaf people were not excluded from economic, religious, educational, social or political activities on the island. However, an example such as this is striking, simply because it is so unusual. In the world today, to be born with or to acquire an impairment raises the chances of being denied an education, being excluded from employment, being rejected socially and religiously, and being seen as a political liability. In short, impaired people are considerably disabled by the attitudes and reactions of others.

From an essentialist viewpoint, the visible differences caused by physical impairment could constitute the 'mark', to which others will react – possibly by stigmatising the individual or groups involved. In many ways this is as obvious a process as are the physical differences which give rise to it, and it may seem inevitable that, given pronounced deformities in a minority of the population, the majority will simply react in ways beyond their control. However, stigmatisation is not simply a behavioural response. As Goffman (1963) has explained, it concerns the attachment of meaning to the mark, a meaning which is itself the result of prior experience, knowledge and assumptions. Such meanings are not fixed, for they are constructed by individuals and, though they may be reified, they can also change.

A good example of the way in which meanings are socially constructed can be found in the work of Bogdan and Taylor (1989), where they examine how the partners of severely disabled people view them. What Bogdan and Taylor found was a level of acceptance which challenged the professional labels ascribed to disabled people. Just as in Martha's Vineyard, on a local family level people were valued for characteristics other than their impairments, although to outsiders they continued to elicit negative responses. While on the one hand it seems clear that familiarity can and does help change the stigmatisation of disabled people, the question of whether it is possible to bring about a more fundamental change in the way disabled people are seen by others still remains.

One of the most important criticisms of theories of stigma came from Finkelstein (1980), who argued that Goffman's comparison of the reaction to disabled people with the treatment of slaves in ancient Greece was fundamentally flawed. What Goffman claimed was that the branding of slaves and others was to signify something bad and unusual, but what he failed to acknowledge was the context within which the stigma or sign had been placed on the slaves by the slave owners (Goffman, 1963). Finkelstein explains that slavery was not unusual but commonplace. It depended upon oppression, and branding the slaves was useful in preventing their escape. Slave owners needed to assert that being a slave was the natural place for certain people, and far from needing to avoid such people, slave owning was in fact very desirable. He goes on:

> It is a distortion to view the person who has been forcibly branded so that he or she permanently carries a stigma as the 'signifier' of a bad moral status. This is to invert the real social relationships whereby the one who assigns the stigma is the 'signifier' and the one who is chained and forced to bear the oppressor's views of himself is the

bearer. To say the bearer of suffering is the 'signifier' of attributes assigned to him is to take the standpoint of the oppressor in the slave/master relationship.

(Finkelstein, 1980: 30)

Spicker makes a similar point in discussing the relationship of stigma within welfare, when he states: 'The idea that stigma is a personal characteristic implies a pathological view of social problems. This use is unsatisfactory. A mark cannot be inherently discrediting; the marked individual is discredited by the interpretation that is put on it. A stigma is socially defined' (Spicker, 1984: 62).

While it is possible to treat this as simply a matter of semantics, Finkelstein was in fact engaged in the development of a new and challenging way of viewing disability. Rather than treating the disadvantages faced by disabled people as simply the natural result of their impairments (in other words, because of a spinal injury this person cannot walk and, because she cannot walk, she cannot work), he was arguing that it was the organisation of society and the attitudes of non-disabled people which imposed these limitations. This 'social model of disability' has become the main theoretical basis for the disabled peoples' movement which has been seeking political and social change for the past thirty years.

Furthermore, as Oliver (1990) has pointed out, the presence of stigmatising attitudes can have very debilitating effects. He considered the questions used by the Office of Population, Census and Surveys in their surveys of disabled people, and questioned the effect of their terminology. In one question they asked disabled people: 'Do you have a scar, blemish or deformity which limits your daily activities?' Oliver (1995) suggested that this question could have been reformulated to ask: 'Do other people's reactions to any scar, blemish or deformity you may have, limit your daily activities?' He argued: 'This reformulation is not only about methodology or semantics, it is also about oppression' (Oliver, 1995: 9).

What Oliver is referring to here is the way in which the process of such interviews reinforced the oppressive treatment of disabled people. Indeed, the very first question people were asked was: 'Can you tell me what is wrong with you?'; making very clear the assumption of the researchers that they perceived the disabled person to be in some way dysfunctional or deviant. This is a long way from the concept of an acceptance of human diversity.

In fact, rather than recognising the heterogeneity of individuals, the process of stigmatising is creating and reinforcing a homogeneity based upon the marks of impairment. This characteristic becomes the one which others decide to use in identifying and labelling disabled people as precisely that: disabled. It may occasionally be possible for certain individuals to be accepted for other attributes of their character, but it is likely that, unless they hide their impairment, they will first and foremost be thought of as disabled. Given that such a category is constructed, not from a full knowledge of the individuals involved, but from a reaction to one particular mark, it is possible to argue that the whole concept of a grouping called 'the disabled' is the construct of others. This is particularly pertinent in terms of the clinical gaze, in which it is the body, and specifically its dysfunctioning, that becomes the overriding concern of doctors, nurses and others connected to the medical profession.

The scientific construction of stigma

The role of stigma in the construction of disability as a category may be far more of a deliberate project than an unwitting social or psychological process. Marks (1999) makes the point that stigma has some of its roots in the classification work of nineteenth-century evolutionary psychologists and phrenologists. This social Darwinist exercise was closely associated with the development of eugenicist policies, which were extremely influential at that time. The popularity of eugenics spanned the political spectrum, but a significant contribution was made to the theories by statisticians such as Francis Galton and Karl Pearson (Pfeiffer, 1994). Statistics played an important part in giving scientific credibility to the classifications which were taking place and hence to the appropriateness of reacting to marks of impairment as both unusual and bad. However, what needs to be considered and questioned here is the basis for accepting the statistical analysis of human diversity as an objective scientific process.

MacKenzie (1979) has explored the rise of statistics in the latter half of the nineteenth and the early part of the twentieth century and concludes that, for Galton and Pearson in particular, their developments in this field were indeed governed by their own political agenda to show that eugenicist, not environmental, reform was the way to improve the British race. They did this by taking judgemental data which could only appear in ordinal scales and treating it as if it were an interval scale, thereby giving scientific credibility to the reactions associated with stigma. This linking of the eugenics project with the classification of undesirable attributes, and hence to the adverse reactions to stigmatising marks, underlines the extent to which we have had, and continue to have, choice in this matter. The ideas may have been reified, but this does not detract from the fact that they have been constructed in order to serve a purpose similar to the aim of the Greek slave owners – the identification and control of particular groups of people.

Financial implications of exclusion

Thus, stigma plays a role in the creation of disablement as a category which will be ascribed to individuals, and as a means by which their membership of that group will be reinforced. However, a pertinent question here is whether this is entirely a bad thing, for it has been through the label of disability that many people have gained access to a wide range of welfare services. The provision of social security benefits and of personal care services, both health and social, has long been organised through the assessment of an individual's dysfunction, so could it not be argued that this is of direct advantage to disabled people?

Within a hegemony of care, such an assertion may well be founded, but care itself has its critics within the disability movement. Many writers, for example Morris (1993) or Macfarlane (1996), have referred to care in terms of the custodial and institutionalised ways in which it has been experienced. Spicker (1984) also provides a wealth of examples of the ways in which welfare is experienced as stigmatising, to the extent that it leads to considerable avoidance of the claimant status by young and old alike. Finkelstein (1980) goes much further, and suggests that it is the hegemony of care which is essential to maintaining the oppression of disabled people. In his view, which has been very influential in disability studies, the maintenance of a welfare system acts to keep disabled people out of the mainstream of society, by giving professional sanction to the notion that it is welfare rather than work, segregation rather than integration, and dependency rather than independence that is in the best interests of disabled people. For Finkelstein, the problem with welfare is not its content, but its very existence. This viewpoint may not be widely shared in its extreme manifestation, but it is pertinent today, given the nature of new modes of oppression, in particular social exclusion.

While the term 'social exclusion' can be and is used in a common-sense manner to encompass a wide range of processes which result in some form of disadvantage, its real significance is as a term to describe the effects that follow from being economically excluded from the global economy. The massive changes that have been taking place over the last few decades, in particular what Castells (1996) has described as an informational revolution, and the globalisation of capital, have led to substantial reformation in the distribution of economic participation within nations and throughout the world. In short, it is now possible for economic activity to transfer relatively easily between nations and continents seeking out efficient and economic labour forces. While there are still considerable geographical barriers to the total transferability of many industrial and agricultural activities, this is not the case for much of the informational economy, and that sector is the one which is growing most rapidly. Castells's (1996) observations of the impact of these changes suggests that particular groups of people are being economically excluded: for example, black people in American inner cities, those in many parts of Central and South America, and those from sub-Saharan Africa. What these groups also have in common is that there is little or no welfare response to their isolation from employment as we might have expected in the past. The results are seen at their most extreme in the mass starvation that periodically takes place in Africa, the development of globalised crime and its alternative economies, and in the rise of resistance movements throughout the globe.

In comparison to this, the position of disabled people as a group singled out for favourable treatment within the welfare system may appear to be somewhat generous, but there are several indications that this may be changing. My own analysis of available data from both the UK and the USA (Sapey 2000) indicates clearly that disabled people, when they are employed, will tend to be located in low-status industrial and agricultural work; and, so far, they appear to be even more excluded from jobs associated with the informational economy. There is an extensive literature in disability studies which points to both structural and attitudinal barriers to the employment of disabled people. Roulstone (1998) argues that these attitudes which focus on the deficits of individuals rather than of the production process are being transferred to new technology industries, and that additional difficulties are creeping in, such as resistance to the use of technologies that might prove of assistance.

Furthermore, Tomlinson and Colquhoun (1995) argue that there is some evidence to suggest that even those low-status jobs are at risk as other groups of people who are economically excluded from the new economies are prepared to compete for that employment. So, despite the potential for technology to make work accessible to disabled people, it would appear that their economic exclusion is increasing.

At the same time the attitude of government in the UK is rapidly changing towards the welfare support of disabled people. The reviews of disability benefits that have occurred since the election of the Labour Party in 1997, and the ongoing reviews such as the integrity project associated with the Disability Living Allowance, have tended to be imbalanced in policy terms. On the one hand they are positively addressing issues of dependence through a recognition that the causal relationship between impairment and unemployment has been misunderstood, but on the other there is little evidence of government attempting to deal with the structural problems of disablism in employment. In short, we appear to be heading towards a situation in which little or nothing is being done to prevent the economic exclusion of disabled people, and at the same time the safety-net of care is being gradually eroded or withdrawn. This process may not have impacted fully as yet, but the indications are that it will unless it is restrained by political and social pressure.

In the twenty-first century, therefore, people who have been disabled, in the sense that they have been economically excluded from the industrial economy and supported through a medical hegemony of care, are likely to find that their exclusion from both the industrial and informational economies increases, and in addition they will be socially excluded because of changing attitudes towards welfare. This poses extreme difficulties for disabled people and a range of challenges for professions engaged in work within the 'disability industry'.

Promoting exclusion through medicalisation

A wide range of medical, therapeutic and caring professions are involved in working with disabled people to provide the care that has been the alternative to economic inclusion. Their activities vary, both in terms of substance and in terms of the acceptability of their practices to disabled people. In substance, doctors may be concerned with a wide range of procedures which are designed to correct physical imperfections. While some of these have been instrumental in increasing the life-expectancy of disabled people (and therefore increasing the prevalence of disability), others have been experienced as intrusive and devaluing of difference. Furthermore, the range of activities of doctors goes well beyond the medical sphere in which they have expertise, so that they are consulted over matters concerning education, employment and entitlement to social security as if these matters become medical as and when they relate to a disabled person.

Physiotherapists also provide an expertise which may assist people to increase their physical agility so as to enable them to be less dependant on others, but they, too, are involved in more controversial practices such as conductive education, which has been perceived by some disabled people as undermining the self-esteem of individuals who gain considerable mobility through the use of wheelchairs (Oliver, 1993). The criticism is that, in order to assist people to walk badly and possibly to little effect, the advocates of conductive education engage in the denigration of wheelchair use. Occupational therapists do not escape criticism from disabled people either, for, despite their role in providing a considerable range of equipment and advice which might enable people to live independently, Abberley (1995) has argued that this takes place in a context which is primarily concerned with the professionalising project of that occupation, and that, in so doing, they seek to individualise problems and place the responsibility for failure on disabled people rather than on themselves.

The disability industry has been primarily concerned with both the care and the rehabilitation of disabled individuals, though in the last thirty years there has been an increasing development of independent living schemes and advocacy services controlled by disabled people. These developments have been a reaction to the experience of segregation within the welfare system and to the dependency that was created by this industry. As Brechin and Liddiard (1981) have said:

Our first concern is that disabled people are faced with impossible social, financial, housing and environmental difficulties, and are then offered a piecemeal welfare system of professionals and services to help them adjust to and cope with their unacceptable circumstances ...

Here is a second major point of concern for us: that the role a disabled person is expected to play in determining his own well-being seems to be an inherently dependent one.

(Brechin and Liddiard, 1981: 2–3)

Implications for the delivery of health and social care services

However, while taking control of some services may provide a model for the way in which they could be delivered, it would be reckless to suggest that healthcare and social care professions are of no future value to disabled people. Indeed, the challenge is for us to change our approaches to disability so that we can make ourselves useful. A good example of this can be seen in the research undertaken by Oliver (1995) into the role of counselling with disabled people. Along with many others engaged in the psychosocial aspects of welfare, counsellors have been subjected to criticism for the pathologising tendencies of their activities. The widespread use of theories of loss, based upon the behaviourist approaches to bereavement which were popularised by Parkes (1975), have been widely criticised for the ways in which they were applied to disabled people without consideration of the meanings that people themselves applied to the experience of impairment (see, for example, Oliver and Sapey, 1999). What Oliver did was to examine the ways in which counselling could be used to assist disabled people to counter the discrimination they were experiencing, rather than to enforce their psychological adaptation to an oppressive world. In many ways this provides a model for the way in which professional skills can be used to the advantage of disabled people by analysing the problems they face from the perspective of a social model of disability. The same approach can be taken to rehabilitation, where we need to examine the ways in which our professional organisation acts to restrict or control people. In other words, part of the assessment or diagnosis of a problem needs to be focused on ourselves and our practice, rather than on the individual involved. This has some resonances with the thinking behind reflective practice.

There are, however, some major obstacles to be overcome for practice to move towards a social model. At a structural level this would involve some action to ensure that the development of welfare is inclusionary rather than exclusionary, while at an institutional level the employers and organisations of welfare professions need to examine their own motivations – whether they are more concerned with the advancement of their own interests over and above those people they purport to serve. Neither of these are possible without a more fundamental change in our personal attitudes to disability. Parkes (1975) says of the disabled people's movement that:

> ... the challenge that it makes to the rest of society is absolutely fundamental .... The whole way that people think about themselves and about their impairment. These things are very significant and they are about changing society very fundamentally.
>
> (cited in Campbell and Oliver, 1996: 139)

Thirty years earlier, Hunt expressed the demand in this way:

> We are asking of people something that lies a lot deeper than almsgiving. We want an extension of the impulse that inspires this, so that it becomes a gift of self rather than the dispensing of bounty (material or other kinds) from above. To love and respect, treat as equals, people as obviously 'inferior' as we are, requires real humility and generosity.
>
> (Hunt, 1966: 158)

It is this fundamental change in the way in which we perceive disability that is key to bringing about other changes in the structure and organisation of welfare. We need to begin to think of difference as something to be valued rather than feared, and not in terms of sympathy. An inclusionary welfare system needs to be based upon the respect of others' rights to participate, and this will mean challenging some taken-for-granted aspects of life in both healthcare and social care services. In nursing, for example, it is necessary for new recruits to have to meet strict health checks, and this is accepted by employers, educators and the professions. And this is not simply about having the physical ability to conform to the current organisation of nursing tasks, but also about the appearance of nurses and what 'marks' might be considered offensive.

When I discuss the disabled people's movement with social work students, a common reaction is to refer to this as a 'user' group. In nursing it might even be thought of in terms of a patients' organisation. These descriptions are flawed in that they betray the extent to which we attribute characteristics of dependency to disabled people – we cannot conceive of such organisations as existing unless it is in relation to the fact that some of their members may be users of welfare services. We perpetuate the world in which there are just two groups of people, citizens and recipients of welfare, those with rights and those without. Changing the way we think about impairment and disability is therefore an essential co-requisite to institutional and structural change.

An inclusive welfare system would probably need to be built on what Holman (1993) has described as mutuality. This would have to incorporate a change of personal attitude, as it would be based upon an assumption that we are all vulnerable and have an interest in collectively protecting each other. Marks (1999: 136) refers to a study in the USA which calculates that, with a life expectancy of 75 years, the average person could expect to spend 13 years with some limited capacity; and Thomas (1999) suggests that a more accurate term than able-bodied might be 'congenitally able-bodied'. Therefore, when those of us who are not disabled talk of disabled people as the 'other', we are in fact referring to a temporal state, and this may have more to do with our own fear of what may happen to us than with a real understanding of the situation of that other person. But if our responses can be understood in terms of interactionism, then they can be modified through our active seeking-out of new experiences which might change our perception of disability and impairment.

The alternative, if we do not address our own attitudes, is that stigmatised groups become socially excluded and the role of both healthcare and social welfare professions will become more overtly one of policing disability. The impact of this on individuals is immense, as Battye has described:

> Somewhere deep inside us is the almost unbearable knowledge that the way the able-bodied world regards us is as much as we have a right to expect. We are not full members of that world, and the vast majority of us can never hope to be. If we think otherwise we are deluding ourselves.
>
> (Battye, 1966: 8–9)

Healthcare and social care workers need to bear in mind Hunt's statement on behalf of disabled people: 'We are society, as much as anybody, and cannot be considered in isolation from it' (Hunt, 1966: 146). Thus, if we, the non-disabled, do not wish to identify with the slave-owners, we must attempt to examine and change our perceptions of disability.

References

Abberley, P. (1995) 'Disabling ideology in health and welfare – the case of occupational therapy', *Disability and Society*, 10, 2: 221–32.

Battye, L. (1966) 'The chatterley syndrome', in P. Hunt (ed.), *Stigma: the experience of disability*, London: Geoffrey Chapman.

Bogdan, R. and Taylor, S. (1989) 'Relationships with severely disabled people: the social construction of humanness', *Social Problems*, 36, 2: 135–48.

Brechin, A. and Liddiard, P. (1981) *Look at it this way: new perspectives in rehabilitation*, Sevenoaks: Hodder and Stoughton.

Campbell, J. and Oliver, M. (1996) *Disability politics: understanding our past, changing our future*, London: Routledge.

Castells, M. (1996) *The information age: economy, society and culture: vol. 1 – the rise of the network society*, Malden, Mass.: Blackwell.

Finkelstein, V. (1980) *Attitudes and disabled people: issues for discussion*, New York: World Rehabilitation Fund.

Goffman, E. (1963) *Stigma: notes on the management of spoiled identity*, Harmondsworth: Pelican.

Groce, N. (1985) *Everyone here spoke sign language: hereditary deafness on Martha's Vineyard*, Cambridge, Mass.: Harvard University Press.

Holman, B. (1993) *A new deal for social welfare*, Oxford: Lion.

Hunt, P. (1966) 'A critical condition', in P. Hunt (ed.), *Stigma: the experience of disability*, London: Geoffrey Chapman.

Macfarlane, A. (1996) 'Aspects of intervention: consultation, care, help and support', in G. Hales (ed.), *Beyond disability: towards an enabling society*, London: Sage.

MacKenzie, D. (1979) 'Eugenics and the rise of mathematical statistics in Britain', in J. Irvine, I. Miles and J. Evans (eds), *Demystifying social statistics*, London: Pluto.

Marks, D. (1999) *Disability: controversial debates and psychosocial perspectives*, London: Routledge.

Morris, J. (1993) *Community care or independent living*, York: Joseph Rowntree Foundation.

Oliver, J. (1995) 'Counselling disabled people: a counsellor's perspective', *Disability and Society*, 10, 3: 261–79.

Oliver, M. (1990) *The politics of disablement*, Basingstoke: Macmillan.

—— (1993) 'Conductive education: if it wasn't so sad it would be funny', in J. Swain, V. Finkelstein, S. French and M. Oliver (eds), *Disabling barriers – enabling environments*, London: Sage.

Oliver, M. and Sapey, B. (1999) *Social work with disabled people*, second edn, Basingstoke: Macmillan.

Parkes, C.M. (1975) *Bereavement: studies of grief in adult life*, Harmondsworth: Penguin.

Pfeiffer, D. (1994) 'Eugenics and disability discrimination', *Disability and Society*, 9, 4: 481–99.

Roulstone, A. (1998) *Enabling technology: disabled people, work and new technology*, Buckingham: Open University Press.

Sapey, B. (2000) 'Disablement in the informational age', *Disability and Society*, 15, 4: 619–36.

Spicker, P. (1984) *Stigma and social welfare*, Beckenham: Croom Helm.

Thomas, C. (1999) *Female forms: experiencing and understanding disability*, Buckingham: Open University Press.

Tomlinson, S. and Colquhoun, R. (1995) 'The political economy of special educational needs in Britain', *Disability and Society*, 10, 2: 191–202.

Part III

Where do we go from here?

27 Manifesto for change

Caroline Carlisle, Caroline Watkins, Tom Mason and Elizabeth Whitehead

Introduction

It seems fitting that any book which presents the reader with the challenges facing healthcare professionals in their role in working with people who may be stigmatised should also present a synthesis of the key issues addressed, together with suggestions for future practice. A manifesto is traditionally viewed as some form of public declaration of policy, but in no way do we wish to prescribe. It is for each professional to reflect on the issues which have been raised in this book and to explore whether their practice could incorporate a different and more equitable approach to those people experiencing physical or emotional illness or disability, or engaged in alternative lifestyles. The manifesto is presented as our ideas for the ways in which practice may be taken forward in a number of areas, including education, research and development and individual professional practice. A number of common themes have emerged from previous chapters in this book and these have helped to identify key issues for reflection.

Emerging themes

In any manifesto the declaration of intent will usually outline the desired goal, or end position, that the manifesto seeks to attain in a particular time-frame. This manifesto is no different. However, in declaring a policy for change we hope to incorporate two considerations that are often missing in documents that drive a course of action. The first is concerned with understanding the current position relating to stigma and social exclusion, and this appreciation is not only rooted in a historical context but is also grounded in contemporary practice. Through a close examination of the chapters of this book we have identified the emergent themes that underpin the practice areas. This exploration has located the basis of any change policy at the clinical interface and will, therefore, set the manifesto in a realistic context. This will help answer a central question relating to any manifesto development, that of 'from what to what?'. The second consideration is, to some extent, the easier to address. Manifestos can be grand narratives that are ideological but, perhaps, not always grounded in realism. They can be utopian and point to an ideal situation, and although this makes for pleasant reading these approaches are unlikely to effect the change that is desired. Therefore, the more difficult aspect is to make the suggestion for change realistic and achievable, and to complete this task we again turn to the practice areas of this book. In exploring these chapters for themes relating to change we hope to have set the policy development at a practical level and accept that this will call for a closer relationship between theory and practice.

The first theme to emerge from many chapters was the tension between professional and patient. Many authors spoke about the conflict inherent in being a professional with the concerns and focus brought by their respective disciplines. However, the contradiction occurred when that particular professional also had experience of being a 'patient'. The status of patient may have been about suffering from a particular disability or medical condition that did not preclude their ability to practise but that gave them a powerful insight into this relationship. In dealing with this middle ground between professional and patient it became alarmingly clear that the experiences of being both was very different from being either one or the other. There was a distinctly clear message that the enterprise of the professional was not always as clear-cut as it seems. Although the role of the professional was to assist, care for, and generally help the patient to overcome their particular ailment, much of their activity actually contributed to disabling them. This may have been achieved subconsciously but nonetheless had the impact of stigmatising and marginalising individuals and groups. Subtle mechanisms were at play which constantly divided and split the roles of professional and patient, and ensured that boundaries were clearly delineated. These boundaries were often socially constructed, but had the practical effect of keeping the states of professional and patient apart. This may have deeper symbolic importance which is beyond the scope of this chapter; however, it is sufficient to say here that the professional activity appeared to operate in order to differentiate between those who are afflicted with a 'disease' and those who are not. The practical consequence of this led to the creation of a hierarchical power structure which enabled the professional to exercise authority over the patient. Although this exercise of power is woven within discourse and practice relating to benevolence, kindness and compassion, there is a veiled negative aspect that is at play. This must be the focus of change in a manifesto policy document that relates to stigmatisation and social exclusion.

The second key theme to emerge concerns the question of responsibility. Inherent in the notion of social exclusion, and the stigma that both drives it and accompanies it, is the idea of accountability. In many of the chapters the authors highlight the issue of blame and culpability, often at an abstruse level but also many times as part and parcel of the process of delivering healthcare. Over the past two decades there has been a closer relationship between the service delivery of healthcare and the extent to which a person is considered responsible for their illness. For example, smokers who refuse to give up smoking, or an alcoholic who will not stop drinking, may not be given a particular medical intervention because they are considered blameworthy. Although this is due, in part, to the growing awareness that the delivery of healthcare is limited by the resources that are available, there is also an increasing ethos of viewing the individual as liable for their condition. This may be by blaming them for their poor diet, lack of exercise, or general way of life. However, we can also see that those who are stigmatised and excluded may also bear the brunt of being considered accountable for their plight. Whether it is homelessness or HIV, teenage pregnancy or drug use, placing the onus of responsibility on them merely adds to the stigmatising process. In this respect, healthcare professionals may not separate their professional role from their socialised status as members of society. Clearly, being a member of society is a condition that the professional enjoyed long before they chose the ideology of their discipline. Thus, we can see that the socialised beliefs of a society may well be stronger than the profession-alised beliefs of a healthcare system. In this scenario, such prejudices as blaming a person for their condition may override the role and functions of professionalism. This, again, needs to feature in a manifesto that is designed to create change.

The third, and final, theme to be discussed here relates to the theory–practice gap. Many chapters dealt with the relationship between theoretical explication and its impact on practice, and paid close attention to the role of healthcare professionals in striving to achieve this. However, the fact that this theme looms so large throughout the book would suggest that it is to some degree not being achieved, at least to the extent that it ought to be. This raises the question as to the feasibility of many professional endeavours to narrow this traditional gap. We believe that most would accept that theory needs to inform practice, and certainly without the development of conceptual paradigms humankind would not have progressed as far as it has. Ideas that change into theories, and which in turn are examined through scientific enquiry, lie at the heart of human curiosity.

Furthermore, through rigorous examination these theories are changed and developed, and become grounded as evidence-based concepts. It is expected that modern-day healthcare practice is based on this evidence and is open to serious criticism if it is not. Herein lie two main problems highlighted in this book. The first concerns the many areas of healthcare care delivery that are not evidence-based and are in fact rooted in, at best, experience and, at worst, myth. This makes many professionals reluctant to change their practice in the face of the dearth of evidence. The second problem is that, even when evidence exists, many clinicians are often hesitant to employ research findings in their practice. This has long been the case in numerous disciplines and is currently a problem for the nursing profession. Thus, the development of a manifesto for changing the process of stigmatisation in healthcare settings must incorporate an educational component for practitioners in order that they can more readily employ theory in their clinical practice.

This leads us to consider the final aspect of this section, which is concerned with pointing us to the future. Although, as with any forecasting into the future, we only have available to us such concepts as prediction and guesstimates, we also have a phenomenological capacity which provides us with the ability to engage in reflexivity. We have the capacity not only to reflect on the world but also to reflect on our own thinking. This highly complex philosophical position has pragmatic consequences for our behaviour and, through reflexivity, we have the potential to change both our thoughts and our actions.

Key areas for change

The themes emerging from this book have helped identify possible areas for change, not only in professional practice but also in the fields of education and training, research and development, and personal reflection.

Changes in the education and training of healthcare professionals

Over a million people work in the National Health Service (approximately 5 per cent of the UK workforce population). Skill acquisition is increasingly becoming the responsibility of the worker, although for healthcare professionals it is generally their professional body that determines the appropriateness of education and training. There is a growing acknowledgement of the importance of continuing professional development (CPD) in order that the individual can continue to refine skills and keep up to date with current evidence for practice. CPD must encompass, among many other things, technical skills and attitudes towards patients, staff and the general population.

Several challenges to education and training in the NHS have been identified. The workforce is ageing, particularly in community nursing staff, and there is an increasing proportion of women in the workforce. For example, more than 50 per cent of medical graduates (Young and Leese, 1999) and more than 33 per cent of hospital doctors are now women (Dowie and Langman, 1999). The differing needs in terms of how training is delivered must be taken into account. Whereas in the past training has needed to cater for people in full-time employment, women frequently require more flexible arrangements, such as career breaks in which to raise a family.

It is therefore apparent that, in order to respond to the ever-changing and increasing diversity of skills required to participate effectively in a highly technological healthcare system, mechanisms for continuing skills acquisition are a necessity (Dargie *et al.*, 2000). Yet it is not solely technical skills that are required. It is becoming increasingly important for staff to provide more holistic care (Lamsa *et al.*, 1994) which requires staff from differing professions to work effectively within a multidisciplinary team. These teams may be ward, acute care or primary care based, and may also require working across areas and with other voluntary and statutory organisations. It is increasingly recognised that formal preparation is necessary for staff so as to ensure true teamwork. We are moving away from the traditional, didactic teaching methods (e.g. lectures) to more student-centred enquiry or problem-based learning methods. These alternative approaches not only develop problem-solving skills and enhance critical thinking, but they may also provide a forum for the frank discussion of issues relating to deviance, difference and dilemmas in healthcare, the subject of this book.

While it is acknowledged that the education and training provided for the development of healthcare professionals is the responsibility of the individual and of the professional body, all education providers must share in the responsibility. That is, issues such as those relating to discrimination, stigma and social exclusion should have been raised within primary and secondary education and this should be clearly defined as part of the National Curriculum. One might even suggest that these issues should be raised in pre-school education, and certainly all appropriate opportunities to include such discussions within adult learning environments should be taken.

Research and development

The past decade has seen a growing policy interest in relation to issues of social exclusion and marginalised groups within society. Much of this work is to be commended, and the reports which have emanated from such groups as the King's Fund have highlighted very practical solutions to real problems: for example, the need for integrated services for homeless people and the launch of the 'Under One Roof' initiative funded by the King's fund. This project brings together resources such as healthcare professionals, social services, housing officers and Benefits Agency staff to provide ready access to all services that single homeless people need. Other policy development includes the National Institute for Clinical Excellence (NICE) which aims to form one part of the solution to remedy current inequalities in healthcare (DoH, 1998a). The work of NICE is complemented by the National Service Frameworks (NSFs) which were set up to address unacceptable variations in services across the country. NSFs aim to bring together the best evidence of clinical and cost effectiveness, with the views of service users, to determine the best ways of providing healthcare (DoH, 1998a). The government's research and development strategy (DoH, 1998b) supports these practical initiatives by acknowledging the need for the investigation of inequalities.

The launch of the government's Social Exclusion Unit (SEU) in 1997 raised the public profile of the needs of disadvantaged and stigmatised groups in our society. The review of the SEU (1999) praises its use of evidence, but acknowledges that the resources it has available to commission customised research is limited in relation to exploring the questions it really needs to answer. The SEU has been successful in contributing to government papers on initiatives to tackle social exclusion. The need remains, however, for the Unit to have access to the best available evidence on issues relating to social exclusion and also to strengthen its ability in the coming years to resource project work on key research priorities.

The Model for Change which we present below highlights the need to achieve social interventions against social exclusion which are based on sound research evidence. The policy documents referred to above acknowledge the value and need for evidence, particularly in relation both to matters of equity in healthcare and to the need to develop interventions which are based on best evidence. Every healthcare professional has a need to keep abreast not only of policy, but also of research and development priorities. Depending on an individual's level of responsibility, this can involve the appraisal of published evidence, the synthesis of available evidence, the development of evidence-based protocols or directives, or indeed the generation of sound evidence for key research questions.

There are many gaps in our knowledge and understanding of social exclusion and stigmatisation in healthcare. It is all too obvious why such marginalised groups as the homeless may not have equitable access to quality health services. But, as we have seen from many of the chapters in this book, there are less obvious areas which require investigation. The generation of evidence in relation to these areas needs to be prioritised, and it should be the responsibility of every healthcare professional to work towards the utilisation of best evidence in their practice with marginalised or disadvantaged groups.

Individual responsibilities

The individual responsibilities for contributing towards a manifesto for change are depicted in the model outlined in Figure 27.1. This model shows that the catalyst for change arises from our own personal beliefs and desires for change. The model involves four stages: (1) personal beliefs, (2) primary action, (3) secondary action and (4) tertiary action. The latter three stages are subdivided into social interactions and social interventions. Although it would be the optimum achievement to complete the process through to the tertiary stage, it is not absolutely necessary, and an individual may cease at any level. Change that is produced at each stage would contribute significantly to the overall process and, if the end product is change at the tertiary level, then that would be an excellent result.

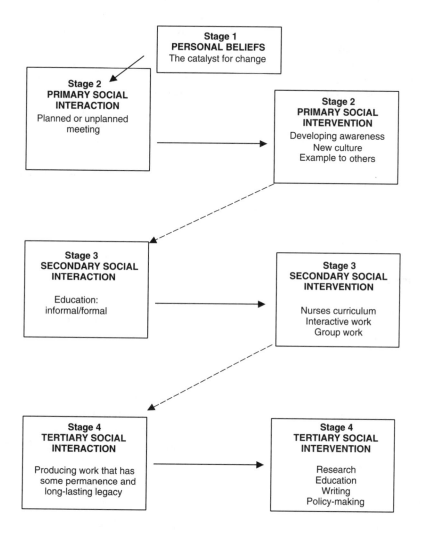

Figure 27.1 Stigma and social exclusion in healthcare practice: a model for change

Stage 1: Personal beliefs

As nurses we believe that a fundamental component of our professional ideology is to promote a practice that challenges stigma and social exclusion in every aspect of healthcare. This section considers how individuals can make a contribution to overcome stigma and social exclusion in healthcare. It is possible for healthcare users to be as equally pro-active and there are many instances of how this has been effectively achieved. An example of a healthcare user working towards reform would be the mother of a child with special needs who, in a predominantly and uncompromisingly stigmatising world, is faced by a whole range of social, emotional and physical problems. This unforeseen and devastating situation is being met by her determination to help not only her own family but also others who find themselves in a similar situation. By working at a local level, this mother offers and shares her experiences, and creates an environment where mutual support is beneficial to families of children with special needs. The community in which she lives now has a greater understanding of children with special needs, and they have the opportunity to pass this empathy on to those with whom they engage in their own lives. This example impresses upon us the impact that one individual can have upon many people. Personal beliefs may be the catalyst for change in small or large projects with the intention of working towards a more socially inclusive society.

Stage 2: Primary social interaction

Primary social interaction is often opportunistic, when an unexpected or casual meeting takes place between two or more people. For example, when the interaction is planned, this may be the result of a booked appointment or a scheduled hospital visit. This section discusses the profound impact of the first interactions that people have with each other. We often talk of the significance of first impressions and how they seem to stay in our memory for what may be a lifetime. Primary social interaction can be an emotional experience, both in terms of the impression we give to others and the impression they give to us. Therefore our primary social interaction has a fundamental effect on outcome of the 'relationship'.

Strategy for primary social interaction

The strategy for social interaction at a primary level is concerned with what individual healthcare workers can do to anticipate social stigma and social exclusion. This will include the following tactical approaches:

- Developing an awareness and sensitivity to the needs of others.

- Creating a culture where 'difference' is accepted, acknowledged and embraced.
- Showing by example our consideration of others.

Stage 3: Secondary social interaction

Our interaction at secondary level is concerned with education. As with the case of primary social interaction, education may be a planned or a spontaneous event. The education may be at a one-to-one level or with several people. The education of social stigma explores personal beliefs and all the levels of social interaction and intervention. Educational sessions should be interactive. Participants draw upon their own experiences and teachers must ensure that adequate time is given to these sessions. In addition, it is equally important that the groups are kept small in number and everyone should have the opportunity to speak. The teacher should also be mindful of the potentially sensitive nature of experiential stigma.

Strategy for secondary social interaction

The strategy for secondary interaction will involve the following aspects:

- The dynamics of social interaction, social stigma and social exclusion (explored in the core curriculum of nurse education).
- Interactive work at pre-registration and post-registration level on how to deal with patients and colleagues facilitates our awareness of social stigma and the impact it may have.
- Focus group and small-group teaching sessions.
- Counselling to address individual issues of a personal and sensitive nature.

Stage 4: Tertiary social interaction

This final section is concerned with how an individual can contribute to reducing social stigma and social exclusion, by making the catalyst for change into a written document that has a permanence and long-lasting legacy. The social interaction and subsequent intervention may involve just one individual, but it is likely to be a group of people working as a team to introduce a hospital policy.

Strategy for tertiary social interaction

Developing our understanding of the complexities of stigma and social exclusion, so as to reach a wider audience and have a longer-lasting legacy, involves the following:

- Developing policy
- Research
- Writing
- Broadcasting through the media.

Thus, we have come full circle. We began this book with a statement regarding man's status as a social animal and yet we have clearly seen some of the strategies of exclusion that occur in modern day healthcare settings. If we are to break this circle of stigma and social exclusion then we must begin with a long hard look at our roles in perpetuating the system and then move towards some form of change strategy. As health-care workers we work with the most vulnerable and socially excluded in society and, if we fail to address their anxieties, then we fail both ourselves and the communities in which we live.

References

Dargie, C., Dawson, S. and Garside, P. (2000) 'Policy futures for UK health, 2000 report', University of Cambridge, The Judge Institute of Management Studies, London: The Stationery Office.

Department of Health (1998a) *A first class service: quality in the new NHS*, London: Department of Health.

—— (1998b) 'Research and development: towards an evidence base for health services, public health and social care', London: Department of Health

Dowie, R. and Langman, M. (1999) 'Staffing of hospitals: future needs, future provision', *British Medical Journal*, 319: 1193–5.

Lamsa, A., Hietanen, I. and Lamsa, J. (1994) 'Education for holistic care: a pilot programme in Finland', *Journal of Interprofessional Care*, 8, 1: 31–43.

SEU (1999) *Review of the Social Exclusion Unit*, London: Social Exclusion Unit.

Young, R. and Leese, B. (1999) 'Recruitment and retention of general practitioners in the UK: what are the problems and the solutions?', *British Journal of General Practice*, 49: 829–33.

Index